David MacGarty • David Not
Editors

Disaster Medicine

A Case Based Approach

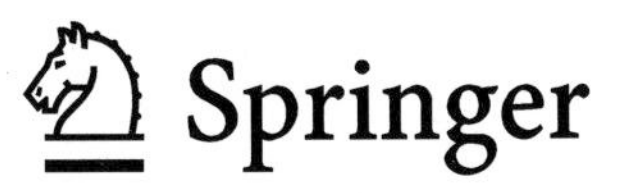

Editors
David MacGarty, MBBS, BSc
FY2 Doctor
Department of Obstetrics and Gynaecology
St Peter's Hospital
Surrey
UK

David Nott, OBE, OStJ, DMCC, BSc, MD, FRCS
Department of Surgery
Chelsea & Westminster Hospital
London
UK

ISBN 978-1-4471-5228-6 ISBN 978-1-4471-4423-6 (eBook)
DOI 10.1007/978-1-4471-4423-6
Springer London Heidelberg New York Dordrecht

Library of Congress Control Number: 2012951638

Printed on acid-free paper

Springer is part of Springer Science+Business Media (www.springer.com)

This book is dedicated to Sarah Houston. As a medical student she was actively interested in Global Health issues and she hoped to pursue this interest in her career. Her determination to help those in need, both at home and abroad, was inspirational and her legacy will remain with all those who knew and loved her.

Thanks to our mums and wives/girlfriends who put up with us while we burned the midnight oil.

Also special mention to: Brother Elio Croce ('bro Elio') – Director of St. Jude Children's Home and Technical Director at St. Mary's Hospital, Lacor (both in Gulu, Uganda) and Tom Hart – Programme Director in Guatemala for the charity Health Poverty Action (HPA).

Disclaimer

Prologue

I am writing this prologue during a quiet spell working as a surgeon for Medecins Sans Frontieres in Northern Syria during the current civil war. It is not just necessary to be able to perform surgery safely and competently in this poorly resourced environment but also to have an understanding of the rules that allow humanitarian interventions to proceed at all. For many of us that work in the developed world, it is difficult to imagine what it means to be involved in a human catastrophe and conflict. In 2010 I met a group of highly motivated final year medical students who wanted to understand the intricacies of health provision in situations alien to their world. To this end, both hard work and time spent talking to experts in their field, it has been possible to put together this book. It is hoped that it will provide the reader with an understanding of the complexities involved from the moment humanitarian aid is required whether it be for war or natural disaster. At the end of each chapter are case studies "putting it all together", which will provide insight into how it all works in the real situation.

In disaster situations, usually the countries affected open their doors to humanitarian aid and more often than not are overwhelmed with Non-Governmental Organizations. This can lead to a complete lack of order and understanding between various aid providers causing multiplication of services and sometimes total confusion. Even though the United Nations should have ultimate overall control, they have little power to stop aid organizations from setting up shop and adding to the mayhem. The overall situation is usually contained as the event occurs once and those injured or made homeless are a group that can be treated and rehabilitated.

The present conflict in Syria exemplifies the problems of war and caring for internally displaced people and refugees. It is ongoing and the situation is constantly changing; it may go on for a very long time and take significant resources both in terms of human cost and infrastructure. Most countries of the world subscribe to the international humanitarian laws as laid down by the Geneva Conventions and upheld by the International Committee of the Red Cross. This conflict demonstrates how difficult it can be for the international community to act without the appropriate signatories. Although Humanitarian Organizations are by nature apolitical, impartial, and neutral, this alone does not appear to provide security for the doctors and nurses and other healthcare workers who increasingly in this conflict are made to feel insecure.

This book will provide insight into these issues and I hope that you will enjoy it.

London, UK David Nott

Acknowledgments

Mr David Nott OBE is a Consultant General Surgeon at the Chelsea and Westminster Hospital specializing in upper GI laparoscopic surgery. He also works at St. Mary's Hospital where he is a vascular and trauma surgeon and at the Royal Marsden Hospital where he performs retroperitoneal and pelvic side wall surgery. He also runs the Definitive Surgical Trauma Skills course at the Royal College of Surgeons of England.

He is an authority in laparoscopic (keyhole) surgery and was the first surgeon to combine laparoscopic and vascular surgery. He was the first surgeon in the world to perform a totally laparoscopic distal arterial bypass and the first surgeon in Europe to perform a laparoscopic abdominal aortic aneurysm repair. He has written over 100 papers on various aspects of General, Vascular, and Trauma Surgery.

David has worked extensively for both Medecins Sans Frontieres (MSF) and the International Committee of The Red Cross. He has deployed to many conflict and catastrophe settings including Bosnia, Liberia, Sierra Leone, Ivory Coast, Chad, Libya (Misrata), Haiti, Sudan (Darfur), Pakistan, Afghanistan, and Iraq. He recently deployed to Syria (September 2012) to provide surgical care for the victims of conflict.

While working for MSF in the Democratic Republic of Congo, David famously performed a life-saving forequarter amputation on a 16-year-old boy whilst receiving instruction via text message. He is a member of the Royal Auxiliary Air Force and has a passion for flying. He holds commercial and helicopter pilot licenses and regularly flies a Learjet45 for a corporate company based in London.

Professor Jim Ryan OBE (OStJ MB BCh BAO MCh FRCS DMCC, Hon FCE) was the first Leonard Cheshire Professor in Conflict Recovery at University College London, serving in that capacity from 1995 until 2007. In 2002, he was appointed International Professor of Surgery at USUHS, MD, USA. In 2007, he was further appointed Emeritus Professor to the Centre for Trauma, Conflict & Catastrophe Medicine at St George's University of London and he is tasked with taking the center forward.

His conflict and catastrophe experience covers military and humanitarian operations in Northern Ireland, Cyprus, the Falkland Islands, Nepal, the Balkans, the Caucasus, and Central Asia. He is a trustee of a number of charities, including the

Swinfen Charitable Trust—an organization that focuses on establishing telemedicine links between hospital-based practitioners in the developing world and medical and surgical specialists who give advice over the Internet. Professor Ryan's research interests include ballistic and terrorist injury, military and conflict medicine.

Professor Kim Mulholland (MB BS, FRACP, MD) is a pediatrician who joined the Medical Research Council (MRC) unit in the Gambia in 1989 where he undertook research into pneumonia, neonatal infections, and vaccine evaluation, which culminated in the pivotal Gambia Hib vaccine trial. Between 1995 and 2000, he was based in Geneva at WHO where he was responsible for research in child health and bacterial vaccines. In 2000, he established the Centre for International Child Health at Royal Children's Hospital, Melbourne (the hospital where he trained). Since 2005 he has held a personal chair in Child Health and Vaccinology at the London School of Hygiene and Tropical Medicine. He is a Professor of International Child Health at the Menzies School of Health Research, Darwin, and at the Murdoch Children's Research Institute, Melbourne.

Dr Michael Brown is an infectious diseases physician at the Hospital for Tropical Diseases, London, and a senior lecturer at the London School of Hygiene and Tropical Medicine. He runs the HIV/AIDS distance learning MSc module and has research interests in HIV testing and in imported infections.

Jane Gilbert is a Consultant Clinical Psychologist based in the United Kingdom. She specializes in workshops/training on psychological and mental health issues in cross-cultural contexts and consultancy to international NGOs. She has worked in The Gambia, Uganda, Lesotho, Ghana, Jordan, and Liberia. Her particular interests include the effects of culture and language on personal identity, and the integration of different cultural understandings in training and mental health services.

Professor Clare Gilbert worked as a clinical ophthalmologist for 10 years and has an MD in Surgical Retina. Following an MSc in Epidemiology at London School of Hygiene and Tropical Medicine in 1995, she worked in the Institute of Ophthalmology, London, from 1990 before joining the London School in 2002. Clare is a professor at the International Centre for Eye Health (ICEH), and has been medical advisor to Sight Savers International since 1995. Since January 2006, Clare has been co-director of ICEH and is a member of the School's Ethics Committee.

Kate Godden is a nutrition expert with 20 years experience with NGOs, UN and donors. She has an MSc from the London School of Hygiene & Tropical Medicine and is a registered Public Health Nutritionist with the Association for Nutrition. She has worked principally in sub-Saharan Africa and Asia and is a member of the capacity development working group of the UN global nutrition cluster. Kate also teaches at the University of Westminster on an MSc International Public Health Nutrition.

Dr Daniele Lantagne is an assistant professor at Tufts University (Boston, MA) who researches and provides technical assistance to organizations on the development, implementation, and assessment of water and sanitation interventions in both developing countries and emergency contexts to prevent diarrheal disease.

Dr Jessi Tucker is an emergency medic at the Royal London Hospital who promotes education and awareness in pre-hospital, wilderness and conflict and catastrophe medicine. She is a member of the Conflict and Catastrophes Forum at the Royal Society of Medicine, the medical cell of the Royal Geographical Society and she lectures at St George's on the BSc module in Leadership in Disaster Medicine.

Dr Rachel Brand is a Clinical Psychologist in south London who works for both an early intervention in psychosis service and a traumatic stress service and is experienced in assessing and treating refugees and asylum seekers in a mental health context.

Drs David MacGarty, Will Barker, Shao Foong Chong, James Houston, and Ed Mew met as medical students at St. Georges University of London in 2007. They developed their passion for pre-hospital care and disaster medicine by attending electives with the HEMS helicopter service at the Royal London Hospital and completing the diploma course in Conflict and Catastrophe Medicine run by the Worshipful Society of the Apothecaries in London. Under the influence of Professor Jim Ryan, they helped in setting up the BSc module in "Leadership in Disaster Medicine" at St Georges. Now FY2 doctors they are all focused on developing their clinical skills with the aim of using them in conflict and catastrophe settings in the future.

Contents

Contributors

Will Barker, MBBS, MPhys FY2 Doctor, St Thomas' Hospital, London, UK

Rachel Brand Doctorate in Psychology (Dclinpsy), BSc St Georges Mental Health NHS Trust, London, UK

Shao Foong Chong, MBBS, MA (Oxon) FY2 Doctor, Department of Emergency Medicine, St George's Hospital, Tooting, London, UK

Clare Gilbert, FRCO phth MD MSc London school of hygiene and tropical medicine, London, UK

Kate Godden, MSc University of Westminster, London, UK

James Houston, MBBS, MEng FY2 Doctor, Department of Surgery, Chelsea and Westminster Hospital, London, UK

David MacGarty, MBBS, BSc FY2 Doctor, Department of Obstetrics and Gynaecology, St Peter's Hospital, Chertsey, Surrey, UK

Ed Mew, MBBS FY2 Doctor, Trauma, Emergency and Acute Medicine (TEAM), King's College Hospital, Denmark Hill, London, UK

David Nott, OBE, OStJ, DMCC, BSc, MD, FRCS Department of Surgery, Chelsea & Westminster Hospital, London, UK

Jim Ryan, OBE (OStJ MB BCh BAO MCh FRCS DMCC, Hon FCE) Emeritus Professor of Conflict and Catastrophe Medicine, Centre for Conflict and Catastrophe Medicine, St George's University of London, Cranmer terrace, London, UK

Jessi Tucker, MBBS BSc Emergency Medicine Department, Royal London Hospital, Whitechapel, London, UK

Michael Brown, BA (Oxon), BM BCh, MRCP, PhD, DTM&H Consultant Physician, Hospital for Tropical Diseases, London, UK

Part I
Disaster Response

Section reviewed by David Nott

Working for NGOs as a surgeon involves frequently deploying to areas of the world that are prone to conflict or catastrophe. Your phone goes off and you agree in principle to go on the mission; but you have to clear it with your family, colleagues, and the hospital managers. Shackles removed the reality of the mission sets in. Other than the work itself the potential risk from the environment and from warring parties are high on the agenda.

Your job is well defined by the NGO and all the hard work involving negotiations between parties to secure your safe travel have been performed by local logistical and headquarters staff. The most dangerous part of a mission is getting to and from the area. The well-marked vehicle you are traveling in should be given free passage but you have to be aware that drug and alcohol fuelled soldiers and bandits do not adhere to the rules. Being stopped at a checkpoint in the Congo and the barrel of a rifle pressed into my neck was a defining moment in my life. I was saved by a patient in the back of the landcruiser whom I had just operated upon because he was of a higher rank than the crazed guard.

As a humanitarian aid worker one needs to remain focused on the job in hand and that job is to help to relieve human suffering. Remember that despite what is happening around you, you have three priorities; yourself, the team, and the patients. Always adhere to the rules. The head of mission has ultimate responsibility but you are a member of the team and everyone has a role in the safe running of the mission, whether it be in a conflict zone, natural disaster, or looking after refugees.

David Nott

Chapter 1
Immediate Response to Disasters

Ed Mew

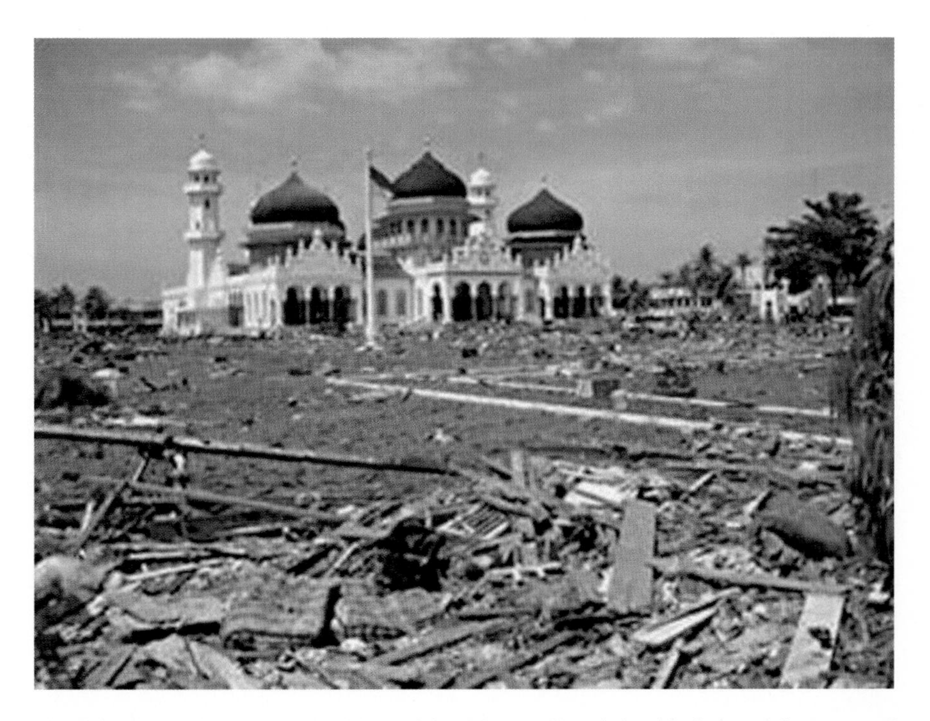

Fig. 1.1 Picture of Banda Aceh with surviving Mosque (Permission kindly granted courtesy of Project Hope/US Navy healthcare team)

E. Mew, MBBS
FY2 Doctor, Trauma, Emergency and Acute Medicine (TEAM),
King's College Hospital, Denmark Hill, London, UK
e-mail: eau.mew@gmail.com

D. MacGarty, D. Nott (eds.), *Disaster Medicine*,
DOI 10.1007/978-1-4471-4423-6_1,

Learning Objectives

- Define and classify disasters, listing conditions commonly encountered in different disasters
- List initial priorities in disaster response in the first 48 h
- Explore how immediate aid is delivered in the immediate post-disaster phase
- Explore key planning issues when considering emergency support work provision, including team composition
- Explore issues in managing the challenges that first responders to disasters face
- Describe acute stress reactions and measures to prevent occurrence
- Evaluate how extra calls for assistance may complicate emergency rescue and relief efforts
- Discuss the shift in priorities as disasters evolve after the first 48 h

Initial Scenario

You are a senior surgical trainee on leave. Switching on the television, your attention is drawn to scenes of devastation on the morning news. A magnitude 9.0 earthquake in the Indian Ocean has caused a huge tsunami. Reports from the area are piecemeal, testament to the widespread disruption. It seems that surrounding coastal areas have suffered catastrophic damage. There is little known about the "on the ground" situation at present. You immediately call a friend who works for a relief charity that you work for, Immediate Action for Medical Relief (IAMR). Despite your experience you have never witnessed post-disaster relief for a tsunami.

Prompt 1: How Are Disasters Defined and Classified?

- Disasters are events that bring about sudden and profound loss of or threat to life, health, property and environment [1].
- They may be divided by cause into man-made and natural causes:

  Man-made:

  - Conflict
  - Famine
  - Fire
  - Explosion
  - Transport
  - Chemical/industrial/nuclear

  Natural:

  - Earthquake
  - Landslide

- Volcano
- Flood/tsunami
- Drought
- Hurricane
- Disease epidemic

Disasters can furthermore be split chronologically into:

- Early phase: <48 h
- Intermediate phase: 48 h–14 days
- Late phase: >14 days up to months or years post event [1]

The rationale behind this split relates to the differing priorities in each disaster phase. Early phase efforts focus on saving victims who will otherwise die quickly from wounds sustained/conditions created from the disaster. The intermediate phase focuses on mediating disruption to provision of basic needs to those affected. Late phase efforts relate to long-term health needs and optimizing the affected area's infrastructure.

Prompt 2: What Conditions Are Commonly Encountered in Tsunamis and Other Disasters?

- The scale of mortality and morbidity encountered depends on the particulars of the disaster (Table 1.1).
- A large death toll should be expected from a tsunami but fewer injuries than in, for example, an earthquake. In tsunamis, there is a lack of time for evacuation, which may result in a relatively high density of victims close to the impact zone [3].
- Specific conditions to be expected in case of tsunami are listed in Table 1.2.

Prompt 3: What Are the Priorities in Immediate Disaster Response?

Disaster response should ideally follow the three-phase model:

Table 1.1 Characteristics of disasters

Disaster	Deaths	Severe injuries	Evacuation
Earthquake	+++	++++	Rare
Flood	+	+	Common
Fire	+	+	Common
Flash flood/tsunami	+++	+	Rare
Chemical	Variable	Variable	Common
Terror attack	+++	+++	Rare
Transportation	++	+++	Rare [2]

Table 1.2 Conditions expected in tsunamis

Disruption	Early phase	Intermediate phase	Late phase
Physical	Drowning Trauma Entrapment Crush injury	Subacute trauma	Psychological
Sanitation		Water-borne disease: cholera, typhoid, hepatitis A	Water-borne disease: cholera, typhoid, hepatitis A
Water and nutrition supply	Dehydration	Malnutrition Dehydration	Malnutrition Dehydration
Shelter	Exposure	Exposure Diseases of overcrowding: typhus, pneumonia, measles, meningitis	Diseases of overcrowding: typhus, pneumonia, measles, meningitis
Healthcare	Lack of prehospital care, lack of definitive care	Malaria Need to vaccinate	Relapse of chronic disease
Infrastructure	Transportation accidents	Transportation accidents, looting and civil unrest	Transportation accidents, looting and civil unrest

Early Phase

- Save and protect human life (including responders) [4]:
  - Search and rescue
  - Triage patients who require life/limb-saving care
  - First aid and ATLS
  - Life/limb-saving surgical and medical care
- Provide:
  - High quantity, reasonable quality potable water [5]
  - Food targeted at children, the elderly, and pregnant/breast-feeding women [5]
  - Emergency shelter, if possible with materials that can be reused as permanent housing [5]
- Contain the emergency: In natural disasters, according to the UNDAC, the speed of response is crucial [5].
- Warn and advise the public appropriately (re: sanitation, etc. [5]).
- Protect property, environment, and existing services.
- Facilitate enquiries [4].

Intermediate Phase

- Involves caring for patients who were able to survive the first days without medical care.

Late Phase

- Represents the transition from a disaster response to a humanitarian response – with development of longer-term healthcare for the population [6, 7]

According to the UK government, eight overarching principles guide every disaster response in every phase and can be applied no matter what stage you enter the disaster:

1. **Anticipation** of future risks and potential emergencies
2. **Preparedness**
3. **Subsidiary** – local agencies forming the response's building blocks
4. **Direction** – coordination of different agencies
5. **Information** management
6. **Integration** of values and objectives
7. **Cooperation** of different agencies toward set aims
8. **Continuity** of response into recovery [4]

Further Information 1

You phone in to check with IAMR. They have liaised with the United Nations Office for the Coordination of Humanitarian Affairs (UNOCHA) and have been asked to help deliver the immediate disaster response to a small coastal town identified by their virtual On-Site Operations Coordination Centre (OSOCC) as particularly badly hit by the tsunami. Your team will provide first aid and definitive medical care to casualties in tented temporary field hospitals. You will be collaborating with search and rescue teams and a task force from the Disaster Assessment and Coordination section of the OCHA. As a long-standing member of IAMR, you have been asked to lead the IAMR team on the ground.

Prompt 4: What Must Be Considered Prior to Undertaking Overseas Emergency Relief?

What Is the Nature of the Disaster?

- Type of disaster – affects the casualty number and resource disruption.
- Scale of disaster – try to ascertain the extent of the destruction in terms of buildings affected (rendered unliveable) and population affected [5].
- Is there a HAZMAT (hazardous materials) element to the disaster? This may prevent you from entering the disaster area if you cannot protect yourselves.
- Distances – if long/by air, consider implications for transporting equipment and cold chain storage for medications.
- Access to disaster area may be limited due to disruption.

- Human elements (like looting and armed conflict) – increase need for security [8].
- You should also take out appropriate insurance for yourself and your equipment – guidance for which can be sought from your organization.

Am I Needed or Wanted There?

- What are the needs of the affected area? Will the health system be able to cope with the surge in medical demand [5]?
- What injury pattern is presenting? This can also be predicted from the type of disaster and will inform the type of care needed.
- What is the baseline medical provision of the area for its population? Lack of prehospital care networks, vaccination coverage under 85 % (90 % for measles), unregulated drug sales, and pre-existing rates of diseases like HIV/AIDS and tuberculosis are, according to UNDAC, important factors to consider [5].
- Needs of the host area come first. WHO recommends that you or the organization you work with should ideally be invited rather than just arrive spontaneously.
- Critically appraise the skill set of yourself and your team. Organizations demand at least 2 years post-qualification experience for doctors – preferably with experience in the emergency department, obstetrics and gynecology, and pediatrics. In reality, overseas work is often carried out by significantly more experienced clinicians.
- Field experience can be hard to gather. There are many courses on emergency coordination and humanitarian practice:
  Redr – humanitarian work training courses [9]
  Diploma in the medical care of catastrophes [10]
  Bsc in disaster management from the University of Coventry [11]
  Diploma in Humanitarian Assistance [12]
  Humanity First – training course [29]

What Are My Sources of Information?

Advice can come from:

- "On the ground" sources.
- Briefing sheets from your organization.
- Local government.
- UK Foreign and Commonwealth Office.
- Virtual OSOCC (On-Site Operations Coordination Centre) and Global Disaster Alert and Coordination System (GDACS) provide real-time global natural disaster alerts and tools to facilitate response coordination [13].
- UNDAC (United Nations Disaster Assessment and Coordination) section of the UNOCHA (United Nations Office for the Coordination of Humanitarian Affairs) provides disaster relief teams within 12–48 h of a disaster's occurrence.

- Reliefweb and the humanitarian early warning service also provide early detection services for disasters [14, 15].

Prompt 5: How Do You Prepare a Disaster Response Team?

Personnel

- Disaster response teams are often drawn up long before they are deployed in disaster relief missions, in the pre-disaster phase.
- Consider applicants' experience, ability to interact in a team environment, and motivation for volunteering.
- Pre-designate individuals to organize communications, health and safety, and logistics. Van Hoving et al. note that downfalls of not having designated logistic manager and operational manager led to ineffective managing and lack of responsibility performing in tasks [7].
- In disaster settings, deploying doctors are often required to function as safety officers, addressing issues like food storage, cleanliness, etc. These tasks may fall outside the remit of most doctors' daily responsibilities [7].

Skills and Accreditation

- Your team members' skills must be up to a suitable standard required for the operation and up to date. A way of guaranteeing this is accreditation.
- Other skills like navigation, survival, and self-protection are bonuses that will give your team members greater flexibility in the face of adverse conditions.
- If taking communication equipment like radios and satellite phones, you should ensure that all team members can use it properly.
- Many larger organizations will provide a pre-deployment preparation course which refreshes key skills and imparts elements of its ethos and mode of operation.

Equipment

- Equipment taken will vary depending on storage capacity and conditions in your destination.
- It is wise to take what your team can carry and little more.
- The following list is adapted from a kit list for emergency responders recommended by the Field Coordination Support Section (FCSS) (Box 1.1):

Health

- Full dental and health check-ups are essential prior to embarking on any foreign mission.
- Make sure you know about all significant conditions in your team members. Finding out about your team member's asthma when he or she has an acute severe attack in the field is the wrong time.

Box 1.1: Suggested Kit List

Austere Living Conditions

- Appropriate robust clothing – preferably as non-military as is possible in conflict situations. Culturally appropriate (especially for women). Clothing to include identifying markings.
- Dust masks
- Sunscreen and 2 pairs of sunglasses (one can go missing easily)
- First aid pack (including sterile needles)
- Documentation – passports, visas, vaccination certificates, certification of blood type, spare passport photos

Lack of Storage

- Backpack
- Daypack (smaller bag for shorter journeys)

Lack of Food Security

- Food supplies (e.g., army-style ration packs)
- Utensils (knife, fork, spoon, bowl)
- Matches

Lack of Sanitation

- Water purification tablets
- Alcohol hand rub
- Toiletries (toothbrush, toothpaste, soap, washing detergent/soap)
- Toilet paper
- Relevant medicines include, if necessary, chemoprophylaxis (e.g., malaria) and mosquito nets. Also, electrolyte replacement oral rehydration solutions, antidiarrheal (e.g., loperamide), antibiotics, anti-mycosis foot cream, sterile syringe, and hypodermic needle

Lack of Shelter

- Tents, roll mats, sleeping bags with liners

Lack of Infrastructure

- Spare batteries
- Torch, camera
- Satellite phone and radio
- Local currency or US dollars
- Pressure cooker (as sterilizer/autoclave) [16]

- Find out what diseases are endemic in the area (e.g., malaria, yellow fever, typhus) and any current communicable disease outbreaks.
- You may need travel vaccinations (with certificates), chemoprophylaxis, and antimosquito chemical-impregnated bed nets. This is dealt with well by travel clinics and by the National Travel Health Network and Centre [17, 18].
- Recommended vaccinations include:
  Tetanus
  Polio
  Hepatitis A and B
  Typhoid
  Meningitis [5]
- Non-communicable conditions will also deserve thought. Envenomation, crush injury from debris, and transportation accidents are all best handled by avoidance. Transportation accidents make up a large portion of the injuries and deaths sustained by aid workers. Adherence to the speed limit, use of seatbelts, avoidance of drunk-driving, defensive driving, and familiarity with local road rules and customs will reduce this risk.

Prompt 6: What organisational issues affect team performance?

Ground Rules

- Setting up clear ground rules is important. Rules exist to pre-empt commonly encountered problems when operating in the field (see Table 1.3).

Objectives and Exit Strategy

- Your team will have set objectives prior to deploying. In practice, as noted by van Hoving et al., these objectives will often be altered or added to by strategic coordinators during your mission [7].
- It is important to have an exit strategy and a secure way of leaving the area once priorities have been achieved.

Table 1.3 Matching avoidable outcomes to ground rules

Avoidable outcome	Ground rule
Loss of direction and purpose	Clear roles and team leadership
Devaluing team members	Equal respect for team members
Breakdown in moral behavior	Intolerance of stealing, dishonesty, sexual violence, physical violence
Unarticulated team grievances	Transparent paths of feedback
Lack of clarity in team process	Regular progress reports

As team leader, your responsibilities are to the team, the "mission," and to yourself.

Responsibilities:

- Responsibilities of team members are to the team, the 'mission' and to themselves with team leaders as organisers and motivators [19].
- Physical and psychological safety of team members is crucially important.
- Effective communication and adhering to specific goals and values are also key responsibilities.
- Team leaders traditionally give direction and considered action in ambiguous situations [19].

Further Information 2

A response team is alerted and assembled, consisting of an engineer, a logistics/communications manager, an emergency medical doctor, a surgeon, and four nurses. The engineer will supervise erection of the treatment tents. Nurses will help to triage casualties and administer first aid. The medical doctor and surgeon will manage complicated medical cases, act as safety officers and ensure waste disposal. The logistics and communications manager will ensure safe passage of your equipment (several tons in total) and will provide communications links with representatives from IAMR, OCHA, and other NGOs.

Your team is adequately supplied for five days (as contingency) and has necessary vaccinations, chemoprophylaxis, and antimosquito bed nets. You have agreed to spend four days in the area and have booked a return flight for your team. You decide to take 2 sharp containers although you are not sure where you will dispose of the sharps when they are filled. Your team gets a final briefing and you fly.

You arrive at your destination. Conditions are worse than estimated by the press and international community. Local transportation, administration and supply infrastructures have been almost completely destroyed. The public works office was located in a badly hit part of town. Relief forces have been mobbed by survivors demanding food, water and shelter, many of whom have been relocated to large camps. Looters are raiding intact stores. The army and relief forces are struggling with handling the huge number of bodies and many are left unburied. There are serious worries about the possibility of epidemics of water-borne diseases like cholera. You and your team feel lost and purposeless amongst this human catastrophe. As your flight was commercial, your supplies of medical oxygen have been impounded.

Prompt 7: What Are the Logistics and Operational Issues Surrounding How Immediate Disaster Relief Is Delivered?

Team Size

- Immediate disaster relief targets the early phase and therefore must be mobile and flexible enough to organize, deploy, and treat within the 48-h period.
- Recent trends have been toward small, self-sufficient teams called disaster medical assistance teams (DMATs) [20]. These are specifically trained to deploy in disaster scenarios, performing triage, emergency medical care, search and rescue, and treatment during patient transport [20].
- Kondo et al. argue that small team size (ideally 4–5) make DMATs able to mount a speedy response to disasters – a principle that Japan has embraced in developing its own network of DMATs (see Box 1.2).
- Disadvantages of many small groups providing rescue, relief, and aid include problems in coordination, cooperation, and integrating operations.
- Also, small groups may lack specialist knowledge that larger groups with more manpower may possess.

Box 1.2: Japan's DMATs

Japan, following the American model, adapted its own DMAT system in the early twenty-first century for dealing with disasters [20]. It found key limiting factors in the effectiveness of emergency response teams related to organization, mobilization, and transportation to the scene. Therefore,

(i) DMATs are pre-trained and drilled on quick emergency response.
(ii) DMATs would be put on standby regardless of the actual disaster outcome or requests for assistance in cases of high intensity earthquake, tsunami alert, or large-scale air crash.
(iii)To increase flexibility and speed of response, Japanese DMATs are under 1/5 the size of American teams (4–5 versus 29).

At time of printing, no major comparisons of effectiveness have been made between small and large team sizes in emergency disaster response.

Field Hospitals

- Field hospitals are mobile, self-contained, and self-sufficient healthcare facility capable of rapid deployment. They are used to provide advanced trauma life support (ATLS) care in early stages of disaster (under 48 h) and follow-up care (days 3–15) or to act as a temporary substitute for damaged hospitals (long term) [21].

- WHO-PAHO guidance notes that, from experience, field hospitals are useful in complex emergencies with elements of conflict but of questionable value in natural disasters [21].

Prompt 8: What Should Be Considered When Dealing with the Challenges of Immediate Disaster Management "On the Ground"?

Adapting to Reality

- The reality "on the ground" often differs markedly from pre-conceived ideas gathered from media and government releases. Even if you do have a good idea of what to expect, the reality of witnessing first-hand the aftermath of a disaster is profoundly unsettling [7].
- As leader of a recently deployed aid team, you must ensure you "hit the ground running" and quickly adapt to life in a disaster zone. This entails heightened situational awareness, propensity to forward plan, and critical appraisal of yourself and your team's operational strengths and weaknesses [22].

Coordination

- According to the UNDAC, coordinating a response can represent some of the greatest challenges in disaster response [5]. Barriers to effective coordination and communication include:
  - Perceptions that cooperation will limit team autonomy
  - Too many actors vying for overall responsibility
  - Differing priorities of what is "best" to do
  - Coordination deprioritized
  - Limited "on the ground" decision-making authority
  - Staff turnover such that new staff are unaware of previous arrangements

Information Gathering

- UNDAC suggests the following sources for "on the ground" information gathering:
  - Local level: local authorities/leaders/village elders, police/fire service, army, NGOs and IFRC/ICRC, religious leaders, UN national staff, evacuation centers, birth/death registration office, and health facilities
  - Capital level: national authorities, UN agencies, geographical institutes, bilateral agencies, NGOs, embassies, and OCHA (if in-country) [5]
- They also recommend grading your information for reliability (A = completely reliable, through to F = reliability cannot be judged) and credibility (1 = confirmed by other sources, through to 6 = truth cannot be judged) [5].

- If information in the acute phase is often contradictory or inconsistent – often due to a combination of factors: differences in perception, access to information, and misrepresentation of facts [5]. Try to scrutinize information gathered and triangulate your information with multiple diverse corroborating sources [5].

Security

- Reports of looting should lead to heightened awareness of the security situation as the security state may be extremely unpredictable.
- Your team must try to gather as much information as is possible on the health, security, and safety situation.
- According to Redmond, relief work can be hampered by civil unrest, with rescuers threatened or held hostage if they do not find relatives [22].
- Your team's organizational emblems may not be acknowledged or respected.

Survivors

- The majority of people who are trapped in disaster situations are rescued by friends and family or not at all [23].
- Survivors often congregate in areas of communal significance – like religious buildings, schools, or hospitals [24]. The individuals in relief camps may therefore represent a small but obvious "tip of the iceberg," with many more displaced individuals elsewhere.
- Search and rescue efforts after the immediate emergency phase often yield few survivors in relation to resources expended but are good for morale [22].

Burying the Dead

- Often, the most important reason to bury the dead promptly after death is for sociocultural reasons. In cases of natural disasters, burying the dead often offers little/no medical benefit to the population [24].
- Dead human or animal corpses will spoil water supplies by introducing fecal matter and so should be stored in areas remote to main water supplies.
- With epidemics of viral hemorrhagic fever, tuberculosis, and certain diarrheal diseases like cholera, extra caution is advised to inhibit the spread of disease [24].
- Your team's focus should be on the survivors and in maximizing their chances of continued survival.

Your Team

- The immediate post-arrival period may be the most stressful and disorientating period for your team.
- You should combat these pervasive feelings by remembering your mission aims and setting small manageable tasks to set up a foundation and build morale with small successes.

Further Information 3

Your team has been working solidly now for over sixty hours without break triaging and treating the survivors. You have established a tented base/treatment area and are now receiving a deluge of casualties on top of those extricated and delivered by search and rescue teams. Your team members have worked frantically to stem the tide of human suffering. Some have started to argue and make mistakes. Others are becoming increasingly introverted and quiet, burying themselves in their work. Your team has received requests from a local hospital, critically damaged in the tsunami, for you to help support their overwhelmed staff or at very least donate some of your equipment.

Prompt 9: What Is an Acute Stress Reaction?

- Acute stress reactions are well documented in emergency field work. An acute stress reaction usually results from direct involvement in traumatic or emergency events.
- Features include disorientation, changes in personality/libido/reaction to stimuli and physical changes in bowel habit/appetite/sleep [25]. In practical terms, this may manifest itself as the team member who distances himself/herself from the group, frequently retreats into a "dream-world" and fails to react to things as one would expect. Symptoms can last from a few days to a month.
- A more pervasive problem is the physical and mental exhaustion that inevitably follows prolonged periods of time in stressful environments with overwhelming humanitarian need and questionable security. Many humanitarian workers that work in the field for prolonged periods of time become jaded, "burnt-out" or engage in high-risk behaviors.
- For this reason, shift work is important as it enforces dedicated rest time, although you may need to literally force your keen team members to take breaks. Of course, the reality of immediate disaster response makes this ideally hard to enact.
- An awareness of your limitations – that you cannot change the world – is vital to prevent burnout. Furthermore, the Headington Institute has identified the following factors as important in personal coping [26]: social support, self-esteem, adaptability, curiosity and aptitude
- Courses like the TRIM course equip practitioners with the awareness and skills to identify the early onset of stress-related reactions.

Prompt 10: How Do Additional Calls for Assistance Complicate an Emergency Response?

- Calls for extra assistance may come in situations like these. It may sound noble to help out with assisting the local services when they are stretched. However, this comes with a serious caveat.

- First, by providing help to the hospital, you will be abandoning your own mission which you have been tasked to perform.
- Astute readers may also note that the safety of the hospital is unknown – as is the scale of the help required. Hospitals in developing countries are often a bottomless pit of need before a disaster strikes – let alone after! It may be incredibly hard to escape when committed [27].
- Similarly, it is advisable to think carefully before responding to requests to donate your equipment as you may need the equipment to accomplish your own aims.

Further Information 4

Your logistics manager liaises with a large NGO and manages to secure some medical oxygen to your team's relief. You put the local hospital in contact with the emergency response coordinator for your sector in the hope that they can arrange a team to help. The tide of casualties continues unabated. At the end of your four-day period, your team is exhausted. A fresh team from IAMR arrives and you prepare yourself to meet the new team leader, leave the disaster area, and come home.

Prompt 11: How Do Priorities in Emergency Management Shift in Passing from the Early to Intermediate Phase?

As disasters evolve past 48–72 h, priorities will shift accordingly. This will depend on the nature of the disaster, specifically whether it is static or dynamic (as mentioned above) with resulting risk of further complications [2]:

Definitive Scene Management

- Scene control and containment, especially relevant in dynamic disasters
- Relieving exhausted rescue crews and re-supply

Needs Assessments

- Once scene safety is achieved, needs assessments can be undertaken to determine exactly what the needs of the affected area are, and therefore what aid it should receive.
- For more information on needs assessments, please see next chapter.

Relief

- Relief efforts, targeted at the needs of the affected population [28]

Starting Recovery

- Frequently underemphasized in disaster plans but crucial for the affected community. Public utilities are re-established, and infrastructure begins to operate effectively [2].

Case Study: Banda Aceh

A magnitude 9.0 earthquake and tsunami reported to be 60 ft in height hit an unsuspecting Banda Aceh on December 26, 2004. The human cost was approximated at 200,000 in Sumatra with almost four times that number internally displaced. The damage caused by the earthquake and resulting tsunami ranged from structural damage to buildings to almost complete destruction of buildings up to 3 km from the coast. Some buildings were still standing but were structurally unsound, presenting a further danger. Interestingly, mosques seemed to survive the earthquake and tsunami well. The initial formal emergency response was organized by the Indonesian government, later joined by local and foreign NGOs. This focused on attending to emergency medical needs; locating, identifying, and burying the dead; and assessing and providing food, water, and shelter. However, weeks after the disaster bodies were still lying unburied and survivors were waiting for medical aid and emergency support. Armed exchanges between the government and separatists added further tensions to and politicized the relief process. There were reports of separatists kidnapping relief workers to only treat their own people. In the aftermath of the relief and reconstruction efforts, Oxfam has criticized foreign NGOs for undermining local operations and a lack of coordination in joined-up disaster relief.

References

1. Redmond A in Hopperus Buma A, Burris D, Hawley A. Conflict and Catastrophe Medicine: A Practical guide. Second edition, Springer 2009, p. 125.
2. Adapted from Australian Emergency Manual Series No. 09 Disaster Medicine (since replaced with Australian Emergency Handbook Series No 2 Disaster Health 2011). Available from: http://www.ema.gov.au. Accessed on 5 Jan, 2012.
3. Australian Emergency Manual Series No. 09 Disaster Medicine (since replaced with Australian Emergency Handbook Series No 2 Disaster Health 2011). Available from: http://www.ema.gov.au. Accessed on 5 Jan, 2012.
4. HM Government Err guidance. Available from: http://webarchive.nationalarchives.gov.uk/+/http://www.cabinetoffice.gov.uk/ukresilience/response.aspx. Accessed on 5 Jan, 2012.
5. United Nations Office for the Coordination of Humanitarian Affairs. UNDAC handbook 2006, 2006. Available from: http://ochanet.unocha.org/p/Documents/UNDAC%20Handbook-dec2006.pdf. Accessed on 5 Jan, 2012.
6. Adapted from American Academy of Pediatrics. Operation Unified Response. http://www.sciencedaily.com/releases/2010/10/101003081443.htm. Accessed on 5 Jan, 2012.
7. Van Hoving DJ, et al. Haiti: the South African perspective. SAMJ. 2010;100(8):513–5. Cape Town.
8. Nott D. The Association of Surgeons in Training Yearbook 2009–2010. The Rowan Group, London 2010. Accessible online at http://www.asit.org/assets/documents/ASiT_Yearbook_2010.pdf. Accessed 5 Jan, 2012.
9. http://www.redr.org.uk. Accessed on 5 Jan, 2012.
10. http://www.apothecaries.org/index.php?page=26. Accessed on 5 Jan, 2012.

11. http://wwwm.coventry.ac.uk/undergraduate/ugstudy/Pages/ugft_disastermanagement.aspx?itemID=982. Accessed on 5 Jan, 2012.
12. http://www.lstmliverpool.ac.uk/learning--teaching/lstm-courses/professional-diplomas/dha. Accessed on 5 Jan, 2012.
13. Virtual OSOCC – www.gdacs.org/coordination.asp. Accessed on 5 Jan, 2012.
14. www.reliefweb.org. Accessed on 5 Jan, 2012.
15. www.hewsweb.org. Accessed on 5 Jan, 2012.
16. Adapted from FCSS recommendations, taken from United Nations Office for the Coordination of Humanitarian Affairs. UNDAC handbook 2006, 2006. Available from: http://ochanet.unocha.org/p/Documents/UNDAC%20Handbook-dec2006.pdf. Accessed on 5 Jan, 2012.
17. http://wwwnc.cdc.gov/travel/content/vaccinations.aspx. Accessed on 5 Jan, 2012.
18. www.nathnac.org. Accessed on 5 Jan, 2012.
19. Adair J. Effective Leadership: how to be a successful leader. Pan Macmillan 2011.
20. Kondo H, et al. Establishing disaster medical assistance teams in Japan. Prehospital Disaster Med. 2009;24(6):556–64.
21. WHO-PAHO guidelines for the use of Foreign Field Hospitals in the aftermath of sudden-impact disasters. http://www.paho.org/english/dd/ped/FieldHospitalsFolleto.pdf. Accessed on 5 Jan, 2012.
22. Relief work can be hampered by civil unrest, with rescuers threatened or held hostage if they do not find relatives. Accessed on 5 Jan, 2012.
23. International Search and Rescue Advisory Group. Guidelines and Methodology, United Nations Office for the Coordination of Humanitarian Affairs, March 2011. Available from: http://ochanet.unocha.org/p/Documents/INSARAG%20Guidelines%202011-Latest.pdf. Accessed on 5 Jan, 2012.
24. http://www.paho.org/English/dd/ped/DeadBodiesBook-ch3.pdf. Accessed on 5 Jan, 2012.
25. Hogan D, Burstein J. Disaster medicine. 2nd ed. Philadelphia: Lippincott Williams Wilkins; 2007. p. 65.
26. www.nmcphc.med.navy.mil/downloads/stress/stressandworkingngo.doc. Accessed on 5 Jan, 2012.
27. Hopperus Buma A, Burris D, Hawley A. Conflict and Catastrophe Medicine: A Practical guide. Second edition, Springer 2009, p. 388.
28. http://new.gbgm-umc.org/umcor/work/emergencies/phasesofadisaster/. Accessed on 5 Jan, 2012.
29. Humanity first, accessible from: http://www.uk.humanityfirst.org/index.php?option=com_content&task=view&id=182. Accessed on 5 Jan, 2012.

Chapter 2
Priorities in Post-disaster Management

James Houston

Learning Objectives

- Describe the role of needs assessments and their different subtypes
- Describe what is included in a rapid needs assessment
- Explore the theory of the disaster management cycle
- Detail sources of assistance and information in disasters
- Describe what is included in a post-disaster needs assessment
- Describe the recovery phase of a disaster
- Understand the role of disaster preparedness
- Understand the role of disaster mitigation (Fig. 2.1)

Initial Scenario

You are a disaster response coordinator working with a large multinational NGO. As you finish the final touches on your latest paper on Disaster Management Theory, news breaks through your contacts abroad of a large earthquake taking place. You switch on the radio and news reports state that an earthquake measuring 7.5 on the Richter scale has occurred in a developing country in the Caribbean. Initial information is scarce, but multiple casualties are expected. After a quick meeting with your director, you are tasked with preparing and organizing a response and making sure it is delivered on the ground. You imagine that this will also eventually involve post-disaster recovery. Your logistics team contacts you asking what the disaster zone requires.

J. Houston, MBBS, MEng
FY2 Doctor, Department of Surgery,
Chelsea and Westminster Hospital, London, UK
e-mail: jameshouston@doctors.org.uk

D. MacGarty, D. Nott (eds.), *Disaster Medicine*,
DOI 10.1007/978-1-4471-4423-6_2, © Springer-Verlag London 2013

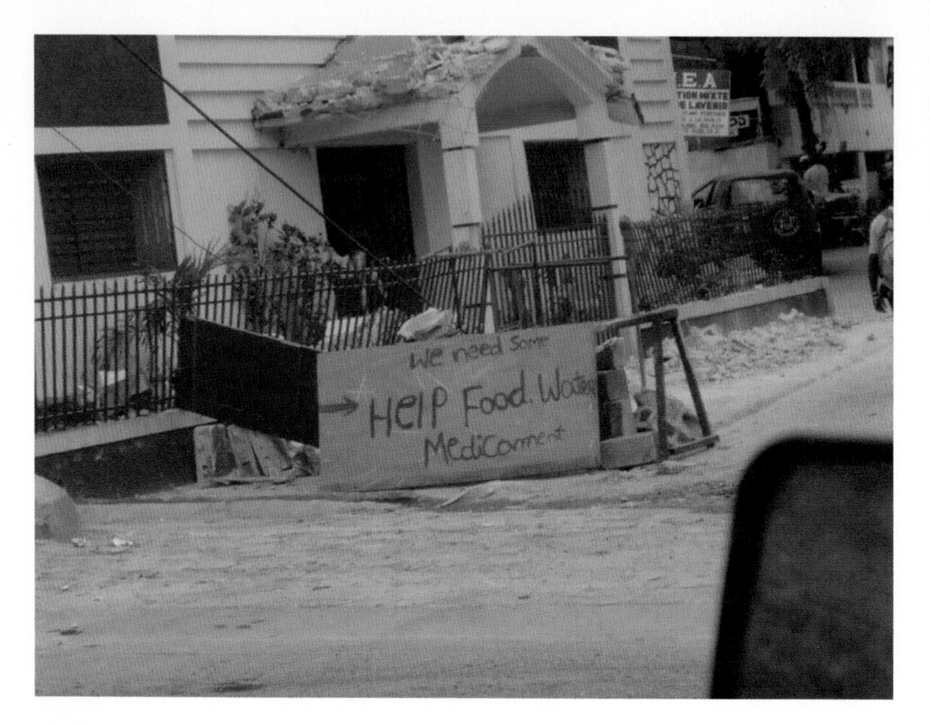

Fig. 2.1 Post-disaster needs in Haiti (Picture by David Nott)

Prompt 1: What Is a Needs Assessment?

Disasters are declared in part when affected people are unable to cope with the situation using their own resources [1]; by definition, they need some sort of external assistance. The aid needs to arrive promptly, but more importantly it needs to be appropriated or *targeted* to what the area needs. Targeted aid must be adjusted to reflect the magnitude and type of disaster. Thus, an effective response requires a timely and specific needs assessment of the affected area. Needs assessments detail requirements from disaster zones and are necessary to provide adequate aid.

Needs assessments are different from damage and loss assessments in that they take into account the ability of the population to cope under certain stressors, the so-called *vulnerability* of a population.

Disaster situations quickly evolve, and, thus, needs assessments are a dynamic concept. They change both over time and in their scope.

Different Needs Assessments at Different Times

Certain information must be prioritized. Needs assessments must not delay adequate aid from arriving. Thus, a rapid assessment should be done, to then be followed by a more detailed assessment.

Needs assessments that evolve over time include:

- Rapid needs assessment – for resource requirement post-event until about 72 h after the disaster. This period is often termed the emergency phase.
- Detailed needs assessment – post-disaster requirements for reconstruction.
- Longer-term needs assessments – these are cyclical and assist development.

Different Assessments for Different End User Requirements

Needs assessments must be done bearing in mind the end user of the information. They must be focused to providing information relevant to their needs.

Prompt 2: What Is Required in the Rapid Needs Assessment?

In the immediate aftermath of the disaster, a needs assessment for the *emergency response* is required. Emergency response broadly refers to the provision of search and rescue teams, basic life support, and security.

A *rapid needs assessment* will thus want to include certain information bearing in mind the following end users:

Search and rescue teams will want to know:

- Type of disaster
- Magnitude of disaster
- Location of disaster
- Number of people affected (including dead and injured)
- Current plans and local capacity to respond to disaster
- Access routes

Providers of basic life support will need to know current:

- Supplies of clean water
- Sanitation
- Food security
- Shelter
- Medical supplies

Security personnel will prioritize the protection of civilians and will need to know current:

- Armed forces – including the rival factions and possible extent of civil war.
- Numbers of refugees or internally displaced persons (IDPs).
- Natural hazards – including flooding, collapsing buildings, and radiation exposure.
- Local crime – widespread looting and violence can take place where there is no effective police force.

Prompt 3: How Might Information Be Gathered After a Disaster?

- Number of people affected
  - Knowledge of this will determine the magnitude of the response from your organization. Past population estimates can be gained from online sources or early contact with local officials on the ground. Basic assessments can be made by examining the number of towns and cities within the radius of the epicenter and the magnitude of the earthquake.
- Severity of injuries
  - This is a product of the energy of the disaster, the density of affected populations, and the resilience of local infrastructure to cope with initial event. For example, an earthquake of high magnitude, affecting a city in a developing country, will be far more devastating than a small event occurring in a rural area in a country that has buildings that are designed to cope with such events.
- Resilience of population
  - A developed country will likely have major incident plans in place in the event of a disaster. Resilience depends much on current infrastructure, training, and experience gained from previous events.
- Supplies for basic life support
  - The *Sphere* guidelines (see next chapter) provide a good measure of what supplies will be needed. These categorize total need by attributing a certain minimum requirement per person. Previous stockpiling of water, food, blankets, and shelters allows rapid shipment in times of need.
- Security
  - Security personnel numbers must reflect need, but not be oppressive. With an overwhelmed police force, it is likely that a temporary military presence may be required to maintain law and order. Forces should be given strict orders on engagement to ensure that no unnecessary confusion and resulting casualties occur. People who are short of food and water can quickly turn into a violent mob. To prevent such events, security must be "seen" to be doing more to help people than contain them.

Prompt 4: What Is the Disaster Management Cycle and What Does It Include?

The overall aim of disaster management is to prevent or reduce the damage caused by disasters in human, economic, and environmental terms. The subject's scope is huge and only a brief overview is dealt with in this chapter. Commonly, disaster

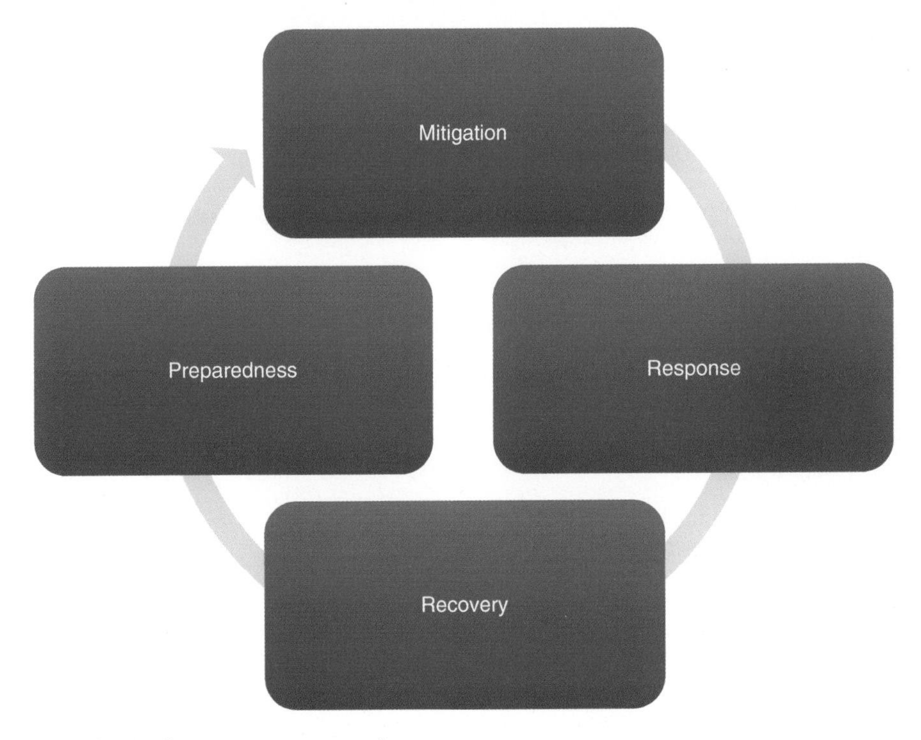

Fig. 2.2 The disaster management cycle

management is divided into the four common areas of response, recovery, preparedness, and mitigation, as seen in Box 2.1.

Box 2.1: The Phases of Disaster Management
Response: The first and initial attempt to provide emergency assistance
Recovery: Focusing on longer-term needs of the population
Preparedness: Planning how to respond to the disaster
Mitigation: Reducing or preventing the effects of the disaster

To fit into the story, this chapter will first focus on response and recovery and will then investigate preparedness and mitigation. In an ideal world, preparedness and mitigation should come before the impending disaster response and recovery!

The four areas can be seen to link together in a cycle as shown in Fig. 2.2. This implies first that overlapping can take place between phases; different parts of disaster management can take different amounts of time, and no fixed transitions exist. Second, disasters can happen in the same place more than once; what can be learned from previous events will hopefully inform future management. The cycle finally implies that disaster management may not even require a disaster to have taken place; adequate planning is an important area of eventual disaster management.

Another word commonly used is resilience, that is, the population's ability to cope in a positive light after the effects of a disaster. It is essentially the opposite of vulnerability.

Prompt 5: Who Might Be Available to Help Following a Disaster?

Broadly speaking, assistance can be thought of as internal and external.

Internal Assistance

This refers to what the affected country can provide for itself. The extent to which internal assistance is available depends on the resilience of the affected region.

- Local emergency services such as police, fire services, and medical personnel.
- A "national guard" whose resources are devoted for assistance in this type of scenario.
- The military who will likely also have access to helicopters and four-wheel drive vehicles. Such equipment can provide better access to disaster-stricken areas.
- Civilian support groups which are often based on volunteers. They can be trained and organized in the time before a disaster.

External Assistance

External assistance refers to help provided from foreign countries. Its presence depends critically on the incumbent government *accepting* help from other parties. This has been refused in some disasters due to political differences or to the government's perception that all is under control.

External assistance can include:

- The United Nations, providing UNDAC (United Nations Disaster Assessment and Coordination) which assists during the first phase of an emergency, and can deploy at short notice to anywhere in the world.
- Humanitarian organizations, many of which have specific emergency response units that are prepared to fly out at a moment's notice.
- Specialist evacuation teams, who will have equipment to get through rubble, and resources such as dogs to help in finding survivors.

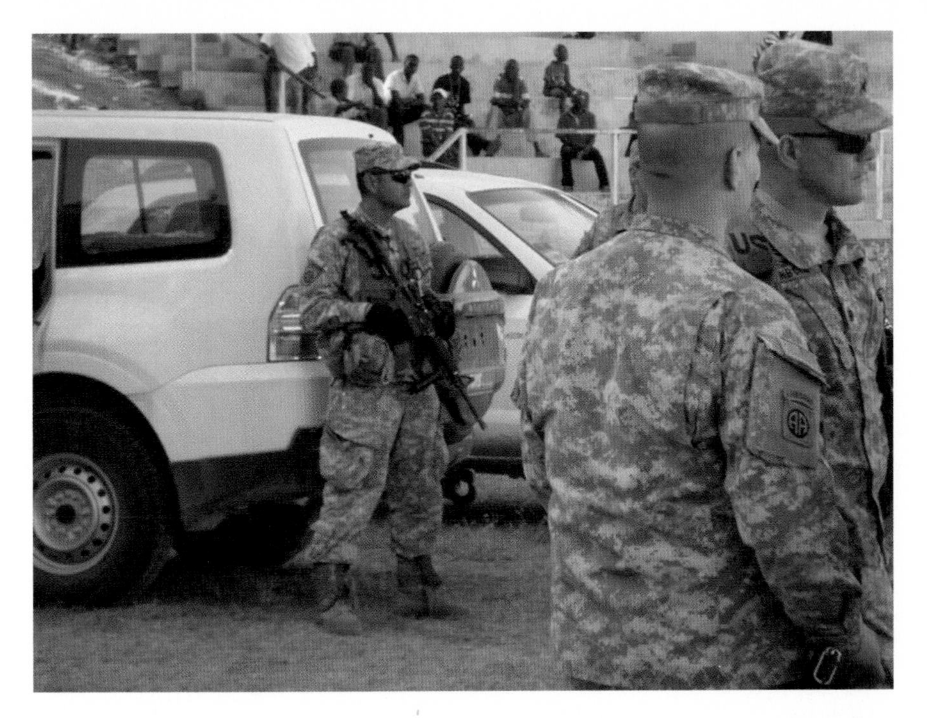

Fig. 2.3 US soldiers deployed in Haiti to help with peacekeeping efforts (Picture by David Nott)

- Foreign military forces, as seen in Fig. 2.3, who can be drafted into help. This may however have political ramifications for the affected government.

Prompt 6: How is Local Information Sourced and Disseminated?

If mobile phone networks are operational, they can be utilized to disseminate crucial information. More recently, social networks such as *Twitter* and *Facebook* have played roles in disaster response, although unverified and unofficial information can also cause problems. Future goals of disaster response will be to maximize their benefit, so that they become a tool rather than a hindrance (e.g., London riots). Traditional methods such as leaflets, public broadcasting, and community networks should not be overlooked for disseminating information.

Satellite imagery and aerial photography can provide a more objective assessment of the size of affected areas. Different imaging modalities such as infrared can pick out both survivors and fires.

Compiling and disseminating such information is one of the most important factors in providing an adequate response. Information should ideally be disseminated publically or at least to relevant aid agencies. However, a combination of poor communication and political interests will often prevent this from happening.

Further Information 1

The earthquake actually measured 8 on the Richter scale. The epicenter of the earthquake was 50 km from a large city, with many smaller towns affected. Most buildings have been unable to withstand the destruction, and widespread collapse has occurred. Around 1,500,000 people are believed to be in immediate need, with an estimated 70,000 killed and 150,000 injured. Many traumatic injuries have occurred and medical teams are currently unable to cope with the number of patients. Little advance plans exist for disaster preparation. While the road from the airport to the city is intact, there are villages in nearby mountains that have been cut off by landslides and require helicopter assistance.

Sphere standards are used to calculate minimum supplies of water, shelters, food and temporary latrines for those gathered on the outskirts of the city. The country has been relatively peaceful in recent years, although suffers from widespread corruption in its police and military. Looting and small pockets of violence have begun to breakout in some areas of the city.

External assistance is requested by the city and national government. Humanitarian teams fly to the scene to help in search and rescue. Shipments of water, food, blankets, and shelter are air-lifted in to the international airport from a nearby stockpiling base abroad. While reluctant to do so, the president agrees to a small external military force to assist in securing the city after looting and violence restricts some of the first aid efforts. A curfew is put in place at night.

The first few days are exhausting work, although your team has helped find many survivors. Better equipment has been made available, but the presence of aftershocks has made work difficult and dangerous. One week later, a large camp has been erected on the outskirts of town. You start to focus on the changing needs of the disaster.

Prompt 7: What Is a Post-disaster Needs Assessment?

The "post-disaster needs assessment" takes a more detailed account of the needs of the population [2]. Provided by the government of the country, it is also governed by legal agreements between the United Nations, the World Bank, and the European Commission. It gathers information that has already been made available but can now take advantage of a more steady state. The assessment will take much longer to put together, perhaps up to 2 months, and reflects the long-term population needs. Alongside the needs assessment, it must also incorporate a damage and loss assessment that includes socioeconomic impact.

A useful way to classify such needs, such as performed in the assessment in Haiti [3], focuses on the impact in three areas:

- Humans – mortality and morbidity, alongside original demographics
- Infrastructure – transport, water, power, schools, and social structure
- Environment – ongoing hazards such as oil, pollution, or radiation

Prompt 8: What Is the Recovery Phase?

The recovery phase aims to address those needs of affected people which were not immediately life threatening during the response phase. Different people can be involved at this point, and a more thorough needs assessment maybe required. There is no distinct difference between the response and recovery phases. Thus, good disaster management should provide assistance more as a continuum rather than in discrete units.

Recovery refers to a return to a state as good as, or ideally improved upon the pre-disaster state. The improvement on the pre-disaster state refers to the fact that plans may now have been put in place to reduce the effect of any future disaster.

For example, short-term repairs may have been initially made to roads to allow access for emergency services; in the recovery phase, more thorough repairs can be implemented to re-enable economic capability.

The recovery phase may contain among other things:

- Infrastructure rebuilding
- Property rebuilding
- Counseling and addressing psychological impact
- Data collection such as TRIAMS described in Box 2.2

Box 2.2: Systems Set Up in Recovery Phases of Disasters: TRIAMS

The *tsunami recovery impact assessment and monitoring system* (TRIAMS) [4] was set up after the 2005 tsunami in South Asia. It aimed to "assist government, aid agencies and affected populations in assessing and monitoring the rate and direction of tsunami recovery in the countries covered over a period of five years." By improving government monitoring of how aid was spent through the setup of this system with key outcomes, efficiency has been increased with less money wasted.

Recovery Phase and Continued Development

Similar to between response and recovery, a smooth transition should be aimed for between recovery and long-term development. Previous disasters have confined themselves to repetition by little investment in long-term schemes that reduce vulnerability. Aid secured for relief efforts should also be ear-marked for longer development options if possible, especially as money is much more difficult to get hold of once the eye-catching photographs and media attention subside.

Further Information 2

The emergency teams move out after a week when a decision is made that no more survivors will be found. A more thorough post-disaster needs assessment is made. Aid agencies are heavily involved in providing basic humanitarian support. As the rubble is cleared and the reconstruction begins, tense negotiations take place. Government ministers and international aid agencies debate about the long-term development of the country. The focus is to try to make sure that nothing like this will happen again.

Prompt 9: What Is Disaster Preparedness?

Disaster preparedness focuses on ensuring that systems can cope as best as possible should a disaster occur. Disaster preparedness is almost synonymous with that of resilience. Many large organizations have major incident plans that come in to place should the inevitable occur, and major humanitarian organizations will have similar plans for coordination of relief efforts.

Central to disaster preparedness are:

1. Disaster plans
2. A workforce ready to carry out those plans
3. Early warning systems
4. Systems and infrastructure that work in austere environments

Disaster plans should:

- Involve all levels of government, particularly those with local knowledge, who will be able to tell if plans are practical
- Have strategic reserves of water and food, alongside blankets and shelter
- Involve logistics operators that take account of strategic placement of stockpiles
- Have up to date information on areas of risk that includes population demographics
- Have some degree of flexibility and use public resources that may not be utilized fully, such as school buses for transport or town halls for emergency accommodation

An Able Workforce

A good plan can only work if people understand what to do if the event occurs; therefore, exercises and training must take place. After this, a full debriefing should occur to evaluate room for improvement. This disaster workforce does not necessarily have to be just made up of professionals; volunteers can provide valuable extra capacity in times of need. This can include helping people to set up areas for emergency shelter, manning helplines to assist those seeking information or wanting to report missing people.

Early Warning Systems

Some disasters such as earthquakes are extremely difficult to predict. Others, such as hurricanes, can be predicted by weather forecasts and satellite imagery that give enough time to spare to evacuate residents. Tsunamis stand in the middle as only hours are given. Warning systems have been set up in both the Pacific and Indian Ocean. Two difficulties exist with these systems: first, can the tsunami be reliably predicted? It is still quite difficult to know which earthquakes will cause tsunamis. Second, can an emergency alert be disseminated in time to those at risk? *CWARN* [5] is an organization that disseminates SMS to members with incoming tsunamis.

Resilient Systems

Systems are placed under extraordinary stress during disasters. While some of their capacity may have been destroyed, communication systems simultaneously experience an increase in demand due to families trying to contact each other. Reliable communication systems are of crucial importance in disasters. Often low-tech solutions are preferable since they have less of a propensity to fail, are often easier to use, and are cheaper to stockpile.

Prompt 10: What Is Disaster Mitigation?

Disaster mitigation refers to either reducing occurrence of disasters or at least reducing the effects of disasters. It primarily addresses risk and can be referred to as either structural or non-structural.

Structural mitigation:

- Building codes for structures to withstand disasters
- Flood barriers

Non-structural mitigation:

- Legislation – public policies to ensure funding or action
- Land Planning – reducing high-density populations in places at risk, not building on flood plains
- Insurance – ensuring people will have capital to rebuild post disaster
- Education – providing people with information so they know what to do in disasters

Some of these policies may prove unpopular and have their costs both economically (e.g., insurance) and environmentally (e.g., flood barriers). Thus, the government must involve stakeholders at all levels to make adequate assessment of risk and provide enough information to convince people of their worth. Most importantly, the causes of the disasters must be addressed where possible.

Further Information 3

A law is put in place to ensure that future buildings must conform to certain structural requirements. Over the following months, a detailed account of all that went on post earthquake is compiled. A team is put together that makes a future disaster plan. Volunteers are recruited and practice exercises in the event of another earthquake. An education program and leaflet are made to inform people of what to do should the same happen again.

Case Study: Haiti 2010
Haiti experienced a catastrophic earthquake in January 2010 whose epicenter was approximately 25 km from its capital Port-au-Prince. Haiti is one of the poorest countries in the world, and the earthquake affected an estimated 3 million people, with up to a quarter of a million people killed. Many important buildings were destroyed in the quake, which hampered initial rescue efforts. Early coordination and leadership was made difficult in these circumstances and made worse with the arrival of thousands of aid organizations. Search and rescue teams came from around the globe with a total of 26 arriving within the first 3 days. They managed to rescue a total of 134 people. In the first 6 months of the response, 4 million people were provided with food aid and 1.2 million with drinking water, 1.5 million received emergency shelter materials and 11,000 latrines were installed [6]. Some existing capacity such as in water supplied was used to some success. Difficulties were present in leadership from the government and the poor humanitarian leadership [7]. A needs assessment was performed which underestimated the magnitude of the disaster.

This led to difficulty in providing adequate sanitation in the post-disaster phase and allowed a cholera epidemic to materialize. While much money has been spent on development, 2 years on there are still streets blocked by collapsed buildings; the situation is no better than it was before the earthquake, and little evidence exists of any disaster preparedness for future earthquakes.

References

1. United Nations Department of Humanitarian Affairs. 1992. Glossary: internationally agreed glossary of basic terms related to disaster management. Available at: http://reliefweb.int/node/21195. Accessed 15 Mar 2012.
2. International Recovery Platform Post Disaster Recovery Needs Assessment and Methodologies, [Home page on the internet]; 2011. Available at: www.recoveryplatform.org. Accessed 30 Nov 2011.
3. Government of the Republic of Haiti, Haiti Earthquake PDNA: Assessment of damage, losses, general and sectoral needs. 2010. Accessed 30 Nov 2011. Available at: www.refondation.ht/resources/PDNA_Working_Document.pdf.
4. WHO: Tsunami Recovery Impact Assessment and Monitoring System (TRIAMS). 2011. Available at: http://www.who.int/hac/crises/international/asia_tsunami/triams/en/index.html. Accessed 30 Nov 2011.
5. CWARN: Worldwide Early tsunami warning system: Available at: www.cwarn.org/. Accessed Mar 20 2012.
6. UNOCHA Evaluation of OCHA response to the Haiti earthquake. 2011. Available at: http://ochanet.unocha.org/p/Documents/Evaluation%20of%20OCHA%20Response%20to%20the%20Haiti%20Earthquake.pdf. Accessed 30 Nov 2011.
7. Grunewald F, Binder A, Georges Y. Global: InterAgency real time evaluation in Haiti: 3 months after the earthquake. 2010. Available at: www.unicef.org/evaluation/files/Haiti_IA_RTE_final_Eng.pdf. Accessed 30 Nov 2011.

Chapter 3
Refugee Camps

Shao Foong Chong

Learning Objectives

- Understand the distinction between refugee and internally displaced people
- Outline the role of the United Nations High Commissioner for Refugees (UNHCR)
- Describe the key components of the Sphere Project
- Discuss the Humanitarian Charter and Minimum Standards in the Sphere Handbook
- Plan appropriate interventions in the post-emergency phase
- Explore issues arising from repatriation and resettlement.

Case Study

Based loosely on real events in a sub-Saharan refugee camp.

Initial Scenario

Following civil war, thousands of people have left their country to escape from war and persecution and have congregated around a town in the neighboring country just across the border. A refugee camp built nearby this border town to originally

S.F. Chong, MBBS, M.A. (Oxon)
FY2 Doctor, Department of Emergency Medicine,
St George's Hospital, Tooting, London, UK
e-mail: shaofoong@hotmail.com

D. MacGarty, D. Nott (eds.), *Disaster Medicine*,
DOI 10.1007/978-1-4471-4423-6_3, © Springer-Verlag London 2013

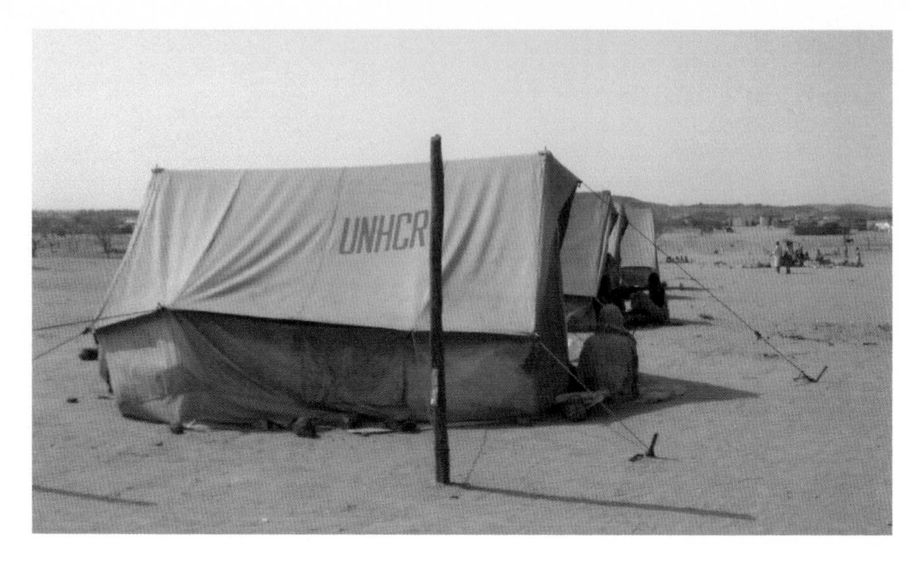

Fig. 3.1 UNHCR tent. Credits: David Nott (Picture by David Nott)

accommodate 20,000, now has over 50,000 refugees (Fig. 3.1). *There were plans for an extension, but the local government has complained that they have not received sufficient funds from the international community. Aid agencies have been deployed for the last few months to manage the crisis; however, their standards and operating procedures vary widely, and arguments develop as to which agency should be in charge. You are the chief advisor to the UNHCR and have been tasked with the long-term management of this refugee camp.*

Prompt 1: Distinguish Between the Terms "Refugee" and "Internally Displaced Person" (IDP)

- Refugees are individuals who have fled their homes and crossed an internationally recognized border in search of sanctuary because of a well-founded fear of persecution based on their race, religion, nationality, political, or social opinion.
- IDPs are people who have involuntarily been uprooted and displaced, often due to armed conflict and human rights violations, but still remain within the borders of their country of residence [1].

Prompt 2: What Is the Legal Status of Refugees and IDPs?

- The UNHCR drew up the 1951 Convention Relating to the Status of Refugees, which mandates state protection of refugees by international law [2]. This includes the principle of *non-refoulement*, which is the right to be protected against forcible return.

Table 3.1 UNHCR statistics: major countries of refugees, end-2010

Countries of origin	Main countries of asylum	No. of refugees
Afghanistan	Pakistan, Iran	3,054,700
Iraq	Jordan, Syria	1,683,600
Somalia	Kenya, Ethiopia, Yemen	770,200

Source: UN High Commission for Refugees (UNHCR). Includes refugees and people in "refugee-like" situations [3]

- However, the international community's ability to assist IDPs may be limited, as they remain within the boundaries of their country and do not hold the same legal status. This unfortunately may marginalize ethnic groups that are deemed unfavorable by their government.
- Over the last several years, humanitarian agencies have tried to meet the needs of both refugees and IDPs where possible. Thus, references to "refugees" in this case should be taken to indicate both categories.

Prompt 3: Who Has Responsibility for the Needs of Refugees?

- Host governments are responsible for the security and safety of refugees.
- The UNHCR ensures the physical needs of refugees are met appropriately by coordinating and monitoring implementation of aid program interventions.
- There may be large numbers of nongovernmental organizations (NGOs) that operate on the ground. An inter-agency approach designates individual agencies to be sector leaders in particular operations, so responsibilities are not missed nor duplicated.

Prompt 4: What Are the Global Trends of the Refugee Population?

- Refugee numbers are at a 15-year high. UNHCR's 2010 "Global Trends" report estimates that the number of people forcibly uprooted by war and natural disasters is 43.7 million, which includes 15.4 million refugees, 27.5 million IDPs, and a further 840,000 people waiting to be given refugee status [3].
- Most refugees live in a country neighboring their own. In 2010, Afghanistan, Iraq, and Somalia were the top source countries of refugees (Table 3.1), while Pakistan, Iran, and the Syrian Arab Republic hosted the largest number.

Further Information 1

The numbers of refugees arriving at the camp are swelling at an alarming rate, and the camp is large and overcrowded. Many of the new arrivals, the elderly and children in particular, who have been walking for days on end alongside being malnourished and affected with gastrointestinal disease. NGOs on the ground report that makeshift settlements have been constructed but in such close proximity that there is a lack of clean drinking water and basic sanitation facilities to share within communities. From the initial assessment, they estimate that, with the current food and water resources and increasingly large population, acute malnutrition is as high as 30 % and people are dehydrated receiving 10 L of water/day, which are causing many case fatalities.

Prompt 5: What Is the Sphere Project?

The Sphere Project

- Launched in 1997 as a response to inconsistencies in basic levels of care and the lack of accountability of humanitarian agencies in disasters.
- A handbook was put together by experts drawn from NGOs, Red Cross, UNHCR, WHO, and WFP to provide common principles and concrete, measurable, minimum standards for humanitarian agencies in order to achieve greater quality and accountability [4].
- The Sphere Handbook is designed to be used in disaster response as well as disaster preparedness and human advocacy. As the principles remain universally consistent, it can be applied in any range of situations – whether there is a famine in rural Africa or a flood that has displaced millions of people from their homes in a large US city.
- The emphasis of Sphere is meeting urgent survival needs of people affected by disaster while asserting their basic human right to life with dignity.

Prompt 6: What Are Sphere's Principles?

- The Humanitarian Charter, the Protection Principles, and the Core Standards reflect Sphere's rights-based and people-centered approach.

Humanitarian Charter

- The charter emphasized the importance of the humanitarian imperative, based on the principles and provisions of international humanitarian law, human rights, and refugee conventions:
  - The right to life with dignity
  - The right to receive humanitarian assistance
  - The right to protection and security

Protection Principles

- Humanitarian agencies have a duty to protect the safety of populations by:
  - Avoiding exposing people to further harm

- Ensuring people's access to impartial assistance
- Protecting people from harm arising from violence and coercion
- Assisting people to claim their rights, access remedies, and recover from abuse

Core Standards

- Emphasizes active participation of local communities, effective coordination and communication between agencies, and continual professional development.

Prompt 7: How Can the Sphere Handbook Be Applied to Provide Minimum Standards of Care in This Refugee Camp?

Minimum Standards

- The Sphere Project has developed a set of universal minimum standards to act as concrete achievable benchmarks in four key areas:
  - Water supply, sanitation, and hygiene promotion
  - Food security and nutrition
  - Shelter, settlement, and non-food items
  - Health action

Water Supply, Sanitation, and Hygiene Promotion [5]

- Provision and adequate quantities and quality of water are essential to population health. Refugees should be provided with at least 15 l/day for drinking, food preparation, personal hygiene, and cleaning. As a result, you have constructed more water distribution points each of which should supply 80–100 refugees to meet the rising needs of the population.
- Basic sanitation and hygiene are important but neglected interventions in refugee camps in emergencies. Information about the lack of minimum standards in this camp is being fed back to donors. It is noted that large volumes of reasonably clean water are preferable to small amounts of pure water. Thus, they pledge to send simple technologies such as bucket and chlorination to treat the potentially contaminated water to mitigate the gastrointestinal diseases that are spreading rife throughout the camp. Those who are suffering are provided with oral rehydration salts and hygiene education by properly trained staff. Culturally appropriate sanitation, bathing, and washing facilities are made, segregated either by sex or by household.

Food Security and Nutrition

- Wasting and micronutrient deficiency disorders such as scurvy, pellagra, and beriberi are very noticeable in the new arrivals. They are provided with micronutrient and caloric requirements of at least 2,100 kcal per person per day. Focus is directed toward key vulnerable groups – i.e., women, children, elderly, disabled, people living with HIV/AIDS, and ethnic minorities.

- There have been logistical problems in distributing food fairly in this camp. Some local leaders distribute food to their own communities and ignore others. This has caused much hunger and frustration in the marginalized groups; thus, you endeavor to ask one of the NGOs to be in charge of distributing food and monitoring whether all groups are receiving them equitably.

Shelter, Settlement, and Non-food Items

- It is suggested that large, densely populated camps over the size of 20,000 should be avoided, and this camp of 50,000 is reaching more than capacity. At the moment, Sphere's minimum standards that 30 m^2 should be provided for living space and 3.5 m^2 for shelter space are not achievable due to the level of overcrowding. You propose to the local government that another camp needs to be made, and that you will free up stockpiles of UNHCR tents and funding for its establishment.

Health Action

- The majority of deaths in refugee camps are normally attributed to diarrheal diseases, acute respiratory infections, malaria, measles, and malnutrition.
- Mortality rates of over 2 deaths per 10,000 per day indicate an emergency health situation. Thankfully you have not reached that level. This may be due to a number of key public health surveillance and outreach information campaigns which have reduced the risk of epidemics. One key intervention included a measles vaccination program, where herd immunity of over 90 % of children aged 6 months to 5 years was achieved.
- Primary health clinics are in the process of being set up at points around the camp with sufficiently equipment, drugs, and trained staff to serve all refugee communities.

Prompt 8: How Has Sphere Been Accepted by the International Community?

- More than 200 major agencies are in consensus with the minimum standards in disaster assistance. The Sphere Project has provided accountability to the attainment of quantitative standards which is pivotal in ensuring interventional projects are successfully achieving their aims amidst the chaos that arises from disasters.
- It has been criticized by some NGOs for being too prescriptive and curtailing creativity in programming. Donors may even misuse sphere standards as being maximum standards. Some argue that there is too much emphasis on the technical aspects of attaining minimum standards, and that other nonquantifiable measures are missed.
- Médecins Sans Frontières (MSF) has not embraced the Sphere Project, as it felt that it would reduce the humanitarian response to a technical exercise of focusing on standards, as instead has its own way of responding to a refugee crisis (Box 3.1).

Box 3.1: Top Ten Priorities for Refugee Health

MSF has listed the following top ten operational priorities for the acute emergency phase of a refugee crisis [6]. These interventions should be rapidly implemented simultaneously to control and reduce the mortality rate and improve the population's health.

1. Rapid assessment of the health status of a population
2. Mass vaccination against measles
3. Water supply and implementation of sanitary measures
4. Food supply and implementation of specialized nutritional rehabilitation programs
5. Shelter, site planning, and non-food items
6. Curative care based on the use of standardized therapeutic protocols, using essential drugs
7. Control and prevention of communicable diseases and potential epidemics
8. Surveillance and alert
9. Assessment of human resources, training, and supervision of community health workers
10. Coordination of different operational partners

Further Information 2

UNHCR camps have provided the refugees with food, housing materials, clean water supplies, sanitation facilities, and health centers. After 8 months, minimum standards of care have, by in large, been attained. However, the population is almost entirely dependent upon outside assistance, as they have few means of cultivating the nearby land, and there is little incentive to do so as aid supplies bring in the vast majority of their needs. A new disaster has occurred elsewhere in the world, and media attention is refocused. Consequently, international aid is less forthcoming, and NGOs start pulling out. Community leaders are complaining of a lack of funds that have dramatically affected the welfare of the camp. Communicable diseases start to become more prevalent, and women and children's health are accused of being neglected.

Prompt 9: Define the Post-emergency Phase

- The post-emergency phase occurs when all the minimum standards have been addressed, and the mortality rate has stabilized to a satisfactory level.
- However, this transition from the acute response to long-term recovery is often plagued with budget cuts leading to a lack of vital supplies and skilled personnel.

Prompt 10: What Are the Longer-Term Objectives During This Phase?

- *Consolidation* – Skills and knowledge need to be transferred to local government and community leaders to maintain low mortality rates, good nutrition, and health status. Aid agencies ought to train up local staff to take over the operational positions of relief programs.
- *Sustainability* – Active involvement of local refugees from the beginning should be encouraged to decrease dependency upon relief aid. This may include agriculture, vocational community-based activities, long-term income generating projects, and cooperative banks.
- *Emergency Preparedness* – The capability to confront potentially new challenges, such as a large influx of new refugees or major disease epidemics, should be thought through. Public health screening and surveillance systems are essential to catch disease outbreaks at an early stage. Community outreach programs can help to combat emerging health problems in refugee camps, such as HIV/AIDS and mental health.

Prompt 11: How Might Interventions for Refugees Cause Conflict with Surrounding Communities?

- Humanitarian agencies that solely focus on the plight of refugees without consideration to the needs of the host community may fuel conflicts and lead to undesirable consequences [7].
- Refugee camps may provide living standards that are vastly better than the national standard where poverty and deprivation are prevalent [8]. This may cause resentment as the new marginal group, the refugees, become more privileged than the impoverished locals. Sometimes local communities are displaced from their normal abode as camps swell in population and a combination of such factors may in turn lead to violence.
- Reducing these inequalities is vital to maintaining peace. Interventions should be offered to all members of the community, refugee, and non-refugee to help long-term integration.

Further Information 3

The civil war has finally settled down, and a peace agreement has been signed. There is much joy and jubilation among the refugee population. Some refugee communities are considering moving out of the camps and returning home, while some are afraid as unverified reports have been spread that their villages and land have been destroyed, leaving extremely poor prospects if they return. A rumor is propagating that a select number of people who claimed to be suffering from ongoing persecution have been resettled in the USA. This has led to a situation where some refugees who were previously prepared to go home are now camping out to wait for resettlement.

Prompt 12: What Are the Long-Term Solutions for Refugees?

- *Voluntary Repatriation to Their Homeland* – Most refugees in the world prefer to return to their countries of origin, rather than seeking refuge elsewhere. However, repatriation is not always feasible due to ongoing conflict, discrimination, or lack of economic opportunity in their homeland. Although this option is actively encouraged, sometimes with substantial relief packages, the number of refugee returns has continuously decreased since 2004 due to humanitarian crises or political situations.
- *Local Integration in Their Countries of Asylum* – Sometimes refugees may acquire citizenship through naturalization by host countries. Policies for naturalization differ between countries, so this can become a very complex procedure.
- *Resettlement in Third Party Countries* – When refugees face an ongoing threat of persecution in their country of asylum, resettlement provides a way to protect their intrinsic human rights. This is a protection tool that is shared by the international community. A minority of countries offer resettlement programs, and often there is a strict annual quota; of the 10.5 million refugees who were of concern, only 1 % of the world's refugees were submitted for resettlement [9]. However, some refugees will wait and remain in refugee camps with the small glimmer of hope of being resettled to a high-income country.

Prompt 13: What Challenges Are Involved in Returning Refugees Home?

- *Political* – Ethnic divisions may still persist, especially after a civil war. Political motives may keep groups of people displaced from their land. Local authority leaders may discriminate and prevent minority groups repatriating.
- *Social* – Lack of access to public services such as education, security, and healthcare which was previously provided by the international community may hinder communities leaving refugee camps.
- *Economic* – After a humanitarian disaster, there may be a lack of potential for agriculture, commercial activity, and entitlement to land. For example, refugees

may find their abandoned houses destroyed in the conflict or have squatters occupying them. Compensation is unlikely to be forthcoming.

Prompt 14: What Repatriation Assistance Can NGOs and UN Relief Agencies Provide?

- *Information* – Unfounded rumors about poor conditions in their home areas or the chances of being resettled in a rich country may hinder repatriation attempts. Thus, NGOs and UN relief agencies are key players in updating local community leaders with accurate information, such as socioeconomic conditions, health services, and nutritional aid. Information should be culturally appropriate, and a range of media may be used such as megaphones, radio, TV, leaflets, posters, and billboards.
- *Relief Package* – This may include transportation, blankets and temporary shelter, water and food assistance, practical help adapted to local needs such as seeds, farming equipment, and building materials, and occasionally financial help. When assisting refugees in repatriation, NGOs must allocate a proportion of their resources to aid the local non-refugee population and to help overcome inequalities that may otherwise cause conflict and resentment.
- *Conflict Resolution* – As persistent conflict or fear of persecution often prevents people from returning to their countries of origin, assistance with peace agreements can greatly help people return home.

Case Study: The Great Lakes Refugee Crisis, 1994–1996

An estimated 800,000 Tutsis and moderate Hutus were murdered in the Rwandan genocide. In the conflict that ensued, millions fled to refugee camps across the border in Tanzania and Zaire. Camps were large, overcrowded, insecure, and infiltrated by the fleeing Hutu Interahamwe militia responsible for the original genocide. Deaths among the refugee population rose alarmingly, and 50,000 died, the elderly and children first, from a cholera epidemic that swept round the camps.

After delayed international media coverage, worldwide fundraising campaigns raised an unprecedented amount of $1.5 billion for the immediate relief operation in these refugee camps. Tents for shelter were constructed, latrines and wells were dug, and clinic and food distribution centers were established to serve the refugee population. Never before had there been so many aid organizations involved in a single humanitarian territory.

However, this vast injection of money and resources created a plethora of activity by the many aid organizations on the ground but resulted in an overall mal-coordinated humanitarian response. Major issues identified were the responsibility of protecting innocent refugees from violence and logistical problems in assessing and prioritizing basic needs of such a large population. It was called the "world's worst humanitarian crisis in a generation." But it was a catalyst for change. The Sphere Project was created to improve organizational and management issues in meeting minimum standards of care and to ensure greater international commitments and accountability in humanitarian interventions.

The return and reintegration of refugee returnees remain massive challenges to Rwanda. Many have not granted any land and access to basic shelter, healthcare, and education. Vulnerable groups, such as orphaned children or victims of physical and sexual violence, have not received the psychosocial support they required. There is an ongoing struggle for Rwanda's refugees to make a livelihood.

References

1. Ryan J, Childs D. Refugees and internally displaced people. In: Conflict and catastrophe medicine: a practical guide. London: Springer; 2002. p. 49–53.
2. UN High Commission for Refugees. UNHCR handbook for emergencies. 3rd ed. Geneva: United Nations High Commissioner for Refugees; 2007. Available from: http://www.unhcr.org/472af2972.pdf. Accessed 22 Aug 2012.
3. UN High Commission for Refugees. UNHCR Global Trends 2010. Available from: http://www.unhcr.org/4dfa11499.html. Accessed 22 Aug 2012.
4. The Sphere Project. Humanitarian charter and minimum standards in humanitarian response. 3rd ed. Geneva: Practical Action Publishing; The Sphere Project; 2011.
5. Noji E. Public health in the aftermath of disasters. In: Redmond A, Mahoney P, Ryan J, editors. ABC of conflict and disaster. Oxford: Blackwell Publishing Ltd; 2006.
6. Médicins Sans Frontières. Refugee health: an approach to emergency situations. Paris: Médicins Sans Frontières; 1997. Available from: http://www.refbooks.msf.org/MSF_Docs/En/Refugee_Health/RH.pdf. Accessed 22 Aug 2012.
7. Healing T, Pelly M. Refugees and disasters. In: Parry E, Godfrey R, Mabey D, Gill G, editors. Principles of medicine in Africa. 3rd ed. Cambridge: Cambridge University Press; 2004. p. 77–86.
8. Cochrane, L. UNHCR policy and practice: confronting calls for change. The Journal of Humanitarian Assistance. Tufts University, Feinstein International Center; 2007. Available from: http://sites.tufts.edu/jha/archives/47. Accessed 22 Aug 2012.
9. UN High Commission for Refugees. A new beginning in a third country [homepage on the Internet; cited 2012 Feb 27]. Available from: http://www.unhcr.org/pages/4a16b1676.html. Accessed 22 Aug 2012.

Chapter 4
Complex Emergencies

Will Barker

Learning Objectives

- Understand various definitions of a complex emergency
- Describe the factors that lead to a complex emergency
- Understand different models of complex emergencies
- Discuss ways relief aid can be sometimes harmful
- The UN humanitarian principles and their role in humanitarian access
- Explore the motives of key stakeholders in a complex emergency
- Define humanitarian intervention and discuss its role in disasters

Initial Scenario

You are a doctor with a medical NGO deployed to provide basic medical care to a camp of internally displaced persons (IDPs) following regional conflict.

A local militia the "Lords Protection Army" (LPA) forcibly displaced the IDPs two years ago as a land grab with tacit approval of the national government. Shortly after another militia, the "National Liberation Army" (NLA) was born claiming to protect from LPA attacks. The protection failed, but new militia became embroiled in conflict with the government army, leading to hundreds more civilian deaths and thousands of displacements.

The ReliefWeb briefing pack your NGO has prepared for you states that the UN is treating it as a complex emergency (Box 4.1).

W. Barker, MBBS, MPhys
FY2 Doctor, St Thomas' Hospital,
Westminster Bridge Road, London, UK
e-mail: willbarker@doctors.org.uk

D. MacGarty, D. Nott (eds.), *Disaster Medicine*,
DOI 10.1007/978-1-4471-4423-6_4, © Springer-Verlag London 2013

Prompt 1: What Is a Complex Emergency?

The concept of complex emergencies arose in the 1980s when it became clear that some relief efforts to disasters were severely constrained by local and international politics.

The term "complex emergency" is used widely to describe when an international humanitarian response is required in a war-affected region. ReliefWeb characterizes a complex emergency as having [1]:

1. Extensive violence and loss of life
2. Massive displacements of people
3. Widespread damage to societies and economies
4. The need for large-scale, multifaceted humanitarian assistance
5. The hindrance or prevention of humanitarian assistance by political and military interests
6. Significant security risks for humanitarian relief workers in some areas

Box 4.1: ReliefWeb
ReliefWeb (http://reliefweb.int/) is the UN website providing information to humanitarian relief organizations. It was launched in 1996 to serve the information needs of the humanitarian community. It contains the latest reports by UN organizations and NGOs and can rapidly generate briefing packs for humanitarian emergencies across the world [2].

Prompt 2: What Definitions Exist for Complex Emergencies?

The Inter-Agency Standing Committee of the UN (the primary mechanism for inter-agency coordination) defines a complex emergency as [3]:

> A humanitarian crisis in a country, region or society where there is total or considerable breakdown of authority resulting from internal or external conflict and which requires an international response that goes beyond the mandate or capacity of any single agency and/or the on-going United Nations country program.

Despite being an important definition (Box 4.2) and probably the most widely accepted, the IASC definition is weak: All humanitarian emergencies go beyond the capacity of a single agency, and often there is not a breakdown of government authority; the government may maintain a perpetual state of conflict as a way of targeting political enemies and unfavoured ethnic groups [4]. "Emergency" also implies that the problem is acute, but most complex emergencies develop for years with relief starting only once a critical stage is reached.

Box 4.2: Why the Definition of Complex Emergencies Is Important?
There is often political infighting for the control of UN missions, for example, between the Office for Coordination of Humanitarian Assistance (OCHA), the UN Office for Displaced Persons (UNDP), and the UN Country Programs. Calling a disaster a complex emergency can change which agencies lead and so therefore becomes political.

A more recent definition by the medical journal the *Lancet* expanded the definition of a complex emergency to include

> situations in which mortality among the civilian population substantially increases above the population baseline, either as a result of the direct effects of war or indirectly through increased prevalence of malnutrition and/or transmission of communicable diseases, particularly if the latter result from deliberate political and military policies and strategies (national, subnational, or international) [5].

The mortality that is typically used is a doubling of the baseline mortality in sub-Saharan Africa, giving a crude mortality rate (CMR) greater than one death per 10,000 people [5]. This includes scenarios where war may not be prominent, but government actions lead to a humanitarian crisis, for example, the famine in Sudan caused by years of poor governance.

Prompt 3: What Factors Lead to Complex Emergencies?

Complex emergencies by definition are entirely man-made or have a major man-made element. This can be in the form of internal conflict, forced displacement of populations, famine, genocide, and violence directed against civilians.

Large-scale genocide continues and has been seen recently in Rwanda, Bosnia, and Sudan. Spontaneous ethnic tensions may lead to violence, but more often ethnic tensions are engineered for political reasons, as was the case in the Rwandan genocide [6].

Complex emergencies are typically reported with simple explanations, for example, "ethnic violence," "societal breakdown," or the actions of a tyrant (Table 4.1). These can be wildly inaccurate and overlook complex political situations and to understand the disasters better, more detailed analysis needs to be made [6].

Further Information 1

You conduct a survey of the camp to address key questions:

- *Is violence being directed at civilians, is it intentionally, and by whom?*
- *What are the motives of the perpetrators of violence?*

Table 4.1 Models of complex emergencies

Model	Explanation	Weakness
Breakdown of authority	Poor governance leads to lawlessness and violence	National governments are often orchestrating the violence
Contest	Conflict fought by rebels against the national government with civilians caught in between	Often the war is directed at civilians with both armies avoiding costly direct conflict This is described as the "sell game" with neither army pursuing victory and both benefitting from continued conflict [6]
Good vs. evil	TV typically portrays the UN and humanitarian agencies as good obstructed by 'evil' dictators	There is rarely international consensus on which side is the good and which the aggressor, e.g., Syria or Iran
Greed	Economic benefit drives conflict and war, economies develop where violence maintains power and generates wealth for political elites	Not all violence is explained by greed as was the case in the Rwandan genocide
Ethnic violence and grievances	Historical tensions between ethnic groups erupt in violence	Ethnic divisions are the intended product of violence rather than the cause and serve political ends
System	Key players benefit economically, psychologically, or politically from conflict. Behaviour is complex but can be predicted and anticipated in relief efforts	Understanding motives is complex and has not been done well in the past. Explanations are complicated and unpalatable by mainstream media

- *What is the function of the displacement of people?*
- *What are the needs of the population?*
- *Is it logistically possible to get relief into the area?*
- *Is it safe for relief operations in the area?*

You find approximately 100,000 people living in makeshift camps with diarrheal disease becoming widespread. A drought has led to food hoarding and price rises, and so food is becoming unaffordable, compounded by supplies being severely restricted by fighting and bad roads. Many aid agencies are already visibly present, although their efforts are uncoordinated and they are underequipped.

Through interviewing people in the camp, you find that the government aims to displace local subsistence farmers to make way for profitable mechanized farms. Conflict between the paramilitaries and government has been concentrated over areas of mineral resource, and minerals are being exported to buy more weapons. There are widespread attacks on civilians from all sides.

Your interpreter warns you that the militia has suspicions you are a government spy, so you cut short your observations and return to the comparative safety of a nearby town.

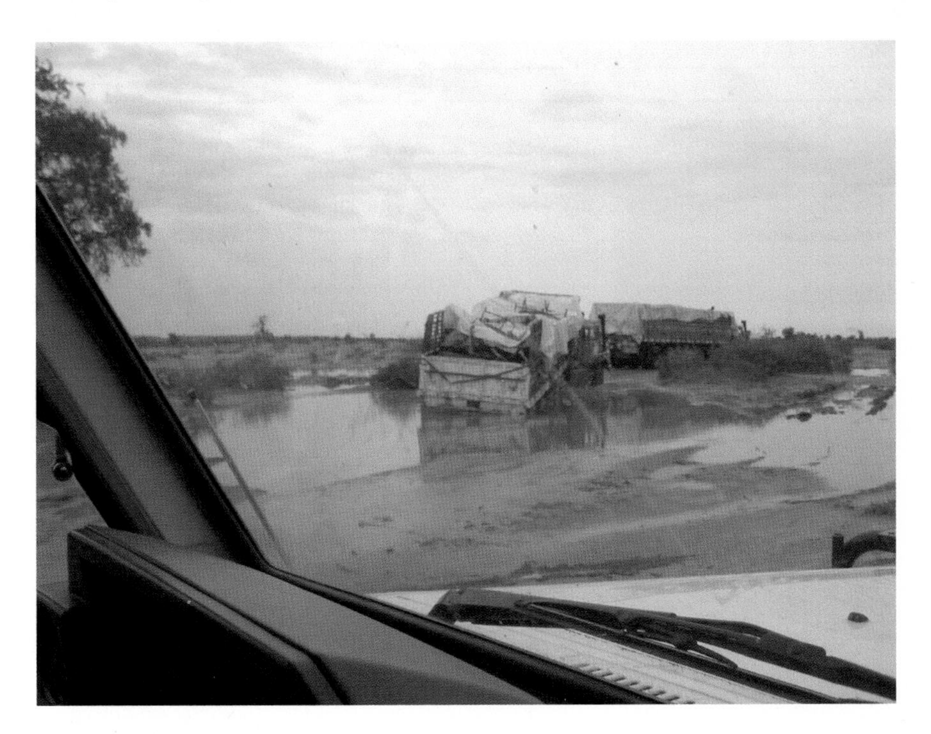

Fig. 4.1 Challenges to access. Chad. Picture by David Nott

Prompt 4: What Factors Can Constrain Access in Complex Emergencies?

Human constraints on access can come from bureaucratic restrictions, diversion of aid, and military operations. Environmental factors can come from difficult terrain, poor or damaged roads/airports, and a target population spread over a large geographical area (Fig. 4.1).

The UN humanitarian principles are intended to overcome the human constraints on access through the principles of humanity, neutrality, impartiality, and operational independence. They are often used as the basis of negotiations for access and clarify the role of humanitarian workers as noncombatants (Table 4.2). They derive from the principles of the International Committee of the Red Cross (ICRC) and are enshrined in history; however, it has been argued that political neutrality may compound some complex emergencies, since humanitarian suffering is not a by-product of war but the objective [7].

The ICRC has been criticized for failing to take a political stance when crimes against humanity have taken place both during the WW2 holocaust and the Biafran War, 1967–1970, the latter being the impetus for the formation of Médecins Sans Frontières (MSF).

Table 4.2 UN humanitarian principles

Principle	Explanation	Discussion
Humanity	Protect life, address suffering and respect human beings	The government receiving aid may overtly agree to the principle of humanity but still willfully direct violence at civilians
Neutrality	Not take sides in hostilities	The key members of the UN, including the UN Security Council, take strategic sides in conflicts
Impartiality	Humanitarian action on basis of need	All governments direct aid to their allies. Even if truly impartial, aid can easily be portrayed as favoring one side
Operational independence	Autonomous from political, economic, military, or other objectives	Most governments implicitly and explicitly align their aid to national security and military objectives, including the UK and USA

Deviating from the humanitarian principles carries risks as well as humanitarians may be seen as political opponents to the army resulting in them being denied access or being seen as legitimate military targets as has been the case in Syria.

Further Information 2

You discover the government is interfering with relief provision. The famine, originally triggered by a drought, is being exacerbated by government controls on the movement of food.

The government is also exploiting aid efforts financially. For your mission, the government insists that you buy expensive visas, local currency at an inflated rate, and use government contractors for supplies. You expect the government contractors to divert significant amounts of aid and know foreign currency may be used to import weapons. Some NGOs have already negotiated access, but there is still a massive shortfall, and there is pressure from your charity head office to quickly get a visible presence on the ground for international media.

You feel that your presence might cause more harm than good, but a showdown with your director is coming.

Prompt 5: What Compromises Need to Be Made for Access?

This is one of the hardest decisions in humanitarianism. By doing nothing, a large number of people will starve, but meeting the government demands may prolong the conflict causing more deaths and famine (Table 4.3). There were a lot of reflections following relief effort to the Great Lakes Crisis in Goma, 1995, following the Rwandan genocide (Box 4.3).

Table 4.3 Humanitarian assistance compounding a complex emergency [6]

Country	Example
Biafra Nigeria	Aid money was used to buy arms
Band Aid Ethiopia	The Band AID song portrayed the famine as being due to natural factors which was incorrect and patronizing since the famine was mainly due to the actions of the Ethiopian government ("Where nothing ever grows. No rain or rivers flow. Do they know it's Christmas time at all") [8]
Operation Lifeline Sudan	UN involvement meant both armies washed their hands of civilian bloodshed, meaning many civilians were attended by humanitarians but killed by conflict, coined by David Rieff "The well fed dead" [9]

Providing aid may be given as an excuse for not taking political action. If aid organizations do not coordinate, the receiving government will choose the ones that benefit their objectives the most and exploit this alliance. Personal conflicts of interest must also be examined. What will benefit your career might be at odds with what will benefit those in need of help.

There is no "one size fits all" solution to complex emergencies, but interference can be expected, and should be planned for, to enhance positive outcomes and minimize negative outcomes [6]. You know the government is keen to force people off their land into camps and will resist efforts to provide aid to stop further displacement and repatriation of refugees.

Early efforts should prevent further violence against civilians, either by civilians means (monitoring, human rights advocacy, and legal challenges) or military (ceasefire agreements, peace zones, formal peacekeeping) (Table 4.4). Humanitarian interventions must be careful not to prolong conflict and there are other risks; merely the presence of humanitarian agencies may detract responsibility from the government and could be exploited to give it credibility, especially the case if NGOs do not publicize atrocities to retain neutrality and access.

Box 4.3: Kevin Watkins, Oxfam: Reflection on the Challenges of Humanitarian Action

"The humanitarian imperative to relieve suffering can involve agencies such as Oxfam in complex moral dilemmas, where the relative merits of action and inaction have to be considered. At what point, for example, does food aid become a means of prolonging a war which is destroying more lives than humanitarian assistance can save? Should aid agencies negotiate access to conflict zones with armed groups who have been responsible for appalling human rights violation?...Sometimes people in Bosnia vent their anger on aid workers, who offer food or clothing but seem to have done nothing to try to stop the war" [10].

Table 4.4 Priorities in a complex emergency

Peace and protection	Seeking agreement from warring groups, protecting people at risk, and creating civilian safe areas
Humanitarian access	Relief work guided by humanitarian principles, with recognized civilian noncombatants to gain consented access to vulnerable people
Political action	Generating the political will and international consensus for peacekeeping efforts, restrictions on arms or trade, and coordinated humanitarian relief

Prompt 6: How Is Coordinating Relief Different in Complex Emergencies?

In complex emergencies, there needs to be much higher level coordination between NGOs, UN agencies, and foreign governments since the host government is not capable of coordinating the relief effort [12]. More experienced staff are required, and typically UN operates a "cluster" approach where one organization accepts ultimate responsibility for a need, for example, sanitation, and coordinates other organizations working in the same field [11]. This clarifies roles and responsibilities, prevents duplication of efforts, and facilitates greater accountability.

The largest cause of mortality in complex emergencies is usually communicable disease, so in famines food aid needs to be combined with measures to check the spread of disease such as water, sanitation, vaccination, and camp planning [12].

Another key difference in complex emergencies is that many stakeholders may be pulling in diametrically opposite directions, complicated by huge differences between their stated and actual aims. A simple generalization can be seen in Table 4.5.

Further Information 3

The famine worsens with over 20 children dying daily, there is a motion for the UN to intervene; however, two members of the UN Security Council veto the motion. Back in the UK, talent shows dominate the television, and you wonder why the media is not covering the disaster more.

Prompt 7: What Is the Role of the Media in Complex Emergencies?

International media is important in raising awareness to create political action, but coverage frustratingly rarely reflects severity of disaster and is often skewed to the host's national agenda. Western media considers audiences to be weary of humanitarian news and is therefore slow to cover disasters. Despite this, issues

Table 4.5 Key stakeholders in a complex emergency

Stakeholder	Explicit/stated aim	Alternative agenda	Consequences
Developed nations' (formerly "Western") governments	Peace Democracy Development	Access to resources and access to markets for corporations. Support friendly regimes, generate military exports, and avoid refugee influxes	Slow to recognize abuses by allies. Containment strategies for refugees driving policy. Partiality in response
Media organizations	Truth, balanced coverage and to raise awareness to issues	Sell newspapers by simple explanations and eye-catching stories. Maintain military relations to embed journalists. Satisfying corporate PR agenda	Visual-based stories, poor explanations, biased coverage based on interest rather than need
Aid organizations	Targeted relief	Appease government donors, publicize success of missions, encourage fundraising. Carve a niche from other NGOs	Positive spin on work covering up mistakes, impartial actions, and poor cooperation between NGOs
Local governments	Peace, willingness to democratic change and development	Maintain grip on power to protect their own financial interests and prolong conflict if beneficial	Targeting of opposition groups and nonsupporters by military, leading to perpetual states of emergency
National armies	Victory, government order, professional	Avoid high-loss conflict and maintain their own status, generating income through corruption or resources	Targeting of disloyal civilians. Military coups if threatened. Autocracy
Local militias if present	Separatist, protecting locals and seeking victory over the government or peace agreements	To avoid high-loss conflict and prolong conflict if beneficial. Often keen to protect interests, either by maintaining share of power or making money. Some may be government agents	Target perceived disloyal civilians. Rarely directly engage the military, control, and exploit local resources
United Nations	Humanity Neutrality Impartiality	National interests, especially the agenda of the Security Council members, USA, Russia, China, UK, and France. This is often conflicting	Failure of resolutions. Failure of impartiality and neutrality when interventions does take place

can capture the attention of Western audiences as was the case with the movie "Kony 2012," leading to calls to bring the Lords Resistance Army leader to justice [13].

Media in recipient country (e.g., state TV, national radio stations) are typically government-controlled and instruments of propaganda in complex emergencies. After disasters, radio and TV can be harnessed for powerful health messages as was the case of Urunana, a radio soap highlighting the issue of HIV in Rwanda [14]. Local newspapers and local radio can easily be overlooked but may be useful ways of informing people about your mission. Increasingly mobile phones and Internet-based networks are starting to dominate communication, as was seen with the influence of Twitter, YouTube, and Facebook in recent uprisings in Egypt, Libya, and Syria.

Prompt 8: What is Humanitarian Intervention?

Humanitarian intervention, despite its benign sounding name, is "*Entry into a country of the armed forces of another country or international organization with the aim of protecting citizens from persecution or the violation of their human rights*" [15].

It is a broad concept with the essential characteristics: (1) Humanitarian intervention involves the threat and use of military forces. (2) It entails interfering in the internal affairs of a state by sending military forces into a sovereign state that has not committed an act of aggression against another state. (3) The intervention is in response to situations that do not necessarily pose direct threats to strategic interests, but is motivated by humanitarian objectives [16].

There are many types of possible humanitarian interventions. For example, UN military forces with a Security Council resolution such as the Unified Task Force in Somalia or other international forces (e.g., NATO or African Union) providing air support such as NATO no-fly zone in Libya.

There will always be debate about the right/duty to intervene in the internal affairs of another country since both action and inaction are risky and may lead to many problematic scenarios. In Libya, it would have been horrendous to see Gaddafi's forces invade Benghazi destroying the popular uprising. However, NATO action risked protracted conflict such as in Afghanistan and Iraq, and raises quesions as to why Libya and not Syria, Bahrain, or Yemen.

Governments invariably proclaim international action is for righteous reasons yet inherently choose options in the national interest. Although the virtuous argument may be stronger in some cases more than others, there is no easy way to separate values and interests in humanitarian intervention (Table 4.6). When there are strong arguments for humanitarian intervention, the five permanent members of the UN Security Council (USA, Russia, China, UK, and France) required to back a motion seldom agree (Fig. 4.2).

Two of the most successful and defensible acts of humanitarian intervention were Rwanda and Cambodia, where lasting peace came about by unilateral military action by a local army and ironically these were actions which were opposed by the

Table 4.6 Humanitarian intervention perspectives (crudely)

In favor	Against
Human rights need to be protected	Implementation is very inconsistent
Intervention can protect political freedom	Intervention may sustain an unjust status quo
There is a "responsibility to protect" by richer countries	Questionable motivations: a pretext for geopolitical goals
Protects internationally accepted rights and liberties	These "rights and liberties" are drawn up by a small clique of "Western" governments
Chapter 7 of UN Charter authorizes countries to act to "restore international peace and security"	The autonomy of sovereign states is a foundation of international law
Humanitarian aid alone in complex emergencies is often ineffective	Humanitarian interventions have themselves had questionable results in complex emergencies

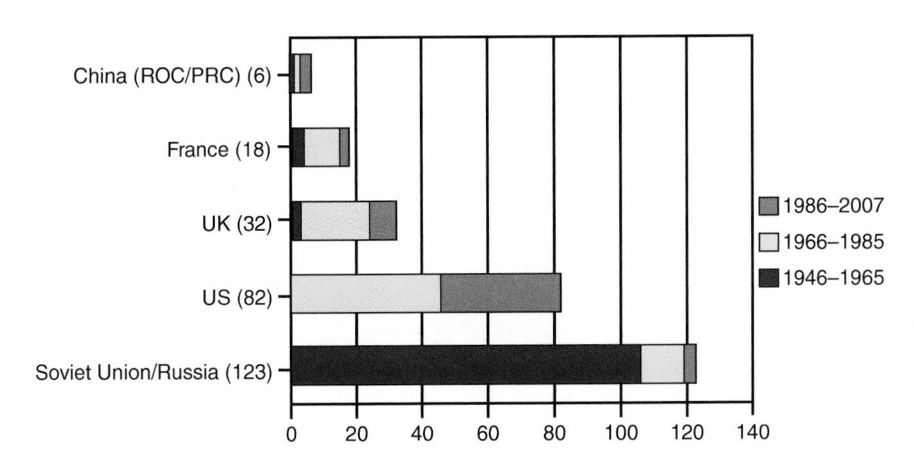

Fig. 4.2 Number of resolutions vetoed by each of the five permanent members of the Security Council between 1946 and 2007

UN at the time [6]. It was only the military victory of the Tutsi Rwandan Patriotic Front that stopped the genocide in Rwanda.

Further Information 4

Finally, images of starving children hit the news leading to public outcry across the world. After protracted negotiations, the UN brokers a peace deal between the militias and government forces.

A peacekeeping force from the UN holds the peace and former militia leaders are given political posts with the promise of elections in the future. Some breakaway militants refuse to sign the agreement, cross the border and take control of a remote border area with mineral deposits. Peace remains fragile.

Evidence emerges which proves the national government sponsored the LPA attacks on civilians; there are calls for the war crimes to be investigated.

Prompt 9: What Compromises Need to Be Made for Peace?

Absolute justice for crimes against humanity may have to be compromised for peace agreements as otherwise military leaders may never agree to peace accords. Truth commissions may be a good compromise to gain recognition for atrocities to allow grievances to be aired and reparations be made.

In "peace" there is often still considerable violence directed at civilains, also there may be less press freedom and personal freedoms as there were in times of conflict (e.g., Guatemala). Sometimes democratic process and elections can be the catalyst for violence.

The needs of the people need to be balanced against the needs of the military. Peace agreements need to accommodate the requests of military leaders on both sides but not forget the needs of civilians. Often, the needs of the civilians are overlooked, sending out a dangerous message that the only way to recognition is through violence, which leads other groups to take up arms. Also, if the military is disbanded too quickly, it will lead to military coups or increase levels of military corruption [6].

Prompt 10: How Do You Prevent Complex Emergencies Reoccurring?

1) **Demilitarize the Country Post War**. Investment needs to be made in disarmament, demobilization, and reconciliation (DDR), getting soldiers to return to peaceful professions. It is usually overlooked and underfunded, but if not done, former soldiers will look for new conflicts leading to wider instability. It is exacerbated by child soldiers who may have known no other life other than carrying a gun. Other professions may not offer the short-term rewards and freedom of military life.
2) **Tackle Root Causes**. UN agencies and charities may be keen to complete their specific missions. However, failure to tackle the original causes of conflict; poverty, inequality, insecurity and persecution, will risk triggering renewed violence.
3) **Find Innovative Ways of Tackling Political Causes of Complex Emergencies**. Freezing the assets of political leaders and preventing arms sales are sanctions that have been shown to be very effective in deterring conflict. Much could be done in securing international agreements to regulate arms trades and flows of capital.

Prompt 11: What Are the Longer-Term Humanitarian Priorities Following Complex Emergencies?

Planning. Develop further understanding of the politics and conflict dynamics and provide early warning systems for new conflict. If there has been a political solution and new government, manage transition toward government management of aid [17].

Funding. Make funding predictable as it is often needed for years to come. Ensure funding is well distributed to provide equitable distribution of assistance across geographic areas. Managing the transition from emergency assistance to long-term development assistance while still maintaining an emergency capacity.

Targeting Aid. Prioritize the vulnerable (women, children, unaccompanied children, and the elderly). Early intervention to prevent communicable diseases. Addressing basic needs of the displaced – food, water, shelter, fuel for cooking, work, services, and household necessities. Allowing for reparation and reunification of communities and strengthening civil society by community involvement.

Case Study: Sudan

Sudan gained independence in 1956 but has been dominated by military regimes and conflict since. The current life expectancy is just 54 years, and one in seven women die in childbirth.

The government of Sudan was formed by a military coup in 1989. Officially, it is a democratic republic with a multiparty system; however, the country's leader President Omar-al-Bashir has created a prolonged state of emergency to gain all executive powers, banned political parties, and ruthlessly executed his political opponents.

Sudan's first civil war (1955–1972) was barely over before the second civil war began (1983–2005). This second war displaced four million and led to two million, mostly civilian deaths. Peace talks eventually culminated in a roadmap which gave the south autonomy leading to independence in 2011.

In the conflict induced famine of 1998, towns where food aid got through rapidly increased in population with large numbers living in poorly planned camps. Poor hygiene and sanitation led to outbreaks of cholera and shigella, and despite the relief efforts, the crude mortality rate remained over 20 per 10000 people per day for several months, 20 times higher than that required to define an emergency [4].

There were three major lessons learned from this emergency: adults and adolescents as well as children are at high risk of death in extreme famines; food aid must be accompanied by public health, water, and sanitation to prevent infectious disease; and only experienced staff should be deployed in the most severe emergencies [17].

Sudan's oil reserves have enticed other countries into support resulting in muted international response against government atrocities and allowing Omar-al-Bashir to amass an estimated personal wealth of $9 billion in foreign bank accounts. In July 2010, he was finally charged by International Criminal Court with genocide for the attacks in Darfur, yet the Arab League, Russia, China, and the African Union have condemned his arrest warrant.

Disasters as seen in Sudan are a massive challenge for humanitarian workers as militias attack civilians and humanitarians with impunity. Operating in such areas is therefore dangerous and yet requires much more experience to coordinate the response [18].

South Sudan faces challenges starting out as a new country. It has wealth from farmland, oil, and mineral wealth but is currently one of the least developed countries, vulnerable to climate change and renewed conflict. For success, aid agencies need to understand the conflict dynamics and involve communities in creating peace.

References

1. Office for the Coordination of Humanitarian Affairs. OCHA orientation handbook on complex emergencies. 1999. [cited 2011 Dec 01]. Available from: http://reliefweb.int/node/21394.
2. Relief Web [Internet]. New York: The United Nations Office for the Coordination of Humanitarian Affairs (OCHA). [cited 2011 Dec 01]. Available from: http://reliefweb.int/.
3. Inter Agency Standing Committee Secretariat. Working paper on the definition of complex emergencies. 1994 Dec; [cited 2011 Dec 01]. Available from: http://www.humanitarianinfo.org/iasc/.
4. Allen T, Schomerus M. Complex emergencies and humanitarian responses. London: University of London; 2008. 2790162.
5. Salama P, Spiegel P, Talley L, Waldman R. Lessons learned from complex emergencies over past decade. Lancet. 2004;364:9447 (13–19) 1801–13.
6. Keen D. Complex emergencies. Cambridge: Polity; 2008.
7. Duffield M. Complex emergences and the crisis of development. Institute of Development Studies Bulletin 25.2. 1994 [cited 2012 Mar 20] Available from: http://www.ids.ac.uk/files/dmfile/duffield254.pdf.
8. de Waal A. Development review. 1995. [cited 2012 Mar 20] Available from: http://www.trocaire.org/resources/tdr-article/humanitarianism-unbound-context-call-military-intervention-africa.
9. Rieff D. A bed for the night. London: Vintage; 2002. ISBN 9780099597919.
10. Watkins. The Oxfam poverty report. 2005. p. 52. [cited 2012 Mar 20] Available from: http://policy-practice.oxfam.org.uk.
11. IASC. Guidance Note on Using The Cluster Approach to Strengthen Humanitarian Response.2006. [cited 2012 Mar 20] Available from: http://reliefweb.int/node/23017.
12. Connolly M, Gayer M, Ryan MJ, Salama P, Spiegel P, Heymann D. Communicable diseases in complex emergencies: impact and challenges. Lancet. 2004;364(9449):1974–83.
13. Kony2012.com [Internet]. San Diego: Invisible Children, Inc. [cited 2012 Mar 20] Available from: www.kony2012.com.
14. Booth I. Urunana – radio soap for health education. 2003. [cited 2012 Mar 20] Available from: http://www.eldis.org/fulltext/rwandasoap.pdf.
15. McLean I, McMillan A. The concise Oxford dictionary of politics. Oxford: Oxford University Press; 2003. [cited 2012 Mar 20] Available from: http://www.highbeam.com/doc/1O86-humanitarianintervention.html.
16. Frye A. Humanitarian intervention: crafting a workable doctrine. New York: Council on Foreign Relations; 2000.
17. Oxfam, World Vision, et al. Joint briefing paper. Getting it right from the start priorities for action in the New Republic of South Sudan. [cited 2012 Mar 20] Available from: http://reliefweb.int/node/444892.
18. OCHA. Humanitarian response review. New York. 2005 Aug. [cited 2012 Mar 20] Available from: http://reliefweb.int/node/414034.

Chapter 5
Security for the Humanitarian Worker

David MacGarty

Learning Objectives

- Outline the recent global trend in attacks on humanitarian workers
- Understand the common approaches to security in the humanitarian setting
- Describe common problems with security provision and their solutions
- Describe the limits of legislation in protecting humanitarian workers
- Explore the motives of those who attack humanitarian workers
- List security threats in the field and explain how they can be mitigated
- Explore the financial realities of providing humanitarian security

Initial Scenario

You are a medical doctor preparing to deploy with an NGO to Afghanistan. The project involves traveling to remote villages in dangerous regions to conduct health needs assessments and provide basic care. Before you deploy, you receive security training and a detailed briefing on the situation. The environment will be hostile and you will have to adjust your mission based on the prevailing security situation. You have gained a basic knowledge about the customs and culture of the country, but the statistics regarding humanitarian safety are worrying.

D. MacGarty, MBBS, BSc
FY2 Doctor, Department of Obstetrics and Gynaecology,
St Peter's Hospital, Chertsey, Surrey, UK
e-mail: dmacgarty@hotmail.com

D. MacGarty, D. Nott (eds.), *Disaster Medicine*,
DOI 10.1007/978-1-4471-4423-6_5, © Springer-Verlag London 2013

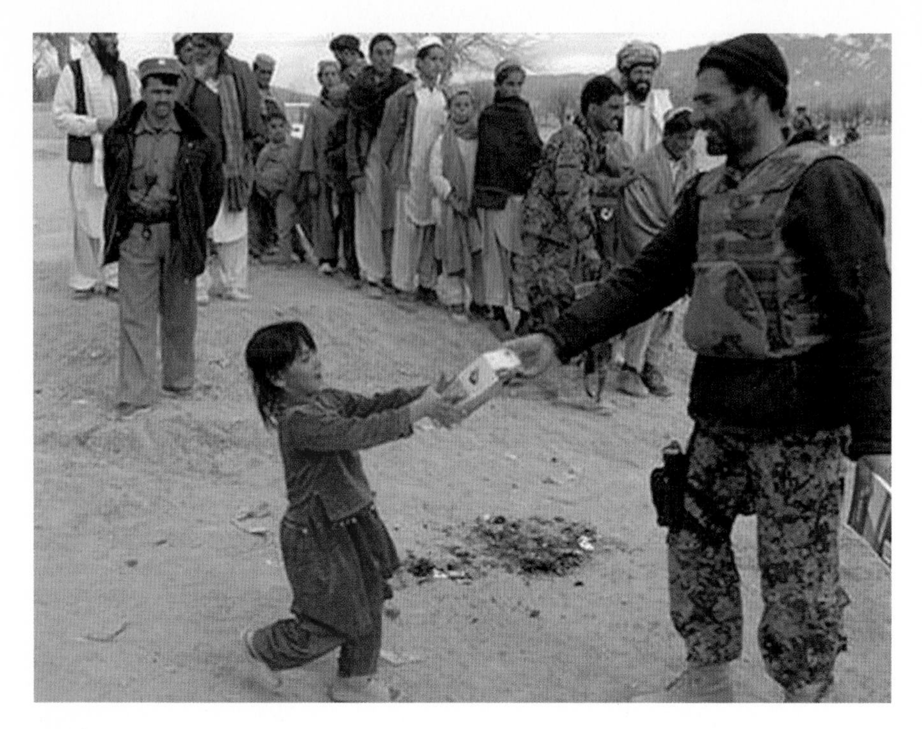

Fig. 5.1 Security and aid provision (reproduced with permission from Afghanistan International Security Assistance Force)

Prompt 1: How Dangerous Is the Situation for Humanitarian Workers?

Since 2006, violent attacks on humanitarian workers have increased. Although more humanitarian workers deploy every year (increasing the number of targets), the growth in the number of incidents is faster than the growth in the number of workers.

The following statistics are taken from the Humanitarian Policy Group Briefing 34 [1] which used data from the Aid Worker Security Database (AWSD). The database records major security incidents affecting the staff of aid organizations working in humanitarian relief.

- Violent attacks against aid workers (murder, kidnapping, and injury) have increased markedly in the past 3 years. In 2008, 260 humanitarian aid workers were killed, kidnapped, or seriously injured in violent attacks. Most deaths of aid workers are due to deliberate violence.
- There are three main categories of humanitarian organization: UN agencies, International Committee of the Red Cross (ICRC), and NGOs, and each employs both national staff and international (expatriate) staff. Of the three, only the ICRC showed a decline in attack rates over the past 3 years. Both NGOs and the

UN saw a rise in attacks relative to their field staff numbers. The rise in casualty rate among international staff was borne primarily by NGOs.

- Aid workers are particularly vulnerable in the first 3 months of deployment with 17 % of incidents occurring within the first 30 days.
- Safety issues rather than security threats still pose the greatest risk to NGO workers. Vehicle accidents, malaria, water-borne diseases, HIV, and other health threats continue to be by far the largest cause of casualties among aid workers [2].

Prompt 2: Where in the World Is the Threat Greatest?

- Three quarters of all aid worker attacks over the past 3 years took place in 7 countries (Sudan, Afghanistan, Somalia, Sri Lanka, Chad, Iraq, Pakistan).
- However, three countries are responsible for the rapid increase in incident rate over the past 3 years: Sudan (Darfur), Afghanistan, and Somalia. Together, these countries accounted for more than 60 % of violent incidents. Clustering like this has never been seen before.
- In the rest of the world (outside the seven mentioned countries), attack rates on humanitarian workers are declining slightly. While this is a positive trend, it exposes the problems in maintaining security in the most volatile areas where humanitarian aid is most needed [1].

Prompt 3: What Security Training Is Available for Humanitarian Workers?

Many organizations (such as RedR) now offer security education courses for humanitarian workers prior to deployment. The aim is to enhance worker skill sets to allow safe and effective work in the field. Most courses incorporate:

- Understanding of security risks in the field environment
- Development of personal- and team-based strategies
- Individual and team risk assessment and management

Further Information 1

You drive from the airport in Kabul to your initial destination. You receive a warning from the Afghanistan NGO Safety Office suggesting the situation is not safe in the region you want to go to. You are told that the security measures in place are not sufficient to ensure your safety on the mission.

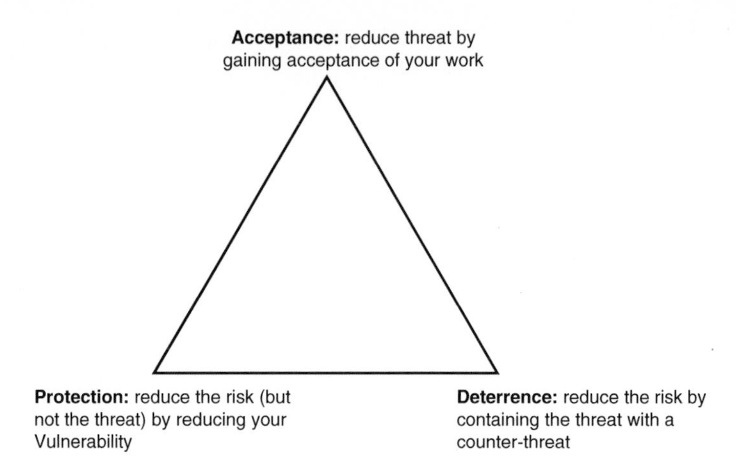

Fig. 5.2 Security triangle paradigm

Prompt 4: Describe the Important Elements of Security for an Aid Organization

The "security triangle" paradigm (see Fig. 5.2) of acceptance, protection, and deterrence remains the conceptual basis for the operational security of aid agencies. The three elements of the security triangle must be balanced in the context of the local security threat.

1. Acceptance – softening the threat
   Acceptance is the degree to which the community in which an NGO is working accepts and supports the NGO's presence. Security grows with increased community acceptance. Acceptance involves encouraging community participation and evaluation of the project. The NGO must be seen as transparent and impartial and act in a politically sensitive manner which can be very challenging (see Box 5.2). Acceptance is the cornerstone of security for NGOs with a development mandate but is often challenged under the timeframes and political circumstances in which NGO relief efforts take place.

2. Protection – hardening the target
   This is the element most readily associated with security (see Fig. 5.1). Protection may involve secure transportation, protective physical infrastructure and clear symbols to identify your agency while avoiding a military appearance. Protection strategies need to be enhanced if conditions deteriorate and acceptance strategies become less effective, but they should never be viewed as an alternative to strong community support.

3. Deterrence – posing a counter threat
   Most NGOs are not appropriately suited to pose a credible counter threat, so the focus of deterrence strategies is the relationships built with larger regional and international institutions. Deterrence strategies can involve political intervention, the use of guards, or the involvement of the military [2].

Prompt 5: What Problems Have Been Identified with Current Security Measures?

The security environment has deteriorated in the past 3 years, and humanitarian organizations have been forced to re-evaluate their security approach and seek improvement. The following problems have been identified:

- There is an over reliance on passive approaches to acceptance where acceptance is assumed rather than brokered and maintained.
- More systematic means of tracking and analyzing security incidents is needed both within and between agencies.
- Security is compromised by high staff turnover and inadequate training, particularly among national staff members.
- There is an insufficient appreciation of the risks posed for local staff and partner agencies.
- There is a lack of criteria for determining when and how programs should be halted when security conditions deteriorate and a lack of clear evacuation plans [3].

Prompt 6: What Measures Have Been Put in Place to Improve Security?

- The International Community of the Red Cross (ICRC) and some large NGOs have made an effort to pursue an active acceptance approach. This has involved spending a considerable amount of time and resources, investing in deeper analysis of the conflict dynamics, and reaching out to forge agreements with potential aggressors.
- Some agencies working in dangerous contexts have either adopted extreme low profile approaches or the use of armed guards and armed escorts. Both these approaches are considered last resort or temporary fixes, and many agencies would prefer to withdraw programs rather than incorporate strong deterrence. However, external financial pressure from donors and internal pressures within the agency to continue aid often compel an agency to remain in operation.
- Remote management is the management of aid from a distance and involves the withdrawal of international staff and transferring responsibilities to national (local) staff (see Fig. 5.1). Most agencies consider remote management as a strictly temporary measure, but in some contexts, it has become the only means of maintaining operations in the long term. Economic incentives can influence the risk which national staff are prepared to undertake. Agencies acknowledge that the importance placed on security risks and the resultant security needs of national staff is still under-prioritized.
- Inter-agency security cooperation has improved in recent years. The UN and NGOs in the field have come together with the "Saving Lives Together" initiative to improve security collaboration, but the initiative has had many problems. More successful field-level security coordination platforms have been generated

by the NGOs themselves. The Afghanistan NGO Safety Office (ANSO) has been particularly successful (see Box 5.1).

- Many agencies have improved policy and procedures and have invested in security risk assessment tools. Reporting, tracking, and analysis of security incidents has also improved [3].

Box 5.1: The Afghanistan NGO Safety Office (ANSO) [4]
ANSO is a field-level security platform which was set up in late 2002 to offer NGOs a range of additional support to their existing security management. It has been very successful in providing up to date security information and improving the capacity of NGOs in dealing with security matters. ANSO is responsible for:

- Convening inter-agency security meetings
- Providing security alerts and undertaking security incident reporting and analysis
- Carrying out risk assessments, undertaking trend analysis by region, and communicating these every 2 weeks in periodic threat reports
- Providing introductory security briefings and technical assistance and advice to individual agencies
- Crisis management support in case of an attack or kidnapping
- Liaison with governmental authorities

Although ANSO has proved popular, it has been difficult to replicate elsewhere as interdependent working does not suit some agencies, and in resource poor contexts, establishing security coordination platforms is difficult to justify financially.

Further Information 2

You consider why the security situation has deteriorated to such an extent. Surely there must be some international law governing security in these environments? Pressures from the donor (supporting your NGO) means you must continue with the mission, but this will necessitate a change in security policy. You liaise with head office and provision is made for an armed escort to the village.

Prompt 7: What Legislation Is in Place to Protect You?

- The Geneva Conventions seek to ensure that people who are part of an impartial humanitarian organization, such as the Red Cross (see Box 5.2), are able to go about their work without the threat of attack or reprisal.

- The Geneva Conventions outline the rights of non-combatants during conflict. These rights include the right to be treated humanely; to have access to food, water, shelter, medical treatment, and communications; and to be free from violence, hostage taking, humiliation, and degrading treatment, and it prohibits collective punishment and imprisonment.
- The conventions do not guarantee access of humanitarian workers to affected areas where aid is needed. Governments and occupying forces may ban a humanitarian agency from working in an area.
- The Geneva Conventions do not require combatants in conflict to guarantee the safety of humanitarian workers. Combatants must not attack non-combatants, but they are not required to provide security escorts, etc. [5].

Box 5.2: The International Committee of the Red Cross (ICRC) [5]
The ICRC was founded in 1863 by Henry Dunant. After witnessing the aftermath of the Battle of Solferino, Dunant became distressed by the suffering of wounded soldiers. He subsequently set up the ICRC with a mandate to protect human life and health, to ensure respect for all human beings, and to prevent and alleviate human suffering without any discrimination based on nationality, race, sex, religious beliefs, class, or political opinion. Red Cross societies are now active in almost every nation, and their history and mandate enable them to occupy a unique neutral position during conflict and disaster.

The ICRC is currently active in Afghanistan, and their support extends to the national and international armed forces, the civilians, and the armed opposition. They have provided basic first aid training and aid kits to both the Afghan security forces and Taliban members. In addition to visiting prisoners of the international forces, they have occasionally had access to people detained by the Taliban.

The ICRC pursues a proactive security management strategy which includes active dialogue with potential aggressors and an emphasis on its unique mandate as an independent and strictly neutral organization. Unlike other actors in the humanitarian setting (NGOs and UN agencies), attack rates on Red Cross workers have declined over the past few years.

However, their impartiality has attracted some criticism by those who question the morality in dealing with perceived unjust aggressors [6].

Prompt 8: Why Is Security Legislation Failing?

- Western humanitarian workers are increasingly perceived as political tools and are thus regarded as legitimate targets by opposition forces. Most humanitarian organizations are determined to be viewed as politically neutral and separate to governments and the military. In the past, this stance has allowed humanitarian organizations to operate safely. However, this "neutral" perception is now fading, and western aid agencies are increasingly seen as an intrinsic part of the "western" agenda [1, 7].

- Opposition forces no longer distinguish between humanitarian agencies and view the aid enterprise as one whole. Statistics support the view that all humanitarian organizations are seen as part of the same agenda [1]. In the recent surge of attacks, organizations which would be expected as popular targets (e.g., faith-based and US-based agencies) have not experienced higher attack rates than the rest of the community [1].
- Increasingly humanitarian organizations and the military work in similar environments. The erosion of the separation between humanitarian and military "space" threatens to blur the important distinction between the two, compromising aid worker security.
- The environments in which humanitarian organizations operate are more unstable than in the past. The wars being waged today are more commonly associated with smaller dissident groups who are less accountable to international laws and conventions than government forces. Indeed, in remote areas, humanitarian workers sometimes represent the only accessible western target.
- Bandits and criminals are increasingly on the fringes of conflict ready to take advantage of the circumstances. Criminals target humanitarian workers for kidnapping and then sell the victim to dissident forces who can then use them for bargaining against the opposition [8].

Prompt 9: Explore the Use of Deterrent Policies to Security

- Strong deterrent policies are required when there is a breakdown in acceptance (in security terms) within the host community. This breakdown may be due to something an aid agency has said or a perceived political agenda, or it may be because the agency provides aid to a perceived enemy.
- There are three facets to deterrence:
  - Diplomatic deterrence is where large international actors exert diplomatic pressure on the NGO's behalf and influence local authorities who either pose a threat to the NGO or are well placed to promote the security of the NGO.
  - The use of guards is a common deterrent strategy used by many NGOs (see Fig. 5.3).
  - Military deterrence is least common and usually appears in conjunction with peace-keeping missions when NGOs formally coordinate activities with external international military forces.
- Humanitarian agencies recognize that strong deterrent strategies can further interfere with community acceptance and undermine the long-term safety of their workers.
- Military deterrent strategies increase the connection between humanitarian agencies and the military and should only be pursued for short periods of time when other elements of the security triangle are clearly insufficient [2].

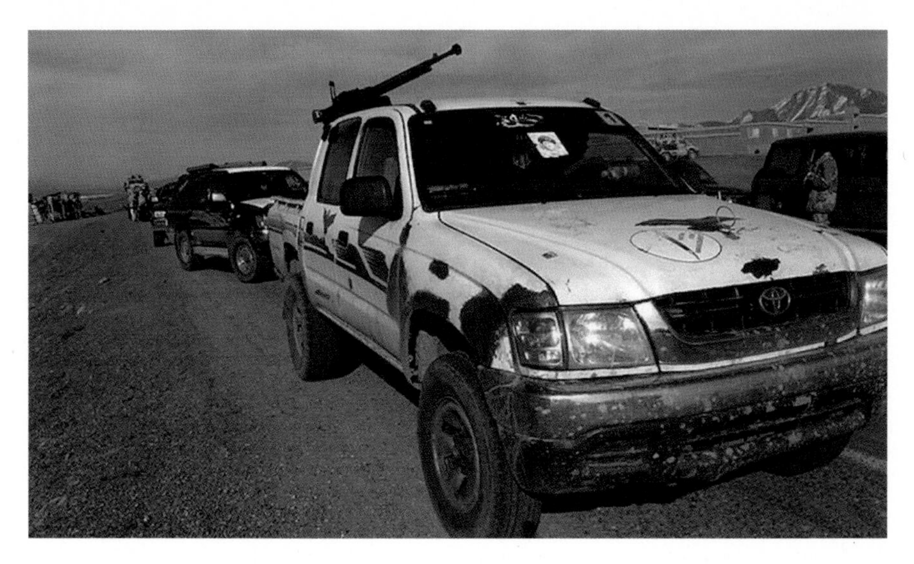

Fig. 5.3 Armed security convoy (Photograph by Sgt. Russell Gilchrest - US army)

Further Information 3

Your convoy sets off on the journey with armed protection from local government forces. After a number of hours on the road, the leading truck stops. You are entering a dangerous area and so you proceed slowly with caution. You suddenly sense a flash followed by a deafening sound and smoke. You are stunned but regain awareness seconds later. You cannot see far out of your vehicle due to the smoke and you cannot hear anything, but you can see that the vehicle in front of you has been blasted apart and is burning.

Prompt 10: Identify the Threats in the Field for Humanitarian Workers

- The most dangerous location for aid workers remains the road with ambushes being by far the most common situation where violence occurs. Indeed, the majority of kidnappings take place while the victim is traveling by vehicle.
- Kidnapping of aid workers has increased by over 350 % in the past 3 years. Kidnappers favor international staff over nationals as victims because they are both more valuable in terms of ransom and make for a more viable political statement.
- Six aid workers were killed in suicide bombings over the past 3 years.
- In Afghanistan and Iraq, improvised explosive devices (IEDs) were used for the first time on aid workers [1, 8].

Prompt 11: What Can Be Done to Maximize Personal Safety When Traveling in Hostile Environments?

Danger to humanitarian workers can be reduced by:

- Quickly adjusting to the new surroundings.
- Being inquisitive and getting as much information on the security situation as you can from sources such as ANSO or other NGOs.
- Avoiding heroics.

In addition, there are a number of considerations which should be addressed prior to any dangerous journey:

- Is the journey absolutely necessary? Risks must be balanced against benefits of travel.
- Plan routes and means of escape if appropriate.
- Get advice from people who know the area about current developments.
- Do not drive off roads/on verges if possible. IEDs are likely to be placed in verges. Also, follow local vehicle routes on roads as they may be informed as to the whereabouts of IEDs and will obviously avoid them.
- Travel in convoys, ideally with protection.
- Use sturdy, robust vehicles that are suited to the terrain and that you are used to driving. Wear a seatbelt – motor vehicle accidents are leading cause of mortality among NGO workers.
- Carry personal protection such as Kevlar (material used in bullet proof vests) if appropriate.
- Carry medical supplies and means for communication in emergencies [8].

Further Information 4

As the dust settles, it becomes clear that the vehicle in front of you is destroyed and everyone inside is dead. You have no option but to pull back from the operation. One of your co-workers has been killed along with three armed guards. You head back to the capital.

After a medical check-up and psychological debriefing, you are asked to attend a meeting with the executives of the NGO to discuss future policy on security. It is agreed that the NGO must attempt a more active acceptance strategy. A proposal is put together for the NGO's donors.

Prompt 12: What Are the Problems with Funding Security?

Providing specific security funding is difficult for two reasons. First, security budgets are difficult to monitor accurately, and, second, security costs may be very high and difficult to justify.

- Monitoring security budgets
  Security costs are very difficult to measure accurately. This poses problems not only for the NGO in their attempt to justify security budgets but also for the humanitarian sector as a whole. The lack of consistent data on security expenditure means there is little guidance available on how much security should cost in different contexts. This hampers security cost planning.

  For instance, if an NGO requires extra security during a mission, they may hire extra vehicles for a convoy. The costs of these vehicles may be placed under the transport budget rather than the security budget.

  Retaining good staff in insecure contexts requires premium salaries and frequent home leave. There is a security component in the salaries of these workers, but again this is difficult to quantify.

  Budgeting practices vary widely even between different field offices of the same NGO, and although the consensus is that donors are responsive to NGO security needs, standardized budgeting practices are needed before larger security budgets can be justified:

- Justification for security spending
  Security spending is problematic for several reasons. Acceptance strategies are widely held as the cornerstone of security management, but they require long-term investment which does not fit the typical short-term donor funding of humanitarian assistance. Cultivating and maintaining acceptance requires investment seemingly incongruent with security spending. Acceptance involves relationship building, often with potential aggressors, involving gifts and hospitality which donors may find difficult to justify.

  Many NGOs themselves have identified problems with increasing security budgets. Those NGOs that are funded by the public have seen their rating on charity watchdog websites decline as their security overhead rises. There is a subsequent disincentive to increase security spending [3].

Case Study: Karen Woo

In 2010, an 11-strong team working with the International Assistance Mission (a Christian charity specializing in health and economic development) set off to provide eye care in the valleys of Nuristan, some of the most remote and dangerous regions of Afghanistan. The team was made up of six Americans, a German, two Afghan interpreters, and Karen Woo, a British doctor. The team completed their mission successfully and were returning to Kabul when disaster struck.

There had been fierce fighting in Nuristan and in an effort to minimize the risk, the group took an indirect route to and from their destination through the safer Badakhshan province. The team traveled in a convoy of three 4 × 4 vehicles without armed security guards. Like many NGOs operating in Afghanistan, they believed their best security would be keeping a low profile and staying on the right side of the local people. The local police chief said the group had been told of concerns about their route.

The team were ambushed by around ten gunmen and were robbed before being shot dead. The Taliban took responsibility for the incident, accusing the team of proselytizing and carrying bibles. This was denied by the director of the International Assistance Mission who said there was no religious agenda, and the team was not attempting to convert anyone [9, 10].

References

1. Stoddard A, Harmer A, DiDomenico V. Humanitarian Policy Group Brief 34, Providing aid in insecure environments: 2009 update.
2. Martin R. NGO field security. Forced Migration Rev. 1999;4:4–7.
3. Stoddard A, Harmer A. Supporting Security for Humanitarian Action: A review of critical issues for the humanitarian community, Humanitarian Outcomes; Commissioned by conveners of the Montreux X conference; 2010. http://transition.usaid.gov/our_work/humanitarian_assistance/disaster_assistance/consultations/fy2010/supporting_security_humanitarian_action.pdf
4. The ANSO report, 1–15 June 2011, Issue 75. Kabul: The Afghanistan NGO Safety Office.
5. International Humanitarian Law and the Geneva Conventions: study guide. Washington, D.C.: The American National Red Cross; 2001
6. The ICRC in Afghanistan, 01/06/2011 Overview, www.icrc.org./eng/where-we-work/asia-pacific/afghanistan/.
7. Lillywhite L. Aid for the aid givers, Chatham House, theworldtoday.org (Feb 2011); 2011. p. 12–14.
8. Lloyd Roberts D. The hazards of the job. In: Matheson JIDM, Hawley A, editors. Making sense of disaster medicine: a hands on guide for medics. London: Hodder Arnold Ltd; 2010.
9. Alderson A, Farmer B. British doctor and nine others killed in Afghanistan ambush. The Telegraph (07/08/10); 2010.
10. Boone J, Thompson T. Karen Woo: Selfless doctor gunned down in Afghanistan's badlands. The Observer (07/08/10); 2010.

Part II
Global Players

Section reviewed by David Nott

Global Players is a section that looks at the international response to disasters and global health. There are so many inequalities in the world, but decisions need to be made about who gets aid and how it is allocated. One of the great success stories of the modern era is how United Nation member states and international organizations have agreed to prioritize several international development goals, but this has not been achieved without controversy.

This section provides a deeper insight into the policies of the Millennium Development Goals to improve infrastructure, rights, and basic standards of living of people in need around the world. It is hoped that readers who are interested in working for NGOs in different healthcare systems will find the cases that explore the practical and theoretical issues of working in such fields extremely illuminating. Controversial debates about the efficacy of aid and perhaps one of the greatest threats to the future of global health and disaster medicine—climate change—are discussed. This is a series of five exciting topics that will confer the reader with a deeper understanding of the international framework when thinking about global players and policies.

Shao Foong Chong

Chapter 6
Global Development: Millennium Development Goals

David MacGarty

Learning Objectives

- Discuss the Millennium Development Goals (MDGs) and their origin
- Identify which parties are responsible for delivering the MDGs
- Summarize the main achievements toward the MDGs
- Explain how barriers to MDG progress are being tackled
- Investigate the importance of gender equality and female empowerment to the MDGs
- Outline criticism of the MDGs
- Explore the future of international development post 2015

Initial Scenario

The heat is oppressive as you exit the aircraft. You consider your classmates arriving to lectures in rainy October, and you are very pleased with your decision to spend a year away from medical school to work with a health-care development charity in Southeast Asia.

The charity works closely with the Millennium Development Goals (MDGs), and despite initial research there is much you do not understand. You are encouraged to visit the UN office in the capital city where you are directed to a local representative for the United Nations Development Project (UNDP). The meeting is very helpful and answers many of your initial questions.

D. MacGarty, MBBS, BSc
FY2 Doctor, Department of Obstetrics and Gynaecology,
St Peter's Hospital, Chertsey, Surrey, UK
e-mail: dmacgarty@hotmail.com

D. MacGarty, D. Nott (eds.), *Disaster Medicine*,
DOI 10.1007/978-1-4471-4423-6_6, © Springer-Verlag London 2013

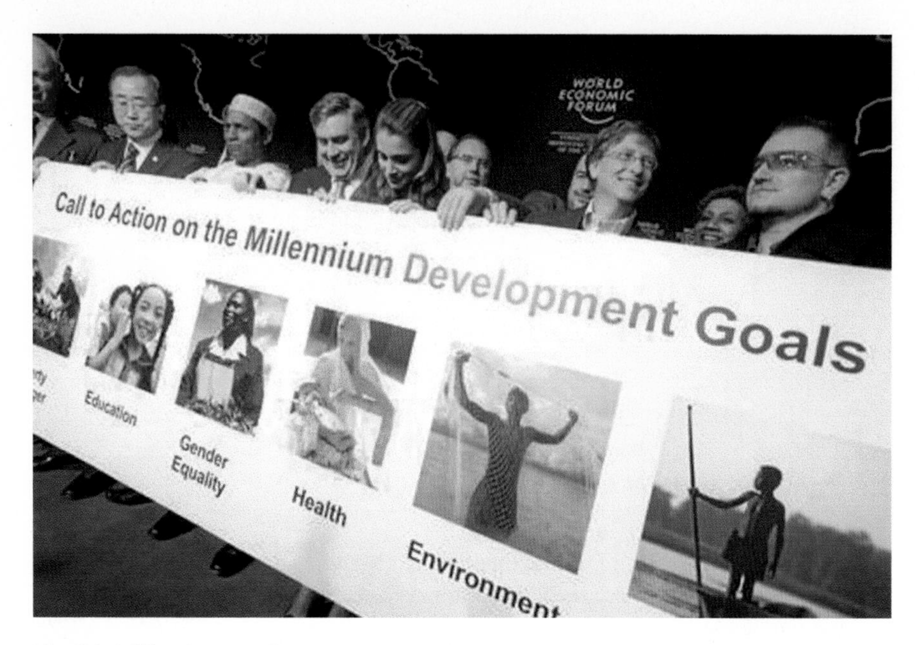

Fig. 6.1 Millennium Development Goals: World Economic Forum Annual Meeting, Davos 2008. (Photo taken by Andy Mettler)

Prompt 1: What Are the Millennium Development Goals?

- In September 2000, world leaders came together at UN headquarters to sign the Millennium Declaration, an international commitment to produce a more peaceful, prosperous, and fairer world.
- Eight Millennium Development Goals (MDGs—see Fig. 6.2) were established from the Millennium Declaration. 2015 was set as the deadline for achieving 21 specific targets within the 8 MDGs using 1990 as the baseline for progress measurement. Progress toward the MDGs is precisely measured with strong monitoring mechanisms in place to ensure that governments are held to their commitments.
- Before 2000, there were many UN conferences and commitments toward global development, but never before had the commitment to achieve them come from the highest political levels. Entire governments, the World Bank, the IMF, regional development banks, and the membership of the World Trade Organization are all committed to achieving the MDGs (see Fig. 6.1).

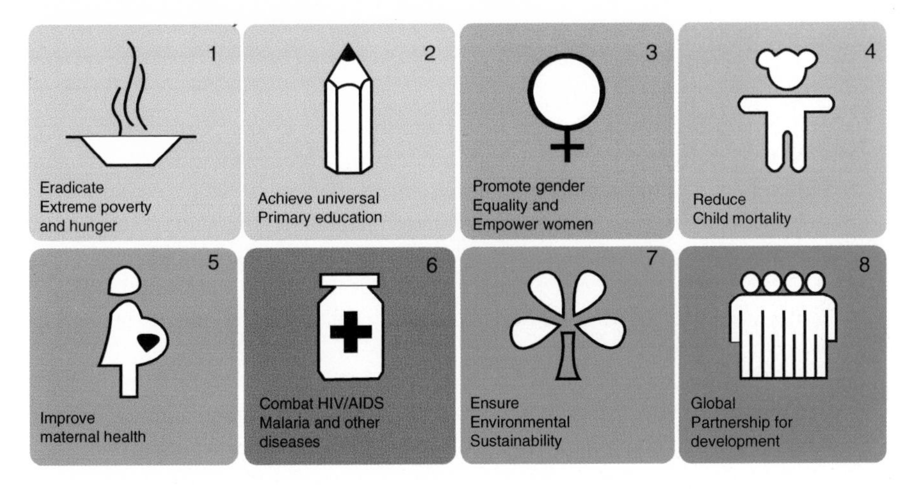

Fig. 6.2 The Millennium Development Goals

- The MDGs support the belief that there exists a "fundamental level of rights and freedoms to which all humans are entitled." It is hoped that by the year 2015, every individual on the planet will have the basic rights and freedoms outlined in the MDGs [1].

Prompt 2: Who Is Responsible for Delivering the MDGs?

- The ultimate responsibility for the achievement of MDGs 1–7 lies with the developing country. The developing country must enable an environment where development partnerships flourish and targets may be met.
- MDG 8 outlines the responsibility of developed countries and international organizations toward achieving the MDGs. Their responsibility is to ensure the adequate provision and opportunity for trade, finance, and knowledge.
- Partnerships between developing countries and donors are key to delivering the MDGs. Donors include bilateral donors (e.g., governments of developed countries), multilateral organizations (NGOs, UN agencies, development banks), and private sector stakeholders.
- The UNDP (see Box 6.1) and the World Bank are responsible for monitoring and reporting MDG progress through national and world progress reports [2].

Box 6.1: United Nations Development Project (UNDP)

- The UNDP is one of many UN agencies such as UNICEF and the UNHCR that report directly to the General Assembly of the UN.
- UNDP is the UN's global development network. It is charged with finding solutions for global and national development challenges and hence helping countries achieve the MDGs. UNDP helps facilitate partnerships by matching appropriate aid organizations with specific development problems.
- The UN has many agencies working in the development field, and UNDP helps coordinate these agencies to ensure collaboration and to prevent working overlap.
- UNDP works with governments and with local communities to provide resources and improve capacity, i.e., improving the skills and competences of local people, enabling them to draw on all the resources available to help them tackle their own development problems.
- UNDP publishes national and regional MDG progress reports, which give an overall picture of MDG progress.

Further Information 1

Working under the regional manager, your initial task is to collect data from local communities to evaluate how much impact the MDGs have made on the health of local populations. Over several weeks, you gather some excellent data from health centers around the region. In one hospital, you meet a doctor who has a keen interest in the MDGs. He tells you that MDG progress in the region has been a mixed bag.

Prompt 3: How Important Is Health to Global Development and the MDGs?

- Health and development have long been thought to be inextricably linked. In 2001, the WHO and CMH (Commission on Macroeconomics and Health) reported: "Health status seems to explain an important part of the difference in economic growth rates (between rich and low income countries) even after controlling for standard macroeconomic variables [3]."
- In all countries, the poor and marginalized bear the greatest health burden. Development can improve health by strengthening health services and reducing inequity [4].
- All 8 MDGs have the potential to improve health. MDGs 1, 4, 5, and 6 directly target health through improved nutrition, maternal health, children's health, and disease eradication. MDGs 2, 3, 7, and 8 indirectly target health improvement through improved education, gender equality and female empowerment, improved drinking water and sanitation, and development partnerships that ensure sustained health development.

Goals and Targets	Africa		Asia						
	Northern	Sub-Saharan	Eastern	South-Eastern	Southern	Western	Oceania	Latin America &Caribbean	Caucasus & Central Asia
Goal1 Eradicate extreme poverty and hunger									
Reduce extreme poverty by half	low poverty	very high poverty	high poverty	high poverty	very high poverty	low poverty	–	moderate poverty	high poverty
Productive and decent employment	very large deficit in decent work	very large deficit in decent work	moderate deficit in decent work	very large deficit in decent work	very large deficit in decent work	very large deficit in decent work	very large deficit in decent work	moderate deficit in decent work	large deficit in decent work
Reduce hunger by half	low hunger	very high hunger	moderate hunger	moderate hunger	high hunger	moderate hunger	–	moderate hunger	moderate hunger
Goal 2 Achieve universal primary education									
Universal primary schooling	high enrolment	moderate enrolment	high enrolment	high enrolment	high enrolment	moderate enrolment	–	high enrolment	high enrolment
Goal 3 Promote gender equality and empower women									
Equal girls'enrolment in primary school	close to parity	close to parity	parity	parity	parity	close to parity	away from parity	parity	parity
Women's share of paid employment	low share	medium share	high share	medium share	low share	low share	medium share	high share	high share
Women's equal representation in national parliaments	low representation	moderate representation	moderate representation	low representation	low representation	very low representation	very low representation	moderate representation	low representation
Goal 4 Reduce child mortality									
Reduce mortality of under-five-year-olds by two thirds	low mortality	High mortality	low mortality	low mortality	moderate mortality	low mortality	moderate mortality	low mortality	low mortality
Goal 5 Improve maternal health									
Reduce maternal mortality by three quarters	low mortality	very high mortality	low mortality	moderate mortality	high mortality	low mortality	high mortality	low mortality	low mortality
Access to reproductive health	moderate access	low access	high access	moderate access	moderate access	moderate access	low access	high access	moderate access
Goal 6 Combat HIV/AIDS, malaria and other diseases									
Halt and begin to reverse the spread of HIV/AIDS	low incidence	high incidence	low incidence	low incidence	low incidence	low incidence	intermediate incidence	low incidence	low incidence
Halt and reverse spread of tuberculosis	low mortality	high mortality	moderate mortality	high mortality	moderate mortality	low mortality	moderate mortality	low mortality	moderate mortality
Goal 7 Ensure enviormental sustainability									
Reverse loss of forests	low forest cover	medium forest cover	medium forest cover	high forest cover	medium forest cover	low forest cover	high forest cover	high forest cover	low forest cover
Halve proportion of population without improved drinking water	high coverage	low coverage	moderate coverage	moderate coverage	moderate coverage	high coverage	low coverage	high coverage	moderate coverage
Halve proportion of population without sanitation	moderate coverage	very low coverage	low coverage	low coverage	very low coverage	moderate coverage	low coverage	moderate coverage	high coverage
Improved the lives of slum-dwellers	moderate proportion of slum-dwellers	very high proportion of slum-dwellers	moderate proportion of slum-dwellers	high proportion of slum-dwellers	high proportion of slum-dwellers	moderate proportion of slum-dwellers	moderate proportion of slum-dwellers	moderate proportion of slum-dwellers	–
Goal 8 Develop a global partnership for development									
Internet users	high usage	low usage	high usage	moderate usage	low usage	high usage	low usage	high usage	high usage

The progress chart operates on two levels. The words in each box indicate the present degree of compliance with the target.The colours show progress towards the target according to the legend below:

- Target already met or expected to be met by 2015.
- Progress insufficient to reach the target if prevailing trends persist.
- No progress or deterioration.
- Missing or insufficient data.

* Red colour refers to insufficient progress (i,e. MMR has declined less than 2 per cent annually).

Fig. 6.3 MDGs 2011 progress chart. Country data are aggregated to the regional level to show overall advances over time. Although the aggregate figures are a convenient way to track progress, the situation of individual countries within a given region may vary significantly from regional averages (Reproduced with permission from un.org)

Prompt 4: What Have the MDGs Achieved So Far?

The MDGs have mobilized public and political support for development, and tremendous progress has been made so far. However, it seems unlikely that all the MDG targets will be met (see Fig. 6.3).

The following statistics are taken from "The Millennium Development Goals Report, 2011" released by the UN in June 2011 [5].

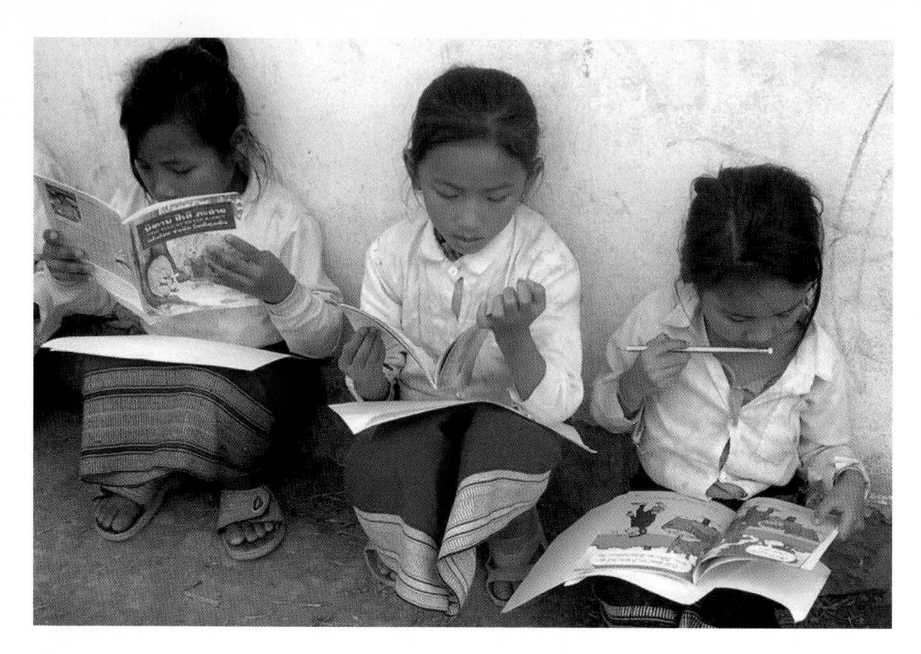

Fig. 6.4 Girls reading outside a school in Lao PDR. This photo was taken after a rural school book party run by "Big Brother Mouse," a publishing and literacy project in Laos, which provides many children with their first books (Photo taken by Blue Plover)

- MDG 1—Eradicate Extreme Poverty and Hunger
  Despite the economic downturn, the poverty-reduction target in MDG 1 is still on track. By 2015, it is expected that poverty will affect less than 15 % of the world's population (well under the 23 % target), but this is largely due to rapid growth in China.

  However, in terms of improved nutrition, the poorest are making the slowest progress with nearly a quarter of children in the developing world underweight. Children living in rural areas of developing regions are twice as likely to be underweight compared with urban children.

- MDG 2—Achieve Universal Primary Education
  Advances in education access have been very successful in some of the world's poorest countries. Between 1999 and 2009, access to primary education improved by 18 % in sub-Saharan Africa.

  However, being poor, female, or living in a conflict zone are the strongest indicators for low school enrolment and attendance. Of all the primary school-aged children that are not enrolled in school, 42 % live in poor countries affected by conflict (see Fig. 6.4).

- MDG 3—Promote Gender Equality and Empower Women
  Women's access to paid work still lags behind men in at least half of all regions. Employment growth during the economic recovery in 2010 was lower for women than for men, particularly in the manufacturing industries.

- MDG 4—Reduce Child Mortality
  The number of deaths of children under the age of 5 declined from 12.4 million in 1990 to 8.1 million in 2009. Between 2000 and 2008, the combination of improved immunization coverage and the opportunity for second-dose immunizations led to a 78 % drop in measles deaths worldwide representing one quarter of the decline in mortality from all causes among children under 5.

- MDG 5—Improve Maternal Health
  Pregnancy remains a major health risk for women in several regions despite major gains in increased skilled attendance at birth. Across all regions, more pregnant women are offered at least minimal care, but not enough women receive the recommended frequency of care during pregnancy. There is unmet need for contraceptives in many regions, with inadequate support for family planning. Reaching adolescents is regarded as critical to improving maternal health.

- MDG 6—Combat HIV/AIDS, Malaria, and Other Diseases
  Deaths from malaria have reduced by 20 % worldwide, from nearly 985,000 in 2000 to 781,000 in 2009. This was accomplished through critical interventions such as distributing insecticide-treated mosquito nets.

  New HIV infections are declining steadily, led by sub-Saharan Africa. In 2009, the number of new HIV cases was 21 % lower than at peak incidence in 1997. The number of people receiving antiretroviral therapy for HIV or AIDS increased 13-fold from 2004 to 2009, and as such, AIDS-related deaths are declining.

  Effective strategies against tuberculosis are saving millions of lives. Worldwide, deaths attributed to the disease have fallen by more than one-third since 1990.

- MDG 7—Ensure Environmental Sustainability
  Every region has made progress in improving access to clean drinking water. In Eastern Asia, access to safe drinking water increased from 69 % in 1990 to 86 % in 2008. Over the same time period, the number of sub-Saharan Africans with access to safe drinking water almost doubled. However, coverage in rural areas lags behind that of urban areas in all regions.

  Improvements in sanitation have been found to neglect the poorest and those living in rural areas. An investigation in Southeast Asia between 1997 and 2008 showed that new sanitation disproportionately benefited wealthy people, while coverage for the poorest 40 % of households hardly increased.

- MDG 8—Global Partnership for Development
  The level of aid being given to developing countries is higher than ever. Protectionism has been averted due to strong international cooperation and tariffs on agricultural products from developing countries continue to fall. Two-thirds of the world's population have yet to gain access to the Internet through high-speed Internet connections, although commercial development by mobile phone companies has benefited development projects.

Independent Lancet Report (2010)

Progress toward the MDGs is described as "patchy" and "uneven," the broad conclusion being that few goals are entirely on track globally, with least progress made in Africa and south Asia. The report concurs that big progress has been made in MDG 1 and MDG 6, but that insufficient progress has been made toward MDG 2, MDG 4, and MDG 5. Progress toward MDG 3 has been slow, and high rates of deforestation are hampering MDG 7. The report claims that Africa is "short-changed" by the aid flows included under MDG 8 and that following the global economic crisis, progress is being jeopardized due to new financial constraints [6].

Prompt 5: What Are the Barriers to MDG Progress?

- In addition to global challenges such as the financial crisis, major natural disasters, and violent conflict, progress is also hampered by local challenges to regional and local community development projects [7].
- Project bottlenecks have been identified by the UNDP as a major impediment to MDG success [7]. "Bottleneck" describes the phenomena where progress of a project is limited by a single or limited number of factors or resources. These factors are often difficult to predict and may be missed in project planning. For instance, if a government works in partnership with an NGO to improve education targets, the NGO may measure their progress with a surrogate marker such as "supply 1 million textbooks." Despite NGO success in supplying books, the schools are too far away for young rural women to justify enrolling. Distance/accessibility to rural schools is a bottleneck to project progress and the books sit in boxes.
- Human capital is a term used to describe the competence, knowledge, and personality attributes of workers within a community. If some of these attributes are absent (e.g., computer literacy), the community may be unable to access resources that have been provided for enabling development. Human capital can be improved through education and experience, but the deficiencies must first be identified.
- Poor and inadequate infrastructure can prevent progress. Development projects require access to energy, storage space, technology, communications, and transport. Workers require food, shelter, and drinking water. The burden of providing these resources may limit community access to development projects.
- In some regions, people lack social and political rights which prevent them from taking part in and shaping development projects.

Prompt 6: What Has Been Done to Ensure Targets Are Met in 2015?

- There are concerns that many of the targets within the MDGs will not be met by 2015. At the MDG Summit in September 2010, the UNDP launched the MDG Acceleration Framework (MAF) to assist countries in maintaining MDG progress in the next 5 years [7].

- The MAF tool was developed to identify bottlenecks in development projects and find solutions through existing country knowledge, experiences, and partnerships. When a solution is found, a shared plan of action is defined between partners with observable outcomes.
- The tool works as follows:
  1. Identify the relevant MDG target and enumerate the key interventions that are considered necessary to reach it.
  2. Analyze the causes of the lack of complete success of each intervention (identifying bottlenecks).
  3. Review feasible solutions and rank them in terms of their impact and feasibility.
  4. Match the bottlenecks with the bodies identified for implementing the solutions (government, development partners, etc.) to constitute an MAF action plan.

Further Information 2

Your data shows that there has been steady improvement in health indicators in local communities since 1990. Although encouraged, you notice several key development areas including maternal health where progress has been slow. A midwife tells you that many women in the region become pregnant too young and have complicated deliveries resulting in frequent injury and death. You read further and find that high adolescent pregnancy rates are strongly linked with low female school enrolment. There is certainly a pattern emerging [8].

Prompt 7: What Is MDG 3 and Why Is It So Important?

- MDG 3 was set to "promote gender equality and empower women" with the specific target of eliminating gender disparity in primary and secondary education at all levels by 2015. The progress and success of MDG 3 is measured through several indicators:
  - Ratios of girls to boys in primary, secondary, and tertiary education
  - Ratio of literate women to men, 15–24 years old
  - Share of women in wage employment in the nonagricultural sector
  - Proportion of seats held by women in national parliament
- Empowering women has been shown to benefit the whole of society as well as directly benefiting the women themselves, and MDG 3 interacts with many of the other MDGs. The elimination of gender disparity in education directly impacts on MDG 2 ("achieve universal primary education"). Educated women and girls are more likely to delay marriage and pregnancy and are better able to make informed choices about family planning, nutrition, and health. Improved education for girls therefore has a direct impact on MDG 1 ("eradicate extreme

poverty and hunger"), MDG 4 ("reduce child mortality"), and MDG 5 ("improve maternal health") [9].
- Furthermore, higher educational attainment has been shown to be a protective factor against HIV infection for women (MDG 6—"combat HIV/AIDS, malaria, and other diseases") [10].

Prompt 8: Why Does MDG 3 Require Special Attention?

- Despite recognition of the importance of MDG 3, progress has been slow. At the 2010 High-Level Plenary Meeting of the General Assembly on the MDGs, world leaders called for action to ensure the equal access of women and girls to education, basic services, health care, economic opportunities, and decision-making at all levels. A single UN entity was set up to advance women's equality and empowerment "UN Women" (see Box 6.2).
- When MDG 3 was written in 2000, several important contributors to women's empowerment were omitted for religious and cultural reasons, such as improving access to sexual and reproductive health services and reducing the prevalence of domestic violence. In 2005, the UN Millennium Task Force on Education and Gender Equality suggested that governments add these additional targets to MDG 3. It was also suggested that governments should target a 30 % share of seats for women in national parliament and reduce inequalities in employment [11].
- It was further suggested that gender specific indicators should be added to every MDG target to ensure national and local accountability on progress toward women's empowerment [11]. However, a UNDP review of national reports argued that this was not feasible, and the review recommended that countries provide sex-disaggregated data and qualitative information on gender issues across goals and targets [12].

Box 6.2: UN Women

In 2010, several UN agencies were amalgamated to form UN Women to provide a strong unified voice in support of gender equality and female empowerment. The roles of UN Women include:

- To support intergovernmental bodies, such as the Commission on the Status of Women, in their formulation of policies and global standards.
- To help UN member states implement the above standards, standing ready to provide suitable technical and financial support to those countries that request it and to forge effective partnerships with civil society.
- To enable member states to hold the UN system accountable for its own commitments on gender equality, including regular monitoring of system-wide progress.

Further Information 3

The more you investigate, the more complex the MDGs appear. Without doubt, the MDG movement has benefited communities in the area, but there is frustration in schools, health centers, and local businesses that the targets fail to address specific issues within the community. Local people feel that important community decisions are made far away by people they have never met. You consider how the chasm between international development agenda and local community action can be bridged. Perhaps a new approach to international development is needed after 2015. You decide to discuss these thoughts with your project manager.

Prompt 9: What Criticisms Have Been Made of the MDGs?

- The biggest criticism pertains to the "top-down" global and national approach to development. Local actors have limited authority and ownership over development projects, and subsequently MDG targets lack direct relevance to many local communities [13].
- The MDGs were not derived from analysis and prioritization of development need but were developed from existing ideas and campaigns from the 1990s. Subsequently, the MDGs fail to address a range of key development issues. A strong case could be made for MDGs targeted at reducing road deaths, non-communicable disease, and human trafficking [6].
- It is argued the current quantification of MDG targets is flawed, and so progress measurement is misleading. Reliable and scientifically valid data are needed [13].
- The MDGs fail to recognize new thinking in the aims of global development such as human "well-being" and a "rights-based approach." As such, the intangible aspects of human progress and development are ignored in favor of quantifiable results [14, 15].
- The MDGs are based on average progress at a national or global level, and so the poorest and most vulnerable will often fall through the net [16].
- The MDGs provide unrealistic expectations for particular regions or countries. They pose a greater challenge for poorer countries that have lower economic thresholds and lower development baselines (e.g., sub-Saharan African countries) [15].

Prompt 10: How Will Global Development Be Managed After 2015?

- Discussion as to what will succeed the MDGs is still at an early stage, and it is feared too much emphasis on the future will derail efforts to meet the current targets.

- The Lancet and the London International Development Centre produced a document in 2010 that suggested principles for goal setting post-2015. They propose that future goals should avoid threshold-based targets and indicators as these may increase inequity. The aim should be to generate well-being for all while taking a proactive, pro-poor approach. They also emphasize that countries should be supported to achieve goals in more diverse ways than simply donor funding. They argue that a high degree of national ownership and ongoing investment in human, social, and physical capital would encourage the sustainability of growth [16].
- Melamed and Scott (2011) argue that any new goals must emphasize the pressing development problems of the day, namely, urbanization, climate change, chronic poverty and the rise in inequality, and jobs and equitable growth. They also suggest new goals should reflect current thinking on development and aid. Traditionally, development has been measured entirely in terms of economic growth, but now there is more emphasis on "well-being" and human rights. It is also argued that the traditional "donor-recipient" aid model needs attention in the current global climate where climate change and global security make international relations more interdependent [15].
- Selim Jahan (Director of Poverty Practice, UNDP) (2009) made the following recommendations for post-2015 goals:

  - There must be more of a focus on national and particularly local needs rather than global needs. Pockets of deprivation within otherwise well-scoring nations must be identified.
  - There must be improved integration of the private sector into government policies and strategies.
  - Policies which improve domestic financial resources must be promoted and supported such as improved tax structures and microfinance solutions. This will empower local communities to take charge of MDG delivery.
  - Buffer systems should be developed to stop country's facing shocks and crises (environmental and financial) from falling offtrack on MDG targets.
  - The data used to measure progress must be improved. Disaggregation must be encouraged, i.e., retaining data along gender, ethnicity, and racial and urban–rural lines. A more harmonized monitoring and assessment framework would encourage increased consistency, robustness, and frequency of data.
  - Increased efforts must be made to tackle country-level capacity gaps, e.g., lack of capacity in strategy formulation, procurement, or in monitoring.
  - If MDGs are to be continued, there must be better collaboration with World Bank poverty-reduction strategy papers (PRSPs) so that convoluted development policy can be avoided.

- The "Beyond 2015 Campaign" involves 140 organizations (including CAFOD, WWF, Christian Aid) in 50 countries and seeks to influence the creation of a post-2015 framework at both the national and international level. They believe this framework should be led by the UN, but that national governments must have primary ownership of and accountability for the framework and its delivery [17].

Case Study: Lao PDR

Lao PDR is a relatively underdeveloped country and ranks at 132 of 157 on the Human Development Index. Although Lao PDR is on track to achieve many MDGs by 2015, the country faces specific national challenges which must be overcome:

- Lack of progress in reducing child malnutrition
- Strong disparities in people's access to opportunities and social services according to sex, geography, and mother tongue
- Women's limited participation in decision-making at the subnational level
- High maternal mortality
- Quick rate of loss of environmental resources

Lao PDR adopted the pilot MDG Acceleration Framework (MAF) in June 2009 with particular attention focused on MDG 3. In order to identify barriers to MDG 3 progress, female access to schooling and female participation in politics were investigated, and a number of bottlenecks were identified for each (see Fig. 6.5).

Identification of these bottlenecks prompted the Lao PDR government to establish the new Lao National Commission for the Advancement in Women (Lao NCAW) aimed at helping to mainstream gender issues across sectors [18].

Intervention Areas	Summary of prioritized bottlenecks			
	Policy and planning	Budget and financing	Service delivery	Service utilization
Ensuring equal access of girls and women to all levels of education	Weak planning capacity leading to lack of prioritization,and failure to reach the most vulnerable;such as girls in remote rural areas	Limited government spending on education and high dependence on donor funding Gender-sensitive budget preparation and implementation limited at province/district levels	Limited individual (service providers) and institutional capacity to provide quality gender-sensitive education. Distance to school, including at higher primary grades, lowers participation of girl students due to time and safety concerns Non-existent and/or inadequate sanitary facilities(e.g., lack of separate toilets for boys and girls) Lack of teaching curriculum and learning materials which are gender-sensitive Lack of promotion of positive discipline and life skills in education curriculum Inadequate number of qualified female teachers coming from remote and ethnic areas	Limited awarness of value of education, and its long-term benefits, especially for girls Poverty, poor health and malnutrition, which limit school participation Language barriers (school language may not be local/ethnic language), high indirect costs for education (uniforms, stationery, transportation) High opportunity costs to send girls to schools, especially among families in remote areas due to their involvement in work at home
Sensitization,including temporary special measures for political participation	Practical steps to ensure gender mainstreaming still a challenge in number of sectors Poor institutional capa city for formulating and implementing policies/ strategies on gender equality Limited awareness and understanding of concept of temporary special measures, including quotas	Limited budget and financing, both from government and donors Poor understanding and skills related to gender-responsive planning and budgeting at national, provincial and district levels	Gender mainstreaming mechanism is in place, but is relatively new and requires institutional strengthening to become fully operational Only a few specialized organizations and programmes available to deliver empowerment trainings targeted to women	Limited awareness of women's rights Prevailing cultural values focus on traditional roles that may not allow for full participation by women in decision-making process Limited time available to women due to heavy involvement in household and care activities Men not involved in awareness programmes on the importance of gender equality and hence unable to support their participation

Fig. 6.5 Summary of bottlenecks related to MDG 3 in Lao PDR (Reproduced with permission from un.org [18])

References

1. United Nations. The millennium development goals report: 2006. New York: United Nations Development Programme; 2006.
2. Asian Development Bank. MDGs and Global Partnership: Working together in pursuit of the goals (http://www.adb.org/poverty/mdgs/about.asp); 2011.
3. WHO. Commission on macroeconomics and health (CMH): Commission report. Geneva: WHO; 2001. p. 24.
4. WHO. Health and sustainable development: meeting of senior officials and ministers of Health, Summary report, Johannesburg; 2002.
5. United Nations. The millennium development goals report: 2011. New York: United Nations Development Programme; 2011.
6. Waage J, Banerji R, Campbell O, Chirwa OE, Collender G, Dieltiens V, Dorward A, Godfrey-Faussett P, Hanvoravongchai P, Kingdon G, Little A, Mills A, Mulholland K, Mwinga A, North A, Patcharanarumol W, Poulton C, Tangcharoensathien V, Unterhalter E. The millennium development goals: a cross-sectoral analysis and principles for goal setting after 2015, The Lancet and London International Development Centre Commission, Published online; 2010.
7. UNDP Report. UNDP's MDG breakthrough strategy: accelerate and sustain MDG progress. New York: UNDP; 2010.
8. Eloundou-Enyegue PM. Population and millennium development: integrating teen fertility and gender-equity programs, public choices private decisions: sexual and reproductive health and the millennium development goals, UN Millennium Project; 2004.
9. Department for International Development (DFID). Gender equality factsheet, Crown; 2008.
10. UNESCO. Promoting gender equality and female empowerment, Global Monitoring Report; 2007.
11. Grown C, Gupta GR, Kes A. Taking action: achieving gender equality and empowering women, UN Millennium Task Force on Education and Gender Equality, UN Millennium Project; 2005.
12. UNDP. Millennium Development Goals: national reports: a look through a gender lens; 2003.
13. Jahan S. The millennium goals beyond 2015: issues for discussion. New York: Director of Poverty Practice, UNDP; 2009.
14. Society for International Development. The MDGs: rhetoric or reality, Washington, D.C.; 2010.
15. Attaran A. An immeasurable crisis? A criticism of the millennium development goals and why they cannot be measured. PLoS Med. 2005;2(10):e318.
16. Melamed C, Scott L. After 2015: progress and challenges for development, background note. London: Overseas Development Institute; 2011.
17. beyond2015.org.
18. UNDP Report. Unlocking progress: MDG acceleration on the road to 2015, Lessons from the MDG Acceleration Framework pilot countries, Published by UNDP New York; 2010.

Chapter 7
Nongovernmental Organizations and Aid

Ed Mew

Learning Objectives

- Explain the nature and classification of nongovernmental organizations (NGOs)
- Explore unique operation and management issues relating to NGOs
- List issues relating to NGO encroachment into an area
- List considerations when choosing an NGO to support
- Explain the UN cluster system and how it relates to NGO organization
- Describe the concept of advocacy and basics of an advocacy campaign
- Explain the aims and methodology of Amnesty International
- List possible future areas of critical change in NGO practice (Fig. 7.1)

Initial Scenario

You are a district administrator in a small low-income equatorial country. Unconstrained logging has decimated much of the rain-forested areas in the country's borderlands with tribes of indigenous people dispossessed from their lands. After a news item on a major international news channel, interest in the area has exploded. Governmental workers find themselves increasingly hounded by calls and e-mails from representatives from international operational NGOs. Some NGO workers have already moved into the area and have started interacting with local people. You are asked to give them a briefing on relevant issues when dealing with NGOs.

E. Mew, MBBS
FY2 Doctor, Trauma, Emergency and Acute Medicine (TEAM),
King's College Hospital,
Denmark Hill, London, UK
e-mail: eau.mew@gmail.com

D. MacGarty, D. Nott (eds.), *Disaster Medicine*,
DOI 10.1007/978-1-4471-4423-6_7,

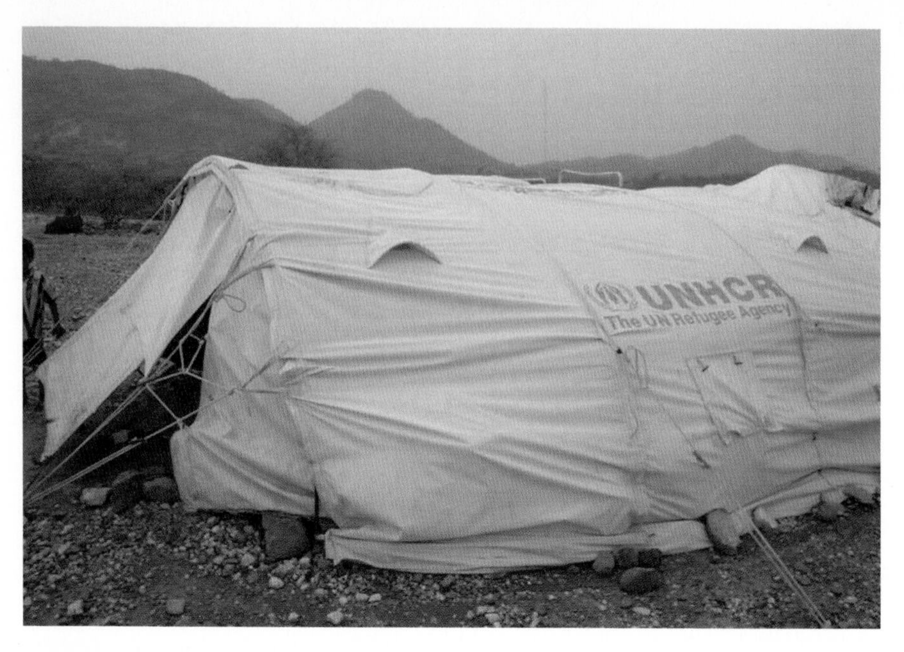

Fig. 7.1 Aid tent (photo courtesy of D. Nott [25])

Prompt 1: What Is an NGO?

NGO stands for nongovernmental organization. Fundamentally, it is any organization that is not government-run and is a legal enterprise. The World Bank definition of NGOs is

> Private organizations that pursue activities to relieve suffering, promote the interests of the poor, protect the environment, provide basic social services, or undertake community development [1].

However, they have attracted an association with charity and benevolent works. Anyone can start an NGO himself or herself, and this is positively encouraged [2]. NGOs are, by this fact, extremely variable in nature and also largely unregulated by international law.

Variety

- NGOs are incredibly heterogeneous. As Storey (1997) notes, "There is no such thing as an NGO 'community'" [3]. Some NGOs operate with multimillion pound budgets, while others comprise a handful of voluntary workers.
- Many religious organizations, charities, environmental groups, lobby groups, and medical associations are also NGOs.

Importance

- NGOs are increasingly important socioeconomic players in the fields of aid, environment, and local policy. Storey (1997) notes that, with the end of the "Cold War" in the 1980s, Western governments became less interested in developing

countries per se, creating a vacuum that left NGOs as chief providers of international public welfare [3].
- Some "NGOs" receive significant funding from governmental sources and are heavily influenced by governmental policies, making the term "NGO" misleading. As noted by the UNHCR, "It is governments, rather than individual donors, that are most responsible for the recent increase in NGO funding. In 1970, public sector funding accounted for a mere 1.5 percent of NGO budgets. By the mid-1990s, it had risen to 40 percent and was still increasing [4]."

Guiding Principles

- Historically, charitable and aid-based NGO operations are heavily influenced by the ethos of humanitarianism (benevolence that is universally applicable).
- The cornerstones of this are humanity, independence, impartiality, and neutrality, operating to help people in a way that does not discriminate between individuals due to political, religious, or social factors. Humanitarian assistance is governed by the Geneva conventions, namely, that it should be neutral and impartial [5].
- How this translates into practice is vague. Cooperation can easily be construed as non-neutral and casual arrangements as implying political allegiance. Storey has noted multiple historical examples of "neutral" NGOs becoming—unwittingly or not—associated with aggressive regimes that committed atrocities in countries such as Rwanda, Cambodia, and Afghanistan [3].
- On the other hand, the obsession with independence has arguably made NGOs reluctant to cooperate with other parties, lest they get accused of losing their impartiality [6].

Prompt 2: How Are NGOs Classified?

It is often difficult to classify NGOs, as their nature is so variable. However, attempts have been made. The World Bank classifies NGOs into

- Operational NGOs—whose primary purpose is the design and implementation of development-related projects. An example of this is Médecins Sans Frontières (MSF).
- Advocacy NGOs—whose primary purpose is to defend or promote a specific cause and who seek to influence policies and practices [1]. An example of this is Amnesty International.

These are further divided up according to the geographical scope of the NGO:

- Community-based
- City-specific
- National
- International

Therefore, for example, Médecins Sans Frontières is an operational NGO that works on an international scale.

Prompt 3: What Unique Organizational and Operational Issues Do NGOs Present?

Funding

- All NGOs need funding from some source—called a "donor." There are many different possible avenues for funding, including public donations, governmental sources, or private companies.
- When analyzing the work and methodology of an NGO, special attention must be paid to its sources of funding as these may influence its aims. See Box 7.1 for an example. Ebrahim (2003) argues that the mutual interdependence of donors and NGOs make both favor short-term, easily measurable activities as opposed to those that may provide the most benefit to the beneficiary area [7].
- Critics argue that NGOs are influenced—often overly so—by their donors. For this reason, funding from governments is controversial as critics say that it reduces the NGO's impartiality. Some NGOs, like Greenpeace, refuse to accept governmental aid.

Box 7.1 Charity Case Study for 2010–2011: Oxfam [8]
Income—£318,000,000
Voluntary 125.6 million, charitable activities 114.3 million, trading 74.4 million, investment 0.9 million, and other 2.8 million
Expenditure—£294,800,000
Generating voluntary income 17.2 million, trading 58.1 million, charitable activities 216.3 million, governance 1.1 million, investment management 0.1 million, and other 2 million

Legal

- Unlike sovereign states, NGOs are not directly subject to international law with the exception of the International Red Cross and Red Crescent. However, they are bound by the legal framework of the country they operate in.
- They are also theoretically constrained by the Geneva conventions which include articles on humanitarian assistance—namely, that it be neutral and impartial [5].

Politics

- As we have explored, it is hard to stay totally impartial. Some NGOs like the International Red Cross and Red Crescent have historical policies of nondisclosure—they cannot be compelled to give evidence in court, perhaps in an effort to remain impartial and thus politically neutral so as not to be denied access.
- However, this move has attracted criticism. Some argue that NGOs in aid-giving roles can never maintain total neutrality, despite their best efforts. In man-made disasters, applying aid without addressing the underlying political causes can be

seen as treating symptoms without curing the disease. Indeed, as with the Pope and Roman Catholic Church in the Second World War, staying politically neutral in the face of atrocities can be construed as indefensible.

- This viewpoint caused French humanitarian workers to form Médecins Sans Frontières in 1971 with the aim that patient need would trump political boundaries and adherence to neutrality.

Prompt 4: What Is an NGO Code of Conduct?

- Increasingly, due to media attention and scrutiny from donors, NGOs are being encouraged to sign up to and operate under a code of conduct. Leader (1999) argues that NGOs often operate in states in conflict and therefore in an administrative and political "vacuum of regulation" [5]. Therefore, codes of conduct are useful as internationally agreed rules that aim to ensure good outcomes in target communities and for NGO workers.
- The first popularized code of conduct was the 1994 Red Cross and Red Crescent Code of Conduct for Humanitarian Work; see Box 7.2 [9]. Codes comprise internationally recognized standards of conduct that inform their operating style. As Leader notes, donors are increasingly using codes as criteria for funding to ensure accountability [5].
- Despite this, signing up to codes is still voluntary, and there is often little discussion of how they are enforced or what happens if they are broken [5].

Box 7.2: The Red Cross Code of Conduct

1. The humanitarian imperative comes first.
2. Aid is given regardless of the race, creed, or nationality of the recipients and without adverse distinction of any kind. Aid priorities are calculated on the basis of need alone.
3. Aid will not be used to further a particular political or religious standpoint.
4. We shall endeavor not to act as instruments of government foreign policy.
5. We shall respect culture and custom.
6. We shall attempt to build disaster response on local capacities.
7. Ways shall be found to involve program beneficiaries in the management of relief aid.
8. Relief aid must strive to reduce future vulnerabilities to disaster as well as meeting basic needs.
9. We hold ourselves accountable to both those we seek to assist and those from whom we accept resources.
10. In our information, publicity, and advertising activities, we shall recognize disaster victims as dignified humans, not hopeless objects [10].

Further Information 1

In the space of a month, over 30 foreign NGOs have set up camp in towns surrounding the rain-forest area, sometimes without any permission from the local authorities. Local reception has been mixed. Some NGOs are seen to be actively pursuing local needs and are keen to involve and empower local leaders. Others take a more controlling attitude, speeding through the countryside in four-wheel-drive vehicles and dictating their preconceived policies to the local leaders without listening to their views.

Representatives from the various NGOs have requested to meet you to discuss the government's assessment of the current situation and opportunities for collaboration. You are struggling to decide which NGOs the government should cooperate with. You note that larger, more powerful NGOs are able to get their points heard the best and can make things happen—however, you express reservations as to how in touch they are with the needs of the local populace.

Prompt 5: What Practical Issues Does Sudden Influx of NGOs into an Area Present?

Invitation

- One pervasive issue in NGO policy relates to whether they should only go to an area when invited or whether there is any moral right to intervene when injustice is identified—no matter what the area or circumstances.
- Often this becomes a political issue. Governments may not welcome any global publicity of situations requiring international attention, and so aid may be badly needed even if not formally requested.
- However, one should also be wary of the perception of NGOs as self-motivated players. NGOs may pursue policies discordant with local needs and appeasing largely foreign donors. For further information on the debate surrounding humanitarian intervention, see the case on complex disasters in Chap. 1.

Access and Competition

- Governmental officials overseeing operations in the locality must decide how many NGOs should be allowed to operate in the area: a decision informed by which NGOs will provide the most benefit to the area with the minimum disruption. Ideally, this is also coordinated by the Office for the Coordination of Humanitarian Affairs (OCHA).
- There may be huge competition between NGOs for giving aid to an area. NGOs often have to compete for funding contracts from donors and so welcome media "exposure" showing their good deeds (and so justifying donor-funding contracts).
- Some high-profile NGOs will "crisis-hop" from one high profile, well-publicized disaster to another, leaving smaller NGOs to "fill in gaps" of development and

service provision when the crisis has peaked [9]. As John Graham from Save the Children notes, "If you don't get starving babies you don't get the money" [24]. On the other hand, it is relatively hard for NGOs to gather support to tackle less well-publicized "forgotten" crises [9], a sad fact that has been prioritized as a major stumbling block for future NGO practice by Jan Egeland, UN Undersecretary General for Humanitarian Affairs and Emergency Relief Coordinator [11].

Agendas

- Many NGOs will have agendas running with their aid. These may represent a precondition to their project, for example, giving aid while spreading a religious message.
- Some NGOs will aspire to project-based aid that may not actually benefit the area as much as simply increasing budgetary funding but is more amenable to advertising and attractive to donors. The needs of the recipient area must have primacy.
- A notable case of "mixed-up" agendas is the case of NGO involvement in areas of conflict and warfare where NGO workers are often grouped into the same bracket of "interfering foreigner" as military forces, leading to suspicion and hostility [6, 12]. This is typified when NGO workers drive around in white 4x4 vehicles and wear military-style clothing.

Prompt 6: What Factors Should Influence Choice of NGOs to Work with or For?

Basic principles will guide your choice of NGOs to support the following:

- Kelly has suggested asking the following questions to determine if it is operating in the humanitarian spirit:

  1. Have they helped out for a good cause before? Previous experience or professional training in the respective field is a useful indicator.
  2. Will they provide aid based on need without discrimination? Heterogeneous staff and founding partners are good signs of the presence of diversity.
  3. Will they carry out operations while separating themselves from political discourse? Scrutiny of an NGO's donors and, if large, who *they* in turn fund and support can elucidate their philosophy [13].

- How effective will it be? Slim notes that NGO credibility comes from three main areas: having skills, having the ability to fit these skills to the current context, and proving you can effectively achieve your stated goals (described as competence, context, and veracity) [14].
- Is the NGO trying to draw attention to the problem or themselves [3]? NGOs that aim to speak "with" the people via creation of partnerships arouse less suspicion than those aiming/claiming to speak "for" the people (outside circumstances where the people are unable to articulate their needs) [14].

- How long-term are their aims? NGOs committed to alleviate suffering should be inquiring where areas of greatest need are and whether needs are being addressed by other groups [3]. An area may have great need but also be oversaturated with NGO attention.

Further Information 2

You meet with the representatives of ten chosen NGOs operating in the area to discuss their agendas, explain your governmental stance, and explore opportunities to collaborate. Some representatives are asking what cluster leads are operating in the area. The NGO camp is bitterly divided between those supporting operational activities and those who argue that advocacy is the only way to ameliorate the lot of the dispossessed. You have the task of mediating between these camps.

Prompt 7: What Is the Cluster System?

The cluster system was created by the UN as a way of coordinating humanitarian support. It aims to provide wide coverage of different aspects (called "sectors") of aid and to guarantee minimum standards. Its aims are detailed below:

- Ensure sufficient global capacity in all sectors of aid in case of new disasters
- Ensure predictable leadership according to agreed standards, working toward common goals
- Ensure accountability of clusters to the UN
- Improve coordination and prioritization

UN agencies are allocated to each aid sector. The relevant aid sectors will change according to the needs of the target community. For the 2010 Haiti earthquake, there were originally 12 aid sectors that were later refined to the following:

1. Protection
2. Water sanitation and hygiene (WASH)
3. Shelter and nonfood items
4. Nutrition
5. Health
6. Logistics
7. Early recovery
8. Education
9. Food aid
10. Agriculture

- The cluster lead takes ultimate responsibility over the area and ensures minimum standards of aid as laid out in the Sphere project. For more information on the Sphere project, see case study on refugee camps and the Sphere project. Examples of cluster leads are the World Health Organization (WHO), World Food Program (WFP), or United Nations High Commissioner for Refugees (UNHCR).
- Under this lead, the actual membership of the clusters is incredibly variable and dynamic. This, in theory, ensures predefined standards (to be upheld by the cluster lead) while maintaining flexibility.
- NGO operatives are expected to understand and work within this framework of clusters [15]. Any new event that requires a multi-sectorial response warrants the employment of the cluster approach to organize the international response.

Prompt 8: What Is Advocacy?

Advocacy is an attempt to influence public policy within political, economic, and social systems. Often associated with humanitarian movements, advocacy may also be motivated by politics, religion, or self-interest. Advocacy is often organized by advocacy groups, defined by Young and Everritt as

> …any organization that seeks to influence governmental policy, but not to govern [16].

Roles of these groups include

- Assisting in development of better public policy
- Ensuring governmental accountability
- Giving a voice to misrepresented citizen interests
- Mobilizing citizens to participate in the political process [16]

Examples of advocacy groups include

- Advocacy international
- Greenpeace
- Children's Rights Alliance for England (CRAE)
- Action on Smoking and Health (ASH)

Conducting a successful advocacy campaign necessitates influencing the thoughts of three key levels of participants: the public, key experts and stakeholders, and decision makers. Ann Pettifor of Advocacy International UK has set out the main stages of advocacy campaigning in her publication "Cutting the Diamond" [17]:

- Survey the political, social, and economic context
- Devise clear aims, your arguments, and to whom you intend to pitch them
- Communicate your arguments clearly using a variety of media
- Have strong institutions to lead your campaign
- Evaluate the impact of your campaign

Further Information 3

The process of advocacy for the dispossessed indigenous people continues. Although public opinion and national experts are increasingly convinced of the need to better the lot of the dispossessed rain-forest peoples, key government members still turn a blind eye—perhaps due to vested interests and lobbying by the logging industry. More advocacy NGOs flood into the country although the situation has not noticeably improved for the local people. You are tasked with streamlining the NGOs to create a profile that is more responsive to the needs of the local peoples. You decide to brainstorm what issues will affect future NGO practice.

Prompt 9: What Issues Will Affect the Future Nature and Practice of NGOs?

Future issues may include the following:

Accountability and Transparency

- As NGOs become more professional with larger workforces and budgets, pressure has been applied for increasing their accountability and transparency. Donors are starting to demand proof of where their funds are going. A more recent trend is toward accountability to the *recipients*.
- Emphasis has shifted toward increasing involvement of beneficiaries in policy decisions.

Core Standards

- New moves are afoot, especially among the larger international NGOs, to ensure core standards in delivery of NGO projects, encompassing higher standards in reporting, audit, and inter-NGO cooperation.
- There is currently much debate in NGO literature about whether they would benefit from adopting more "business-orientated" models of management.
- The emergence of "for profit" players is a new but significant factor in the humanitarian community, according to Ferris. Before the ceasing of hostilities, USAID awarded US$900 million to private nongovernmental companies to undertake reconstruction activities, including areas like public health and education [9].

Shifts in Participants Working for or Collaborating with NGOs

- Historically, representatives from industrialized nations delivered aid to developing or transitional areas. With pressure from the international community, this pattern is gradually changing to a preponderance of more grassroots movements that are more locally involved.

- This has the benefit of greater community integration and perhaps a greater understanding of how aid can be tailored to the local community.
- As a middle class emerges in countries going through the economic-demographic transitional phase like India, NGOs are emerging as community-based organizations. Kumar notes that palliative care is delivered effectively in Kerala using community networks. 80 % of funding is locally derived, and coverage is near 70 % [18].
- An interesting parallel can be made with China with NGOs now enjoying relative operational freedom after years of state control yet still largely state-dependent, a situation that Lu calls "dependent autonomy" [19].

Flexible Funding

- Egeland of the Humanitarian Affairs section of the UN has called for increased flexibility in receiving funding. Taking the East Asian tsunami as an example, Egeland argues that funding at times outstripped NGO demand and that funds could have been better diverted elsewhere [11].
- Projects have evolved in the early twenty-first century like the Good Humanitarian Donorship initiative [20] that prioritize issues like funding based on need [11], flexibility of donor channels, and involvement of beneficiary countries in deciding where aid is directed to.

Governing Relationships

- Ideally, diverse relationships with other NGOs, the private sector, governmental organizations, and target communities will increase NGOs' flexibility of operations and policy.
- The boundaries of civilian and military providers of aid and relief are being blurred. Operational aid/relief-giving NGOs will have to negotiate their relationships with the military in aid provision [6, 21].

Case Study: Goma

Goma is a border town in the Democratic Republic of Congo. Its name has won international notoriety as it was the theater for a huge humanitarian crisis during and after the Rwandan genocide in 1994. Around the time of the genocide, a stream of displaced persons flocked over the Rwandan border to Congo. Over 250 foreign NGOs, 8 UN departments, and 20 government donors were quick to respond to such a well-publicized international crisis. Eyewitnesses described the ensuing scene as an "aid agency supermarket" in which aid agencies "blare out their names and logos like soft drinks manufacturers" [22]. Competition was fierce with international NGOs competing for publicity to drive fund-raising back at home. Meanwhile, supposedly neutral refugee camps were becoming de facto safe havens for Hutu militias who recruited from the refugees, imported arms, and organized military training [23]. In such a volatile situation, inter-NGO competition undercut any potential cooperative efforts to ameliorate the situation, arguably contributing to a huge humanitarian disaster [23]. Some international NGOs estimate that militias stole up to 60 % of aid supplies meant for the dispossessed populace [24]. The end result, some have argued, was a perpetuation of the misery and conflict that many of the NGOs were striving to end.

References

1. Duke University Libraries, World Bank and NGOs. Taken from World Bank website: Nongovernmental Organizations and Civil Society/Overview. http://wbln0018.worldbank.org/essd/essd.nsf/NGOs/home. Accessed 8 June 2001 (no longer available) Accessible via: http://library.duke.edu/research/subject/guides/ngo_guide/igo_ngo_coop/ngo_wb.html. Accessed on 5 Jan, 2012.
2. Global Research Development Centre. Starting an NGO. Accessible via: http://www.gdrc.org/ngo/start-ngo/index.html. Accessed on 5 Jan, 2012.
3. Storey A. Non-neutral humanitarianism: Ngos and the Rwanda crisis. Dev Pract. 1997;7(4):384–94.
4. Office of the United Nations High Commissioner for Refugees. The state of the world's refugees. Oxford: Oxford University Press; 2000. p. 194.
5. Leader N. Codes of conduct: who needs them? Humanitarian Exchange Magazine. March 1999, issue 13. Accessible via: http://www.odihpn.org/report.asp?id=1065. Accessed on 5 Jan, 2012.
6. Roberts N. Spanning 'bleeding' boundaries: Humanitarianism, NGOS and the civilian-military nexus in the post-cold war era. Public Adm Rev. 2010;70(2):212–22.
7. Ebrahim A. NGOs and organizational change. Discourse, reporting, and learning. Cambridge: Cambridge University Press; 2003.
8. Taken from charity commission website, accessible from: http://www.charitycommission.gov.uk/index.aspx. Accessed on 5 Jan, 2012.
9. Ferris E. Faith-based and secular humanitarian organizations. Int Rev Red Cross. 2005; 87(858):311–25.
10. International Committee of the Red Cross. Code of conduct. Principles of conduct for the International Red Cross and Red Crescent Movement and NGOs in Disaster Response Programs. Accessible online from: http://www.ifrc.org/Docs/idrl/I259EN.pdf. Accessed on 5 Jan, 2012.
11. Egeland J. Humanitarian accountability: putting principles into practice. Humanitarian Exchange Magazine. Issue 30; June 2005.
12. Tomb N. Humanitarian roles in insecure environments. Monterey: Center for Stabilization and Reconstruction Studies, Naval Postgraduate School; 2005.
13. Kelly J. When NGOs beget NGOs: practicing responsible proliferation. J Humanitarian Assistance. Apr 2009. http://sites.tufts.edu/jha/archives/451.
14. Slim H. By what authority? The legitimacy and accountability of non-governmental organizations. Oxford: Oxford Brookes University; 2002. Accessible from: http://www.jha.ac/articles/a082.htm. Accessed on 5 Jan, 2012.
15. Hopperus Buma A, Burris D, Hawley A. Conflict and catastrophe medicine: a practical guide. 2nd ed. London: Springer; 2009. p. 36.

16. Young L, Everitt J. Advocacy groups. Vancouver: University of British Columbia Press; 2004.
17. Taken from Advocacy international website. Accessible from: http://advocacyinternational.co.uk/?page_id=328. Accessed on 5 Jan, 2012.
18. Kumar S. Learning from low income countries: what are the lessons?: palliative care can be delivered through neighbourhood networks. BMJ. 2004;329:1184.1.
19. Lu Y. Non-governmental organisations in China: the rise of dependent autonomy. London/New York: Routledge; 2009.
20. http://www.goodhumanitariandonorship.org/gns/principles-good-practice-ghd/overview.aspx. Accessed on 5 Jan, 2012.
21. Welling D, et al. Seven sins of humanitarian medicine. World J Surg. 2010;34:466–70.
22. http://www.independent.co.uk/news/world/battle-of-logos-and-tshirts-rages-in-refugee-camps-aid-agencies-scramble-for-cash-1446538.html. Accessed on 5 Jan, 2012.
23. Brown M, et al. New global dangers: changing dimensions of international security. Cambridge: MIT Press; 2004.
24. Polman L. War games: the story of aid and war in modern times. New York: Viking Press; 2010.
25. Aid tent. Photo courtesy of D. Nott.

Chapter 8
Developing Healthcare Systems

James Houston

Learning Objectives

- List different types of health systems
- Identify the goals of a health-care system
- Describe the components of a typical health-care system
- Identify the costs associated with different global systems
- Describe how to evaluate a developing world health-care system
- Describe the role of primary healthcare and its goals
- Explain the Alma Ata declaration including its successes and failings
- Discuss the problem regarding the shortage of health professionals in the developing world (Fig. 8.1)

Initial Scenario

You work for a development NGO in the capital of a fledgling sub-Saharan African country. Having been impressed with previous work, you are called one morning by a government official to help to set up a functioning health-care system. The country has a difficult recent history, being rather slow to recover from previous decades of internal strife and civil war. However, recently things have been looking more positive; peace has reigned for the last couple of years, and a sense of optimism is currently held by those working within the government. While the politicians understand that such projects take many years to implement, they would like some groundwork done and some preliminary proposals for a new health-care system.

J. Houston, MBBS, MEng
FY2 Doctor, Department of Surgery,
Chelsea and Westminster Hospital, London, UK
e-mail: jameshouston@doctors.org.uk

D. MacGarty, D. Nott (eds.), *Disaster Medicine*,
DOI 10.1007/978-1-4471-4423-6_8, © Springer-Verlag London 2013

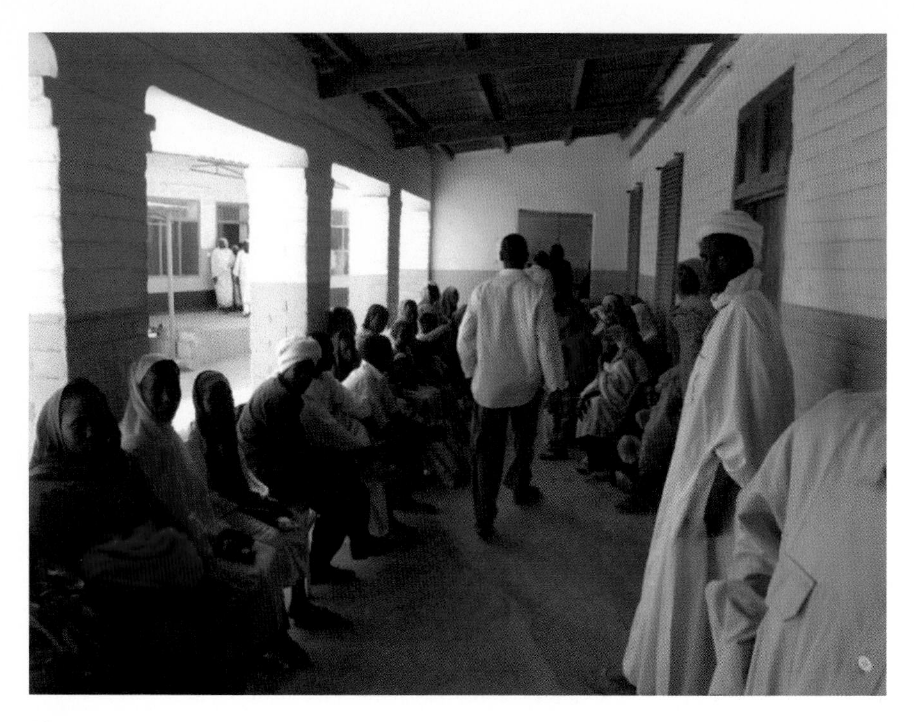

Fig. 8.1 Locals wait with their families at a treatment centre (Picture by David Nott)

The current system is 80 % funded by direct payments, paid out of pocket by people when they are ill. The rest is subsidized by the state. State and private hospitals exist, although both are in short supply. Many government officials are aware that the state hospitals are chronically underfunded, being little more than places poor people go to die. At the same time, private hospitals remain unaffordable for most.

You begin by examining health-care systems in surrounding countries, discussing with the minister philosophical goals of a health system and identifying a structure within the health system.

Prompt 1: What Different Types of Health-Care Systems Exist?

Most countries will have a combination of some of the systems below:

Public Systems: Funded out of general taxation, which may have to be higher as a result. These systems may be free at the point of care or incur a nominal charge to see a practicing clinician. Such systems will treat people regardless of their income or disease profile. Due to fixed resources, not every condition can be treated, and difficult decisions must be made to prioritize some medical care over others, for example, the National Health Service (NHS) in the UK.

The NHS is currently free at the point of care and funded out of general taxation. While it is fairly comprehensive in terms of funding emergency treatment, difficult and emotive debates exist over the funding of expensive drugs, particularly in cancer therapies. To establish which drugs will be publically funded, NICE (National Institute for Health and Clinical Excellence) has been set up to evaluate the treatments in terms of cost-effectiveness.

Insurance Premium Systems: Funded by individuals paying a certain amount every month. This can be to a central government organization, which may subsidize the care given, or to a private provider, for example, healthcare systems in Germany and the United States.

As income is given every month, the prohibitive costs of acute care are avoided. However, in many countries, insurance can be prohibitively expensive in itself. As many employers pay for health-care insurance, redundancy can leave people effectively without health-care provision.

Charitable Systems: While these do not spread over an entire country, hospitals that are funded by charities form a significant, non-politically motivated area of healthcare in the developing world.

Private Systems: Paid by the individuals receiving their healthcare. While every condition can be treated in part, patients pay at point of delivery, and, thus, treatment depends on a patient's ability to pay for it. Although there is no payment occurring when people are healthy, the prohibitive, "upfront" cost of care means that many people cannot afford treatment. A retrospective study [1] found that over 60 % of bankruptcies in the United States were due to medical costs.

Prompt 2: What Are the Goals of a Healthcare System?

The WHO defines the goals of health systems [2] as

- To improve and protect public health
- Responsiveness to the expectations of the population
- Fair financial contribution

In order to last, the system must be

- Self-sustainable in terms of personnel and funding

Good health is a nebulous term; it may be described as an individual's ability to carry out the functions of daily life or by the absence of disease or, in the case of the WHO, "a state of complete physical, mental, and social well-being." Thus, depending on your definition of health, your health system may focus more on mental illness, more on promotion of health, or more on physical disease. While obtaining "holistic well-being" may be an ideal, this may well be impractical within governments with scarce resources. Thus, most systems focus primarily on alleviating medical problems through pharmaceutical or surgical treatment.

Expectations in the population may depend on previous experience, what an individual is paying, education, and health-system accountability. Expectations may well be raised via the media, which can illustrate particular inequalities between regions or countries. Likewise, expectations may well increase co-currently with improvements in the health service. The ability of the health service to respond will depend on its flexibility and availability but also due to the treatment outcomes of diseases in question.

Fair financial contribution can be assessed both in terms of equity and efficiency. Should people who are more able to afford healthcare be charged more, or should those who heavily use the system be charged the highest rates?

Health equity refers to a lack of systematic disparities in health between different social groups [3].

Equity changes dramatically between different countries with different health systems. Most often the issue is compounded by the fact that those who are most in need of healthcare are those least able to afford it. Likewise can illness be seen as something that can be prevented through rational action or something that happens to people by chance? Even if an indisputable link could be shown between lifestyle choices and disease, sociological factors present in that person's life may well make it unfair to charge them for their resulting condition.

Self-Sustainability – Employees: This refers more specifically to retention of employees. Should a system spend much money on training its workforce, it must also retain them to help pay back the investment. However, many staff from poorer countries may move to work in better funded health-care systems abroad due to better pay and quality of life.

Economy: To remain sustainable, a system will have to budget for the long term. It must thus bear in mind the potential costs incurred when committing to any new policy.

Prompt 3: What Different Components Should Make up a Health Service?

A robust health service should consider comprising of the following:

Primary Care: Often described as the gateway to all other health provision. Primary care may provide treatment for common and noncomplex conditions. Vaccinations may be provided alongside the dissemination of medicines for chronic conditions. Primary care can consist of, among others, general practitioners, community nurses, mental health practitioners, and midwives.

Secondary Care: These hospitals are a referral center for more complex cases and will carry out routine operations. They will often be based in larger towns or cities and may well have emergency admission units.

Tertiary Care: These hospitals stand as national referral centers. They will likely be based in large cities and will have significant research and teaching arms attached to them. While the overall number of patients they treat may be small compared to the number treated in primary care, these hospitals may carry politically important kudos and prestige.

Public Health: While healthcare may often be seen in terms of treatment of disease, a great importance should also be attached to disease prevention. Public health bodies form an important part in educating populations. They also gather epidemiological data to inform future health priorities. While many public health offices are based centrally in large cities, it is important they serve those that need them most, often based in poorer educated, rural areas.

Pre-hospital Care: This includes the initial treatment and resuscitation of patients prior to transferring them to a more definitive point of care. These systems may be privatized or run as part of the public health provision.

Further Information 1

The minister is impressed with your ideas. He would like a system that is available to those that need it most but is concerned about funding. A plan for insurance-based healthcare is suggested with a subsidy for those that are from the lowest income groups. The private groups will continue to serve those that can afford it, although laws are designed to make such companies offer more affordable care packages to those in middle-income brackets. Offices are established for a public health department, and links are set up with NGOs. Emphasis will be on improving primary and secondary care. You stress that while improvements can be made, much more information is required. You debate with the minister an economic basis for committing funds, as improved health may also increase the GDP of the country. You both agree that some measures of system assessment need to be designed for accountability.

Prompt 4: What Information Needs to Be Collected Before Setting up a Health-Care System?

Health-Care Demographics: Some idea of the basic health needs is essential. However, the extent to which such information exists varies much in developing countries. Where possible, estimations also need to be made of future health-care needs. This will help in predicting service demand and more efficient allocation of resources.

Health-Care Priorities: This differs from demographics as it implies a political dimension. Politicians may have their eyes set on a prestigious project that may bring a visible, if not useful legacy. In reality, lower profile rural clinics may benefit more people. Likewise, some health-care decisions, such as spending money on drugs and alcohol addiction, may prove less popular with voters who are not directly affected.

Table 8.1 Total healthcare spending per capita in different countries

Country	Total healthcare spent per capita/per annum (2007) [6]
United States	$6096
Germany	$3171
United Kingdom	$2560
Zimbabwe	$139
Tanzania	$29
Democratic Republic of Congo	$15

Economic Viability: Providing healthcare is an expensive business, and funding is difficult to find, especially in countries with many other economic priorities. Systems may thus be reliant on overseas aid. Preconditions on such aid may make things more inflexible. Withdrawal of aid can leave dependants with nowhere to go. Decisions will also need to be made on medicine provision, in particular whether certain more expensive drugs can be afforded. Countries such as the UK have established bodies such as NICE [4] which help to make such decisions.

System Currently in Place: The system does not need to be built from scratch. Much information will likely already be available regarding demographics and disease profiles. However, the most comprehensive data may originate from those hospitals that are the best funded; endemic issues in poorly funded institutions can easily be overlooked.

Prompt 5: How Expensive Is Healthcare Globally?

Health-care costs vary enormously around the world. Its expense depends upon many factors including the cost of labor, equipment, medicines, and administration.

Much basic medicine can be provided very cheaply, but providing similar standards of care and accommodation compared to the developed world can soon become prohibitively expensive.

As medicines and technologies become more expensive, developed countries are spending more and more on healthcare as a fraction of GDP.

Demand is increasing for healthcare as age demographics shift to larger percentages of older people, who are proportionately greater in need of health-care provision.

As a general rule, countries aim for fixed proportions of their GDP to be spent on healthcare. However, this figure and its levels when worked out per capita differ widely between countries. The USA currently spends almost 15 % of its GDP on healthcare, with most developed countries spending around 10 % [5]. When including all countries across the world, a weighted average reveals spending to be at 6.2 % of GDP. When investigating healthcare spending like this on a per capita basis, even greater disparities are seen as seen in Table 8.1. Likewise, more money needs to be spent in developing countries as seen in the WHO announcement detailed in Box 8.1.

Box 8.1: WHO Announcement Asking for More Money to Be Spent per Capita on Health [5]

Recent estimates of the money needed to reach the health Millennium Development Goals (MDGs) and to ensure access to critical interventions, including for non-communicable diseases in 49 low-income countries, suggest that, on average (unweighted), these countries will need to spend a little more than US$ 60 per capita by 2015, considerably more than the US$ 32 they are currently spending.

Prompt 6: How Do You Determine Whether the Health System Is Functioning Well?

The WHO focuses on five points that determine if a system is functioning well and achieving its goals of responding to a population's needs and expectations [7]:

- Improving the health status of individuals, families, and communities: This can be measured by crude mortality and morbidity rates or by working out numbers of days lost to certain conditions in terms of disability adjusted life years (DALYs).
- Defending the population against what threatens its health: This infers that a public health group exists to monitor current and predict future epidemics. It also requires vaccination programs.
- Protecting people against the financial consequences of ill-health: The system must have safeguards in place to insulate people from the costs of treatment. Ideally, a social welfare system might exist to provide support for them and their families when they are not able to earn.
- Providing equitable access to people-centered care: It is a sad fact that healthcare is often not equitably spread across individual countries. Better coverage is often seen in higher socioeconomic areas. Incentives need to be made to encourage health-care professionals to move to areas where their skills are most needed.
- Making it possible for people to participate in decisions affecting their health and health system: This refers to a change from the "paternalistic" model of medicine where doctors would decide unilaterally on what is best for the patient. A more modern model incorporates patient choice into the equation. While this may be good in theory, it can only really be practiced if different options are available and the patients are informed about them. Furthermore, this model also places responsibility onto the patient for their own health; education must be available for the patients to understand about the lifestyle choices that they make.

The points above are quite subjective to measure and thus will have political influence on their interpretation. Much criticism is made of "top-down" targets in developed countries' health-care systems. Open communication channels between policy makers and clinicians must exist to make sure that good intentions from politicians for improving patient's care have corresponding practical solutions implemented.

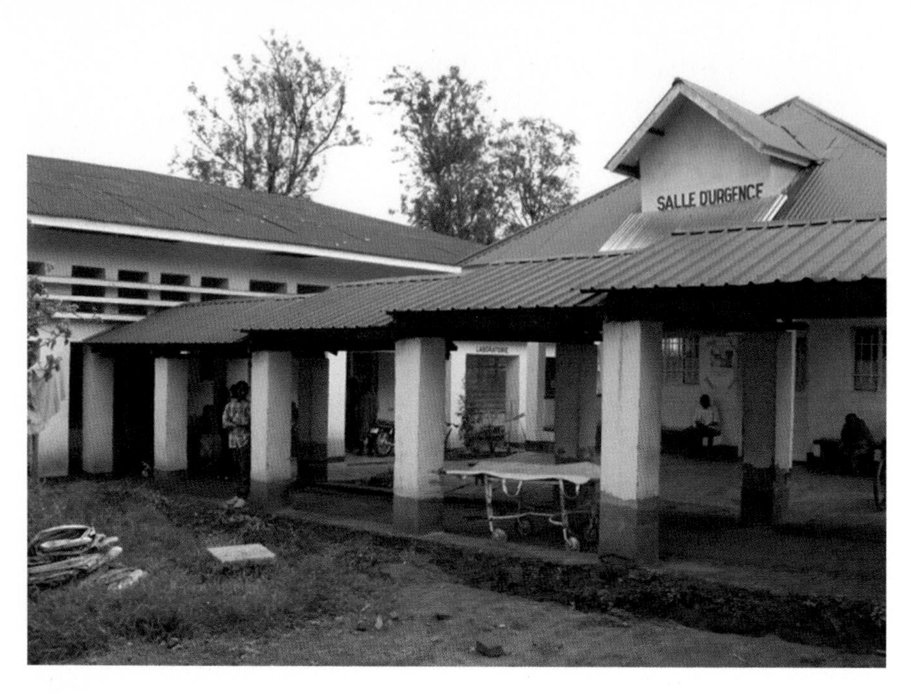

Fig. 8.2 A rural hospital in the Congo (Picture by David Nott)

Further Information 2

You liaise with the Ministry of Health and set to work, trying to pull some figures together. While information is fairly scarce in some areas, you collaborate with another NGO, obtaining some data regarding health demographics. Work with a university department pulls together estimations of how demand might evolve over the coming decade. Difficult negotiations begin regarding funding between government officials and foreign donors.

While everyone has similar overriding interests of improving health, many people seem to have different agendas. Some people believe that the cities are where most of the input is required while others insist that the rural areas are the most impoverished. You are also told of the difficulty in retaining medical staff in rural areas. Likewise, nobody can agree on what conditions the money should be spent on, ranging from malaria to maternal issues to mental health. The most senior politician only really shows interest when another aide suggested naming a new teaching hospital after him. You are most convinced about the need for adequate primary care in the rural areas. You are aware of the political difficulties in getting primary care messages across and of all the hype, followed by lack of progress from previous international conferences (Fig. 8.2).

Table 8.2 Aspects of primary healthcare

Education	Teaching communities safe practices such and infection control, safe sex, and good nutrition
Water/sanitation	Access to safe drinking water and adequate toilet and cleaning facilities
Maternal/child	Monitoring pregnancy, access to births, medical attendance for births, and prevention of childhood diseases
Family planning	Access to contraception to allow birth spacing and manage fertility rates
Immunization	Implementing routine vaccinations and vaccination campaigns
Prevention/control local diseases	Addressing specific local infectious diseases
Treatment of common diseases/injuries	Treating minor injuries that do not require hospital
Provision of essential drugs	Managing acute and chronic conditions

Prompt 7: What Is Primary Healthcare?

Primary health-care services are central to a local community and are the first point of contact for patients. As detailed in Table 8.2, it is wide ranging, can be practiced by a physician or an associated health professional, and relies heavily on preventative medicine and patient education.

Prompt 8: What Is the Alma-Ata Declaration?

The Alma-Ata Declaration was from the 1978 International Conference on Primary Care and has been accepted by WHO as being the key to achieving "Health for All." Its main aims are detailed in Box 8.2.

Primary healthcare is still seen as the best way to implement universal healthcare, as reflected by the 2008 World Health Report: primary healthcare now more than ever [8].

The Declaration of Alma-Ata 1978 defines primary healthcare as

> Essential healthcare based upon appropriate and acceptable methods and technology, made universally accessible to individuals and families in the community through their full participation and at a cost the community and country can afford to maintain in the spirit of self-reliance

Box 8.2: Excerpts from the Alma-Ata Declaration [9]

- Health is a fundamental human right
- Gross inequalities in health are politically, socially and economically unacceptable
- Economic and social development is key to health

- Governments have a responsibility for the health of their people which can be fulfilled only by the provision of adequate health and social measures
- A main social target of governments, international organizations and the whole world community in the coming decades should be the attainment by all peoples of the world by the year 2000 of a level of health that will permit them to lead a socially and economically productive life
- Primary health care is the key to attaining this target as part of development in the spirit of social justice
- Primary Care Includes at least: education concerning prevailing health problems and the methods of preventing and controlling them; promotion of food supply and proper nutrition; an adequate supply of safe water and basic sanitation; maternal and child health care, including family planning; immunization against the major infectious diseases; prevention and control of locally endemic diseases; appropriate treatment of common diseases and injuries; and provision of essential drugs

Prompt 9: What Have Been the Issues in Primary Healthcare Since Alma-Ata?

Sustained progress toward universal healthcare has not been met. Many countries are now dismantling their social protection mechanisms in health as opposed to making them more inclusive.

Health-care systems do not naturally gravitate toward primary care, as three worrying trends identified by WHO [8] illustrate

1. Health systems focus disproportionately on a narrow offer of specialized curative care.
2. Health systems focus a command-and-control approach to disease control, focused on short-term results, which fragments service delivery.
3. Health systems where a hands-off or laissez-faire approach to governance exists allow unregulated commercialization of health.

A number of reasons have been identified for this:

- Political reasons: Insufficient political prioritization of health. Political doctrine may assume that increased national wealth will lead to improved health for all, where rising inequalities has left the poor more vulnerable.
- Poor governance: Leading to corruption and over commercialization.
- Decreased in spending on health: Heavily indebted countries often spend more on debt relief than healthcare.
- Lack of investment in correct services.
- Lack of training people for the personnel required complicated with "brain drain" as skilled workers emigrate.

Prompt 10: What Needs to Be Done to Improve Global Primary Care?

- Improving universal coverage: Removing user fees to protect individuals from uninsured costs. Services to rural communities.
- Access to essential drugs.
- Tailoring priorities of health-care funding especially to maternal health, newborn and child health, and family planning.
- Incorporation of healthcare with other factors responsible for reducing mortality, such as better water, sanitation, nutrition, food security, and control of HIV.
- Use of evidence-based medicine for more efficient allocation of resources.
- Improve research: Developing countries are particularly poorly reknown for their production and utilization of research [10].

Prompt 11: What Factors Lead to Shortage of Health-Care Workers in the Developing World and How Can It Be Tackled?

- There is a critical shortage of health-care workers worldwide, meaning 1 billion people are without healthcare [5].
- Africa has 2.3 health-care workers per 100 population, while the Americas have 24.8 health-care workers per 1000 population [11].
- However, there is still a global lack of doctors; if every doctor that migrated from Africa returned, the WHO estimates it would only solve 12 % of the problem.
- Health-care professionals emigrate because of both "push and pull" factors. These refer to reasons why you want to leave the country such as poor postgraduate training (push) and reasons why you want to go to other countries such as better remuneration (pull).
- The problem of migration of skilled workers will probably increase as developing countries like India and China become wealthier.

Solutions include training staff for specific local roles, investing training in training health-care workers in developing countries, ethical recruiting strategies in developed countries, and self-sufficient training levels.

Further Information 3

A field trip illustrates firsthand the inequalities between the modern hospitals in the city and the decrepit outposts in the country. Glimmers of hope are seen in some new government works that have built new clinics that specialize in maternal and reproductive health. These areas have seen a concomitant reduction of maternal deaths and unwanted pregnancies. Incentives are given to those workers to remain in the rural areas and local employment drives continue. The health system is clearly a work in progress requiring continued funding and input at all hierarchical levels. You leave the office with a wry smile on your face when the minister returns, offering to name a small rural clinic after you as an acknowledgement of your legacy.

Case Study: Cuba

Cuba is an interesting example of a public health system that provides great results against the odds. While the Cuban GNI per capita ranks its 50th in the world ($5,520) [12] and spends roughly 10 % of its GDP on healthcare, it spends approximately $550 [13] per person per year on healthcare. This is in comparison to the USA which spent $6096 per capita in 2007. This said, Cuba has a better life expectancy (79.1 years vs. 78.5 years) and child mortality (6/1000 vs. 8/1000 live births) compared to the USA [14]. Part of this must be due to the way the health system is set up and run. Cuba has one of the highest ratios of doctors to population in the world. It also offers healthcare that is almost completely free to its citizens. While some people are cynical that much of the hype about Cuba may be down to suppression of dissenting critics [15], others are much more positive. In an address in April 2000, Kofi Annan stated that Cuba "should be the envy of many other nations, [Cuba] demonstrates how much nations can do with the resources they have if they focus on the right priorities - health, education, and literacy" [16]. Much of the health-care system is focused on preventing disease rather than just treating it, which includes regular checkups and promoting exercise and hygiene. While staff are paid less, doctors come from all over the world (including the USA) to train in Cuba. Many medicines are also in short supply – something not helped by the presence of US embargoes.

References

1. Himmelstein DU, Thorne D, Warren E, Woolhandler S. Medical bankruptcy in the United States, (2009) 2007: results of a national study. Am J Med. 2009;122(8):741–6. Epub 2009 Jun 6. PubMed PMID: 19501347.
2. World Health Organization. World Health Report 2000 - Health systems: improving performance. Geneva: WHO; 2000. http://www.who.int/whr/2000/en/index.html. Accessed on 30 Nov 2011.
3. Braveman P, Gruskin S. Defining equity in health. J Epidemiol Community Health. 2003;57(4): 254–8. Review. PubMed PMID: 12646539.
4. National Institute for Health and Clinical Excellence; www.nice.org.uk. Accessed on 30 Nov 2011.
5. World Health Organization. The World Health Report – Health Systems Financing: the path to universal coverage; 2010. http://whqlibdoc.who.int/whr/2010/9789241564021_eng.pdf. Accessed on 30 Nov 2011.

6. United Nations. Human Development Project. 2007. Available at: http://www.hdr.undp.org. Accessed on 30 Nov 2011.
7. World Health Organization. Key components of a well functioning health system. Geneva: WHO; 2010. http://www.who.int/healthsystems/EN_HSSkeycomponents.pdf. Accessed on 30 Nov 2011.
8. World Health Organization. Primary health care now more than ever. Geneva: WHO; 2008. www.who.int/whr/2008/whr08_en.pdf. Accessed on 30 Nov 2011.
9. World Health Organisation. Alma Ata Declarations. 1976. www.who.int/publications/almaata_declaration_en.pdf. Accessed on 30 Nov 2011.
10. Sabri AA, Qayyum MA. The problem of evidence-based medicine in developing countries. CMAJ. 2006;175(1):62. PubMed PMID: 16818915.
11. Naicker S, Plange-Rhule J, Tutt RC, Eastwood JB. Shortage of healthcare workers in developing countries – Africa. Ethn Dis. 2009;19(1 Suppl1):S1-60–4. PubMed PMID: 19484878.
12. World Bank. World development indicators 2011. Washington, D.C.: World Bank; 2011. http://data.worldbank.org. Accessed on 30 Nov 2011.
13. UNDP. International human development indicators. Available at: http://hdrstats.undp.org/en/countries/profiles/CUB.html. Accessed on 30 Nov 2011.
14. UNDP. International human development indicators. Available at: http://hdr.undp.org/en/data/profiles. Accessed on 30 Nov 2011.
15. Hirschfeld K. Re-examining the Cuban Health Care System: towards a qualitative critique. Cuban Affairs. 2007;2(3).
16. Kofi Annan, April 11, 2000, From Uriarte, Miren. Cuba: social policy at the crossroads: maintaining priorities, transforming practice. An Oxfam America report. 2002, p. 6. Available at: http://umboston.academia.edu/mirenuriarte/Papers/647928/Cuba_social_policy_at_the_crossroads_maintaining_priorities_transforming_practice, Accessed on 30 Nov 2011.

Chapter 9
International Aid

Shao Foong Chong

Learning Objectives

- Define and classify types of international aid
- Describe the major global partnerships in aid
- Discuss the international commitment in providing aid and development
- Evaluate the effectiveness of aid
- Analyze the criticisms of aid
- Discuss the political and economical factors that influence aid
- Outline the major international agreements on aid effectiveness
- Recommend how the provision of aid can be improved

Case Study

Negotiation of an international aid package between a recipient and donor country

Initial Scenario

In your country, large proportions of the population live in squalor, lacking basic access to schools and hospitals. Parents work from the break of dawn to nightfall to take home a pittance to feed their children. The Treasury itself is in a poor situation with huge debts carried over from excessive spending from previous governments, where a large amount of the gross national income is spent paying off the interest

S.F. Chong, MBBS, MA (Oxon)
FY2 Doctor, Department of Emergency Medicine,
St George's Hospital, Tooting, London, UK
e-mail: shaofoong@hotmail.com

D. MacGarty, D. Nott (eds.), *Disaster Medicine*,
DOI 10.1007/978-1-4471-4423-6_9, © Springer-Verlag London 2013

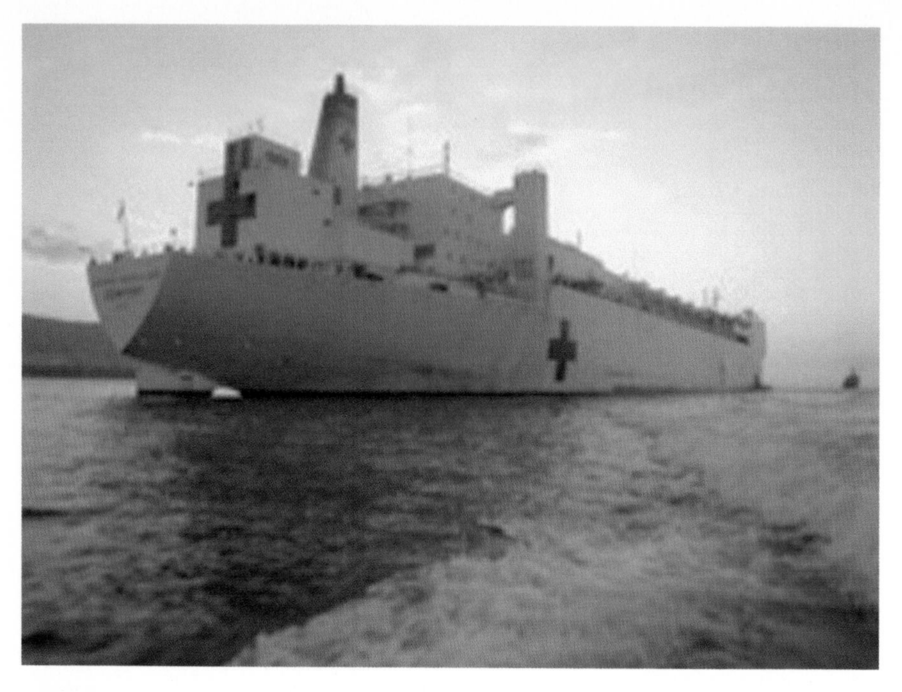

Fig. 9.1 Aid ship (Picture by David Nott)

of these debts. You, as a civil servant in the Ministry of Health, have the opportunity of lifetime; a representative of a major donor country is flying over to negotiate an aid package for your country (Fig. 9.1). *As part of the negotiation team, you have a discussion about some fundamental concepts of aid.*

Prompt 1: What Is Aid?

- Aid, also known as international aid, overseas aid, foreign aid, or official development assistance (ODA), aims to promote economic development welfare of developing countries. ODA is a commonly agreed definition of international aid flow from donor government agencies to developing countries and multilateral organizations. Moreover, at least 25 % must be given as a grant element [1].
- The total aid volume of official development assistance in 2010 was $128.7 billion, over a third of this to sub-Saharan Africa [2].

Prompt 2: Describe Different Types of Aid

The US government gives the largest absolute amount of economic aid to other countries but when calculated as a percent of gross national income is the smallest contributor among the major donor countries [3]. Its foreign policy categorizes them as such:

- *Humanitarian assistance* – Material or logistical assistance during humanitarian crises, such as man-made or natural disasters, is given to people in immediate distress. The main aim is to save lives, alleviate suffering, and maintain human dignity in the short term. The generosity of $12.8bn from donor governments and $4.1bn from private contributions helped to fund the international humanitarian system according to the Global Humanitarian Assistance Report 2010 [4].
- *Development assistance* – Support for health, education, and other development programs in order to alleviate poverty in the long term. Development assistance funds are split between bilateral assistance to countries and multilateral assistance that are often channeled through international organizations.
- *Economic political/security assistance* – Designed explicitly to support geostrategic interests of the donor country, such as access to strategic natural resources or military bases. From the end of WW2 until early 1990s, the rationale for providing foreign aid was to have strategic bases in countries to be seen as defeating communism. Over the last decade post the terrorist attacks on September 11, 2001, aid has increasingly been used as a national security issue to fight the war on terror in Iraq and Afghanistan.
- *Military assistance* – Provision of weapons, equipment, training, and peacekeeping funds. The USA accounts for a vast proportion of the global export trade in military equipment, particularly to its friends and allies [3].

Prompt 3: What Are the Major Global Partnerships in Aid?

- *Bilateral donors* – Bilateral agreements between donor countries and recipient countries are designed to develop economic progress and social stability. Projects include economic restructuring and private sector development, environmental protection, and support for treatment of HIV/AIDS and other diseases. The UK is the second largest bilateral humanitarian donor, after the US government [4].
- *Multilateral donors* – Contributions aggregated from donor nations help to finance multilateral organization, like the United Nations Children's Fund (UNICEF), United Nations Development Program (UNDP), and multilateral development banks (MBDs), such as the World Bank. They provide aid packages and loans to encourage sustainable growth and development.
- *Global health initiatives* – Humanitarian programs are targeted at mitigating diseases and strengthening health systems. Increasingly, we are seeing more international organizations cooperate and pool into large vertical funds to tackle specific infectious diseases. These initiatives include The Global Fund to Fight AIDS, Tuberculosis and Malaria that has a budget of US $177 million to help millions have access to antiretroviral drugs, TB treatment, and insecticide-treated bednets or the GAVI Alliance with US $897.7 which focuses on increasing

access to immunization [5]. There are also major philanthropists such as Bill & Melinda Gates Foundation that have had a profound difference in financing long-term health projects.

Further Information 1

You are extremely excited about the prospect of gaining a substantial financial aid package to help meet the Millennium Development Goals in your country. Enthused, you spend endless nights putting together a case presentation for the Minister of Health. He smiles, takes a puff of his cigarette, and turns his chair to the window looking out to the country which had so much potential when independence was declared in his youth. He doubts whether the aid will come from the international community as they have broken so many promises in the past.

Prompt 4: Have Developed Countries Delivered on Their Aid Commitments?

- The United Nations target for donor countries to commit 0.7 % of gross national income (GNI) as ODA was endorsed in 1970 to promote global development and security. The largest donors by volume are the United States, Japan, France, Germany, and the UK. However, by proportion, most governments, with the exception of a handful of northern European countries, have failed to reach the 0.7 % target [6].
- The world is changing, and as the BRIC (Brazil, Russia, India, China) economies grow, they will play an increasingly involved role in humanitarian emergency responses, particularly in their neighboring regions. China, for example, was an important actor in the response to the Pakistani floods at the end of 2010. It is possible that these countries will take more international responsibility from traditional donors, especially with news that the US Congress is considering whether to significantly reduce its humanitarian assistance budget for food aid and disaster response [5]. Meanwhile, 15 countries in the European Union have bravely committed themselves to increasing their aid budget to 0.7 % of GNI by 2015.

Prompt 5: What Is Global Health Watch and How Does It Encourage Aid Pledges to Be Delivered?

- Global Health Watch is a watchdog that has reported the international community's failure to deliver on aid commitments and commented on how money is not being used effectively to make the desired impact [7]. Moreover, they analyze

and publish reports on government policies in tackling global disease, inequalities, poverty, and climate change, holding them to account.
- It is a forum where health professionals and activists can advocate for the vulnerable or lobby national governments and international financial institutions. They suggest there are undermining power imbalances between donor and recipient countries, and they call for a new model for international development that rebalances the relationships between the richer and poorer countries of the world [7].

Further Information 2

The meeting lasts all day long with arguments running back and forth. The representative has strong criticisms of your previous government stating that even with all the aid packages and multitude of NGOs operating in your country over the last two decades, there is a lack of a coherent national health and education service. He believes that aid so far has not been effective. Furthermore, he demands that if debt relief and international aid is to be provided, major policy changes are required from the current government. Suggestions include increasing competitiveness by privatizing public industries, increasing interest rates, and reducing export prices.

Prompt 6: How Effective Is Aid?

- *Aid effectiveness* – It refers to the impact that aid has in reducing poverty and inequality, increasing growth, building capacity, and accelerating achievement of the Millennium Development Goals set by the international community.
- *Micro-macro paradox* – Although donor agencies regularly report the success of their projects at a "micro" level, there has been no consistent empirical evidence to demonstrate that international aid has a positive effect on economic growth at a "macro" level. This may be the case because aid tends to encourage consumption rather than investments and is often used for humanitarian assistance rather than long-term development goals.
- Consequently, *Burnside and Dollar* [8] argue that aid is effective only if developing countries have sound institutions and economic policies, which include good governance and open free markets. Where countries lack these key attributes, aid has no or even a negative impact on GNI. Thus, they advocate that aid should be selectively allocated to countries conditional upon the quality of state institutions and policies.
- Donor countries are therefore very interested in aid effectiveness by grading international organizations and NGOs according to their ability to produce results and deliver value for money. The Bilateral and Multilateral Aid Reviews [9] produced by the UK Department for International Development have assessed various organizations according to their results and provided the best performing agencies

with more multiyear core funding from the UK taxpayer. Multilateral agencies that score highly are UNICEF, GAVI, the Private Infrastructure Development Group, and the Global Fund to Fight AIDS, Tuberculosis and Malaria. This report is an important step in linking country-level funding to performance.

Prompt 7: What Are the Criticisms of Aid?

- *Lack of harmonization of aid agencies* – There is a lack of coordination and coherence among donors and global health institutions leading to multiple organizations working on the same disease-specific initiative. Funds are often spent unproductively on poorly conceived development projects. For example, political advantage and legacy may be gained in building a brand new hospital with state-of-the-art equipment rather than investing in primary health-care professionals that can help a much greater proportion of the population [5].
- *Administrative bureaucracy* – Donor organizations may require government ministries to monitor their aid projects by producing extensive reports to be accountable for the money they spend. Although this is important for the transparency that donors desire, it also increases the bureaucracy. Large numbers of civil servants are hired just to deal with paperwork rather than helping to produce policies.
- *Redistribution of the health budget* – Some countries may cut their domestic health-care expenditure when given developmental assistance. This allows governments to free up money to invest in other priority areas like education and infrastructure, but may also be used to fund the military.
- *Local corruption* – Large amounts of aid are allocated to financing aid projects, but the precise recipients of this money are not always guaranteed, and the projects themselves are not always realized. In Afghanistan, for example, it is not unusual to find an international NGO passing over the implementation of an aid project to a local NGO, perhaps in response to Taliban attacks on Western humanitarian aid workers [10]. But then, they might subcontract it to a local company, who then asks his uncle to gain the materials for the job, who might use cheap, inferior materials, resulting in a substandard end result. Moreover, at every stage of further subcontracting, each player takes a significant cut of the overall budget allocated toward the aid project.
- *Aid as a weapon of war* – Linda Polman argues that humanitarian aid has become a massive industry, where the beneficiaries of war zone operations are more likely to be the perpetrators of conflict rather than the most needy victims. Local politicians, military, and business leaders may only allow international NGOs access to conflict zones in return for a large proportion of the value of aid supplies. In Liberia, the president demanded 15 % of the value of aid to be paid to him in cash. Reconstruction projects after the tsunami in Sri Lanka were only possible after surrendering money to the Tamil Tigers, which were otherwise labeled as import duties on aid supplies. In order to gain access to areas of

Afghanistan, a significant proportion of food aid and agricultural supplies was passed over to the Taliban. The degree of this corruption poses an important challenge toward all humanitarian agencies who negotiate barriers to assistance as they may fall guilty of prolonging conflict [10].

Prompt 8: How Do Politics and Economics Influence Aid Partnerships?

Third World Debt

- Many developing countries are crippled by the burden of debt that was incurred through the legacy of colonialism or odious debt.
- These countries that may want to invest in social programs to reduce poverty lose a vast proportion of their GNI paying off the interest on decades of accumulated external debt.
- The Heavily Indebted Poor Countries (HIPC) initiative has helped to provide debt relief and low-interest loans to cancel or reduce external debt repayments to sustainable levels. Assistance, however, is conditional.

Conditionality

- The International Monetary Fund (IMF) and World Bank provide debt relief conditional to a number of structural adjustment reforms.
- Structural adjustment programs include trade liberalization, currency devaluation, increased interest rates, privatization of industry and public services, and restrictions on social welfare expenditure. With sound economic policies, economic growth should follow, according to Burnside and Dollar's research [8].
- However, these reforms have been heavily criticized. Often, these changes benefit donors and large multinational corporations and may be to the detriment of the poor. For example, privatization of public utilities may raise the cost of services beyond the citizens' ability to pay.

Selectivity of Aid Partners

- Assistance is more likely to be orientated toward donor countries' foreign policy rather than recipient countries' level of poverty.
- US foreign aid has been disproportionately connected with the Middle East in the fight against terror, Japan in the Asia-Pacific region, and Britain and France to former colonies.

Tied Aid

- Refers to aid tied to goods and services supplied exclusively by the donor country. For example, money may be given for a hospital on condition that a company based in the donor country builds it or that permission is given for a natural resource.

- For donor countries, tying aid in such a way creates local jobs and businesses, promotes exporting industries and services, and exposes domestic firms to these foreign markets.
- Tied aid may encourage donor countries to focus more on their commercial objectives than the needs of recipient countries [11].
- A total of 25–30 % of aid is tied in bilateral agreements.

Further Information 3

The Health Minister is frustrated with the current terms and conditions of the proposed development assistance package. He feels that it is insulting to be told by the West what to do by and suggests that they listen to the recommendations proposed by the Paris Declaration of Aid Effectiveness.

Your minister expounds your presentation that deals with way that aid effectiveness can be improved. Moreover, he persuades the representative that there are other ways beyond aid of improving his country's development. Trade for one is key, and protectionist policies that arise in developed countries create barriers to entry.

Prompt 9: Outline Important International Agreements on Aid

- *Aid partnerships* – A new paradigm for aid as a partnership that depends on mutual accountability, rather than the tied one-way relationship between donor and recipient.
- *Paris Declaration on Aid Effectiveness (2005)* – Donor and developing country governments, multilateral organizations, and MDBs met to address problems with aid development projects [12].
- They found the aid process was still too strongly led by donor priorities and administered through donor channels, making it hard for developing countries to take the ownership. An international consensus has been pledged to allow developing countries formulate their own strategies for poverty reduction, improve their institutions, and tackle corruption, while donor countries align behind these objectives and use local systems to manage aid.
- Furthermore, aid was considered too uncoordinated, unpredictable, and untransparent. Thus, donors committed to harmonize their development work better to avoid duplication and pool aid toward strategies directed by the recipient country, such as a national health plan rather than multiple fragmented health projects. Finally, donors and recipient countries emphasized the need to develop tools to measure the impact of aid and account more transparently their use of aid funds.

- *Accra Agenda for Action (2008)* – Surveys showed that progress had been made, but new global challenges, such as rising food and fuel prices and climate change, required developing countries to take the lead in improving the impact and effectiveness of aid [12].

Prompt 10: What Other Factors Beyond Aid Are Important for Development?

Economic Growth

- There is broad agreement that aid alone is not enough to alleviate developing countries from poverty. Some argue that the most effective form of foreign aid is no aid at all; what really matters is economic growth. Good macroeconomic policy and stability is a significant determinant of growth.
- It is argued that China and Asia-Pacific countries have improved healthcare and reduced poverty through economic growth, not aid and development support [5].

Trade

- Developing countries need to get access to investment and trade flows to promote economic growth [13].
- Trade costs can be significantly reduced through trade facilitation programs and investing in economic infrastructure projects.
- Promoting closer cooperation between trade, finance, and development officials in government should enhance the capacity of government to participate effectively in international trade negotiations.
- Increase incentives for the private sector to trade and export by reforming policies to improve the growth of small and large businesses and create employment for the population.

Policy Incoherence

- Policy incoherence limits the development prospects of poor countries.
- Encouraging developing economies to develop their agricultural industries will not work if trade deals exist where donor or developed countries heavily subsidize excess stockpiles of food to sell on international markets or have high rates of import tax; this results in unfair competition that makes developing countries' food exports economically unattractive.
- The World Bank estimated that 2.55 million people or 40 % of the world's population were living below the "$2-a-day" income poverty line in 2004. Meanwhile, the European Common Agricultural Policy (CAP) provided a daily subsidy of $2.7 per cow [14].
- Training up skilled health-care professionals is undermined by migration policies that support a brain drain of doctors and nurses from lower income countries to higher income countries.

Prompt 11: What Measures Can Be Implemented to Improve Aid Effectiveness?

- Any increases in aid should be clearly dedicated to achieving existing development goals, and not on other priorities like counterterrorism.
- Further debt cancellation and development assistance with no ties or conditions attached.
- Economic restructuring should take into account the social welfare needs of the poorest people and not require the privatization of public services and industries as a condition of development assistance.
- Promote trade and investment, not merely aid, to increase economic growth and reduce poverty.
- Developed countries too must to open their markets to goods from the developing world and reduce subsidies to their own exports.

Further Information 4

The negotiation table closes, and there is much work yet to be done. It is agreed that a substantial aid package will be provided now to kick-start some of the government's projects that aim to improve the health-care infrastructure especially in rural areas but will release the rest of the funds when they have evidence showing the impact of aid a year later.

Case Study – Foreign Aid to Haiti

The 2010 Haiti earthquake killed an estimated 316,000 people and left over a million people homeless. The massive disaster provoked an extraordinary outpouring of generosity from private individual donors and governments around the world who gathered at New York donors' conference pledging a total $5.3 billion in aid.

However, the international media questioned where all this money was going; much of this aid bypassed the Haitian government in favor of UN agencies and NGOs, while many Haitians continued to endure very poor living standards.

While much of the aid bought food, improved health-care needs and long-term development projects, it did so with strings attached. Highly subsidized US rice farmers undercut local producers, driving them out of business and making Haitians lose self-sufficiency in food production. Many NGOs conducted their projects without coordinating their roles with the Haitian government. The international relief effort fell short of meeting the Haitian people's needs.

References

1. OECD. Glossary of statistical terms, Official Development Assistance (ODA). Available at: http://stats.oecd.org/glossary/detail.asp?ID=6043. Accessed 22 Aug 2012
2. UNCTAD. United Nations, Geneva. World Investment Report; 2008: transnational corporations and the infrastructure challenge. Available at: www.unctad.org/en/docs/wir2008_en.pdf. Accessed 22 Aug 2012
3. Congressional Research Service. Foreign aid: an introductory overview of U.S. Programs and Policy; 2009. Available at: http://fpc.state.gov/documents/organization/124970.pdf. Accessed 22 Aug 2012
4. Department for International Development. Humanitarian emergency response review (HERR); 2011. Available at: http://www.dfid.gov.uk/Documents/publications1/HERR.pdf. Accessed 22 Aug 2012
5. Crisp N. Unfair trade (2) – importing ideas and ideology. In: Crisp N, editor. Turning the world upside down: the search for global health in the 21st century. London: Royal Society of Medicine Press; 2010. Chapter.
6. OECD. Statistics on resource flows to developing countries. Table 1 – DAC Members' Net Official Development Assistance in 2010. Available at: www.oecd.org/dac/stats/dcrannex. Accessed 22 Aug 2012
7. Global Health Watch. Global Health Watch 2 – an alternative world health report. London: Zed Books; 2008. Available at: http://www.ghwatch.org/sites/www.ghwatch.org/files/ghw2.pdf. Accessed 22 Aug 2012
8. Burnside C, Dollar D. Aid, policies, and growth. Am Econ Rev. 2000;90(4):847–68.
9. Department for International Development. Statement by the Secretary of State for International Development: the bilateral and multilateral aid reviews; 2011. Available at: http://www.dfid.gov.uk/Media-Room/Speeches-and-articles/2011/BAR-MAR-oral-statement/. Accessed 22 Aug 2012
10. Polman L. Aid as a weapon of war. In: Polman L, editor. War games: the story of aid and war in modern times. London: Viking; 2010. Chapter.
11. Ehrenfeld D. Foreign aid effectiveness. Political rights and bilateral distribution. J Humanitarian Assistance; 2004. Available at: http://sites.tufts.edu/jha/archives/75. Accessed 22 Aug 2012
12. OECD. The Paris Declaration on aid effectiveness and the Accra agenda for action, 2005/2008. Available at: http://www.oecd.org/dac/aideffectiveness/43911948.pdf. Accessed 22 Aug 2012
13. World Trade Organization. Aid for trade and LDCs: starting to show results. OECD/WTO; 2011. Available at: http://www.wto.org/english/tratop_e/devel_e/a4t_e/a4t_ldcs_e.pdf. Accessed 22 Aug 2012
14. Sharma D. Farm subsidies: the report card. Share The World's Resources; 2005. Available at: http://www.stwr.org/imf-world-bank-trade/farm-subsidies-the-report-card.html. Accessed 22 Aug 2012

Chapter 10
Future of Global Health

Will Barker

Learning Objectives

- Appreciate climate change as the greatest current threat to human health
- Outline the challenges of food security
- Discuss other major threats to global health
- Discuss the sustainability and consequences of population growth
- Discuss demographic transition as a model of development

Initial Scenario

You are a doctor taking a year out from specialist training and applying for a health post with a charity in Senegal (Fig. 10.1). *Currently, Senegal is experiencing a major drought for the second year running with water shortages restricting agriculture. There is a talk that extreme weather may be the result of man-made climate change.*

Prompt 1: What Is the Current Evidence for Climate Change?

Science has now provided overwhelming evidence that global temperatures are increasing and this change is attributed to human actions [2–4]. Current scenarios predict an increase of global temperatures of more than 2 °C over this century which will cause famine, migration, conflict, death, and disease, all on an unprecedented scale [5, 6] (Fig. 10.2).

With thanks to Mr David Nott.

W. Barker, MBBS, MPhys
FY2 Doctor, St Thomas' Hospital,
Westminster Bridge Road, London, UK
e-mail: willbarker@doctors.org.uk

D. MacGarty, D. Nott (eds.), *Disaster Medicine*,
DOI 10.1007/978-1-4471-4423-6_10, © Springer-Verlag London 2013

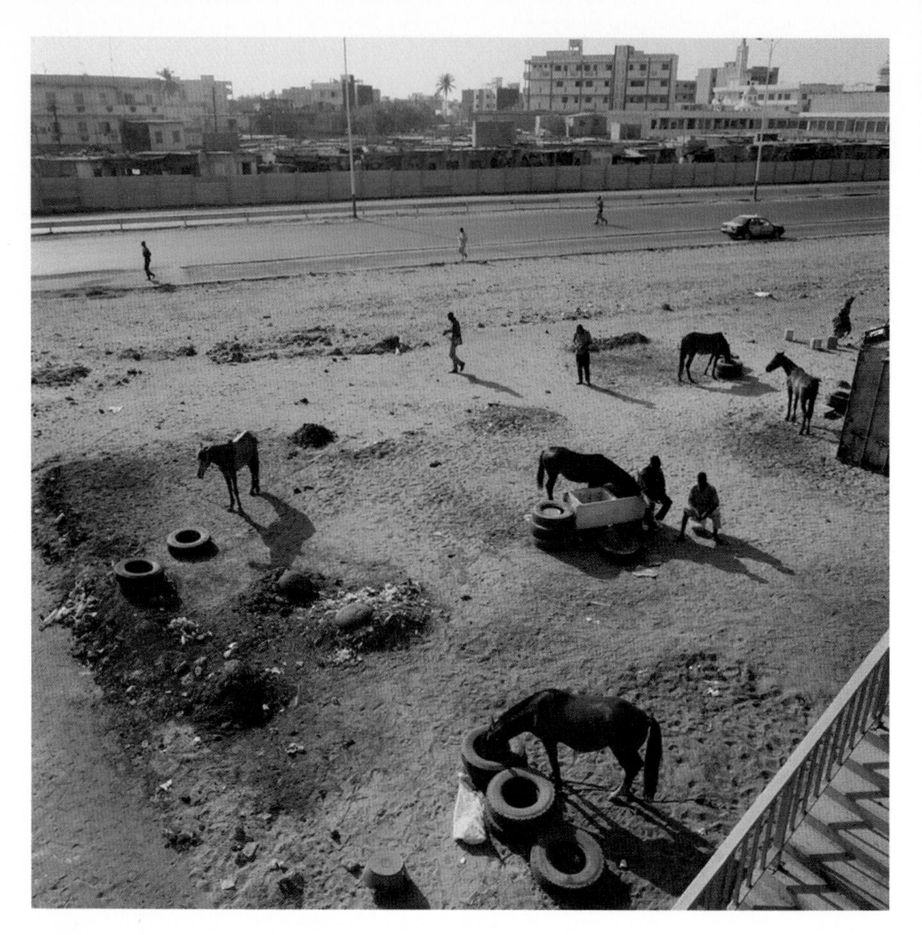

Fig. 10.1 Informal horse garage on the side of the new toll highway under construction in Dakar, Senegal (Part of "En Route To Dakar" series by Mimi Mollica [1]) (Picture by David Nott)

Climate change will hit the most vulnerable people in the developing world hardest with potentially one billion losing access to sufficient, clean water. All the progress made in areas such as child and maternal health could be reversed (Table 10.1). Urbanization and increased density of population could compound the effects of extreme weather; it is therefore not surprising that the healthcare community is beginning to wake up to climate change.

> Climate change is the biggest global health threat of the 21st century
> 2009 Lancet and UCL Institute for Global Health. [4]

> The greatest risk to human health is neither communicable nor non-communicable disease, it is climate change
> 2011 Fiona Godlee, Editor BMJ. [5]

Nitrogen and oxygen which make up 99 % of the atmosphere are transparent to heat, but trace gases (carbon dioxide, water vapor, methane, and others) play a critical role preventing heat from the sun being radiated back into space. The levels of

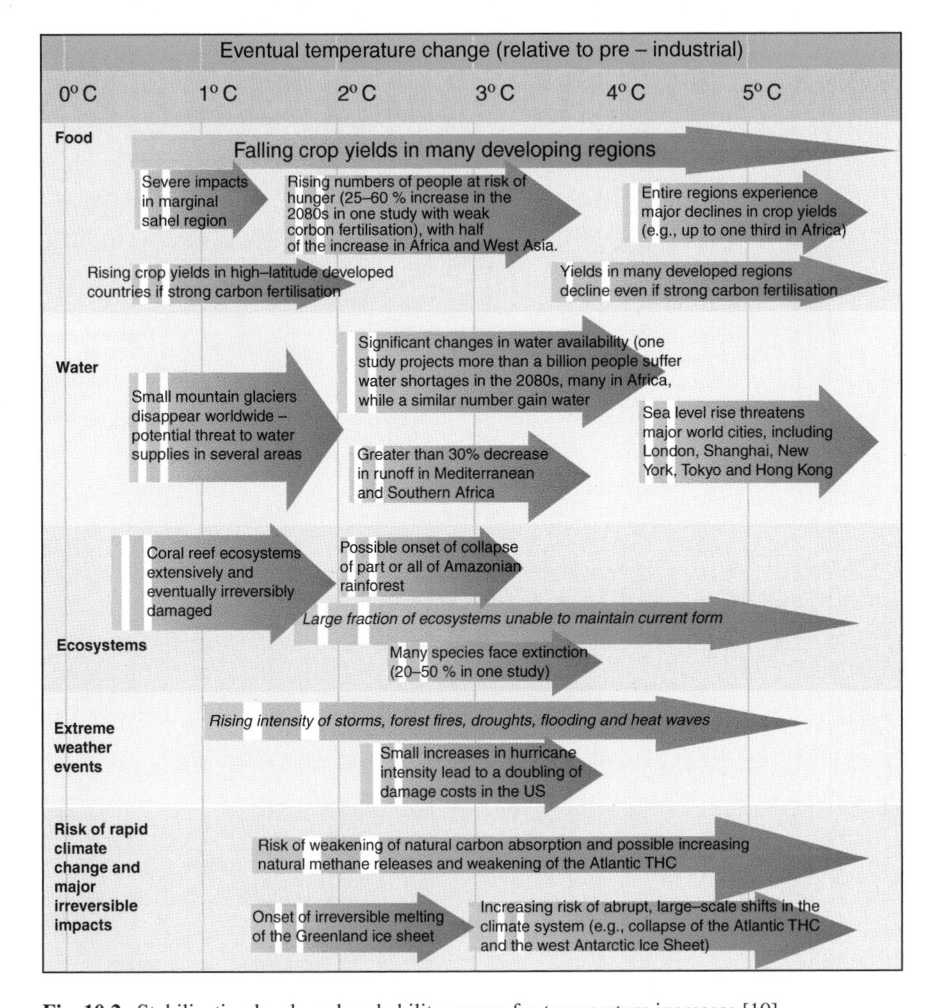

Fig. 10.2 Stabilization levels and probability ranges for temperature increases [10]

Table 10.1 Health risks from climate change [9]

Types of health risks	Examples
Immediate and direct risks	The impact of extreme weather events, heat waves, floods, and droughts
Indirect risks	Disruption to ecological systems affecting food yields and range and activity of disease vectors (Lyme disease, malaria, schistosomiasis, etc.)
Deferred and diffuse risks	Risks associated from rural to urban displacement. Mental health impacts of extreme weather. Anxiety among young people about the future
Risks associated with conflicts and environmental refugee flows	Wars in Africa have peaked in hot and dry years. Demand for water may lead to regional conflicts. There may be refugee flows from famine-stricken areas exposing people to infectious disease

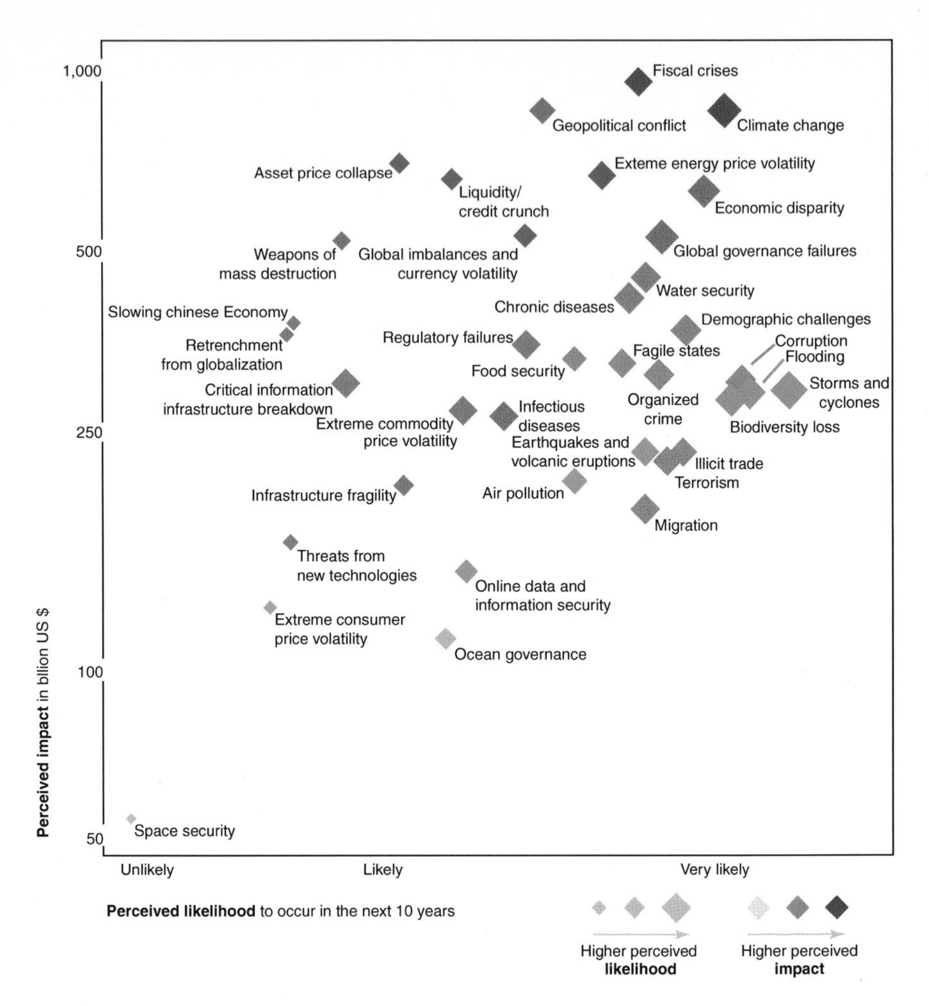

Fig. 10.3 Global Risks Landscape 2011: Perception data from the World Economic Forum's Global Risks Survey [8]

these "greenhouse gases" therefore play a disproportionate role in average global temperatures, and carbon dioxide released from the burning of fossil fuels has already increased global temperatures [7]. Developed countries are largely responsible with the richest 15 % of the world's population producing 50 % of global carbon dioxide waste; methane which is produced by farming livestock also contributes.

China and India make up one-third of the world's population. As their economies develop, their energy demands have accelerated. Currently, their per capita "carbon footprint" is still a fraction compared with most developed countries. However, development models based on low-carbon economies are urgently needed to mitigate the consequences of their industrialization.

The World Economic Forum ranked climate change as the biggest global economic risk as it is both very likely and of huge consequences adding weight to the argument for urgent action now [8] (Fig. 10.3).

Table 10.2 The Stern review criticisms

Criticism	Response
Future predictions are hard to make. Some think the report exaggerated the harmful future effects of climate change	People take out insurance against small risks of catastrophic events, which is a good way of thinking about a low-carbon economy
Some economists think the report underestimated the costs of taking action. This includes the rate of "economic discounting" whereby benefits in the future are reduced to get their present value	Many actions would carry additional benefits such as human-powered transport, diets low in red meat, and decreased air pollution improving health. Traditional measures of GDP fail to include costs of harm inflicted on society by industry such as deforestation
The report does not take into account rebound effects of actions on climate change and adaptations to increased temperatures	Actions to mitigate for climate change should be planned; however, this may be hard as climate change could accelerate as melting permafrost releases gases. By the point of major change, it will probably be too late to reverse the effects
The report favored carbon pricing which would allow emissions to be traded. However, this could hinder fair development, preventing the industrialization of poor countries	A fairer system would be "converge and contract" whereby all nations converge their per capita emissions and reduce them to sustainable levels
Without US, China, or India making decisive commitments, action by a single country will impair its economic competitiveness and probably be unsuccessful	Northern hemisphere countries are responsible for most emissions and should lead the change and promote greener industries. A "green revolution" could create new industries for countries involved (e.g., solar power, electric cars)

Prompt 2: What Was the Stern Review, and How Was It Received?

The Stern review was commissioned by the UK government in 2006 to gather the best evidence available on climate change. It recommended early decisive action to limit carbon emissions, and its actions were broadly accepted by the UK government, charities, and some business leaders. The key points are identified in the executive summary (Box 10.1) [11].

Even before the Stern report, there was overwhelming scientific consensus on climate change. Now this is almost unanimous with 97 % of climate experts agreeing humans are the causative factor [12]. The risks of climate change and the need for urgent action are often disputed in the media which disillusions the general public (Table 10.2). Political lobbying of oil, gas, aeroplane, and other industries also plays a significant role in preventing legislation to reduce carbon emissions and protect self-interests. A breakthrough would require major political momentum and sacrifices shared by society. Ninety percent of all known reserves of oil, coal, and gas need to stay in the ground to avoid catastrophic temperature rises greater than 2° [13].

Box 10.1: Stern Review 2006 Executive Summary (Key Points Abridged)

- The benefits of strong, early action on climate change outweigh the costs.
- Climate change threatens the basic elements of life—access to water, food production, health, and use of land and the environment
- The damages from climate change will accelerate as the world gets warmer.
- The impacts of climate change are not evenly distributed—the poorest countries and people will suffer earliest and most. If and when the damages appear, it will be too late to reverse the process
- Emissions are driven by economic growth, yet stabilization of greenhouse gas is feasible and consistent with continued growth.
- The review estimated the annual costs of stabilization to be 2 % of GDP in 2008.
- The transition to a low-carbon economy will bring challenges for competitiveness but also opportunities for growth.
- Policy to reduce emissions should be based on three essential elements: **carbon pricing**, **technology policy**, and removal of barriers to **behavioral change**.
- Adaptation policy is crucial for dealing with the unavoidable impacts of climate change, but it has been underemphasized in many countries. Adaptation efforts in developing countries must be accelerated and supported, including through international development assistance.
- An effective response to climate change will depend on creating the conditions for international collective action.
- Curbing deforestation is a highly cost-effective way of reducing greenhouse gas emissions.

Further Information 1

You find national food prices have doubled over the last 6 months triggered by drought and decreased regional production. The economy has been faltering, and wages for manual workers have failed to keep pace with food prices, meaning food is now becoming unaffordable for poorer families. You are starting to see severely malnourished children in the local clinics for the first time in years.

Population growth meant the country recently became a net importer of food for the first time. Two years ago, food price increases led to widespread riots, and trouble is brewing again. You investigate approaches to increase ***food security*** *for the poor.*

Prompt 3: How Will Population Growth Impact Global Health?

The world's population is expected to increase by 50 % between 2000 and 2050. This increase is almost exclusively in developing countries due to decreasing levels of infant mortality, high fertility rates, and longer life expectancy. Even if fertility rates stabilized now at two children per couple, increased life expectancy would make the global population increase 50 % i.e., 9.5 billion by 2150.

The world-carrying capacity is how many people the world can sustain. It is not a fixed number, but depends on production (cultivatable land, climate, climate change), distribution (minimizing waste, food being available where it is needed), and diet (farming meat requires ten times as much grain input than vegetarian foodstuff).

So far, the growth in food production has kept up with the growth in population avoiding a "Malthusian catastrophe" (chronic famines occur when population growth exceeds food production). Blame for unsustainable population growth should not be upon "over breeders" of the developing world, such as Africa, but on the overconsumers of the developed world. The poorest 50 % of the world are only responsible for producing 7 % of greenhouse gas emissions. A child born in the West will consume nine times more resources than one born in Africa and will therefore take a much greater share of the worlds carrying capacity and make a much larger contribution to climate change.

The trend for urbanization continues to shape our communities with half the world's population dwelling in cities in 2007 [14]. This presents opportunities as cities provide new opportunities for sustainable living as well as the challenges for providing food and resources for a larger population. Technology such as improved farming and diets with efficient protein sources like fish may be part of the solution of feeding a larger population.

Prompt 4: What Is Food Security, and Why Is It Important?

Food insecurity ranks second only to climate changes as a threat to human health. In 2003, the UN Food and Agriculture Organization (FAO) estimated that 850 million people were chronically hungry and 2 billion lack food security due to poverty [15]. Since food price crises of 2007 (Box 10.2), food security has been high on the global agenda with less confidence in the ability of global markets alone to feed the hungry.

Food security can be defined as:

> When all people at all times have access to sufficient, safe, nutritious food to maintain a healthy and active life. [15]

It requires three elements:

1. **Food availability**: Sufficient quantities of food available on a consistent basis
2. **Food access**: Having sufficient resources to obtain appropriate foods for a nutritious diet

Table 10.3 Challenges to food security

Population growth	Population growth is a major factor increasing food demand and has been responsible for the long-term declines in the per capita food production in Africa
Increased demand of high-input food	Growth in demand for meat and refined foods means grain production will need to double by 2050
Market discrepancies	In the UK, only 9 % of disposable income is spent on food, but in developing countries, this may be closer to 100 %. These economics combine with free trade to allow food to flow away from the hungriest
Land degradation	Greed and ignorance mean large amounts of agricultural land are losing topsoil and becoming unsuitable for further agriculture
Depletion of water resources	Water tables are falling in China, Australia, India, and the USA threatening production of food. More disputes are expected between countries over water
Climate change	Climate change will accelerate land degradation, depletion of water resources, with increased frequency and severity of natural disasters including both floods and droughts
Fossil fuel dependence	Oil prices look likely to continue to rise with knock on effects on the cost of agriculture
Land diversion for cash crops/export food	Cash crops decrease self-sufficiency with much of the wealth generated diverted to wealthy countries. The relative value of cash crops can fall compared with food imports leading to increase levels of poverty
Intellectual property, loss of seed stocks	Biotechnology promises higher yield crops, but the seeds are often infertile and so not reusable. Farmers become dependent on biotechnology companies for seeds, and biodiversity is lost
Crop disease	Decreased biodiversity could increase risk of crop disease such as wheat stem rust which is currently spreading through Africa and Asia destroying crops
Economic crises	Financial shocks expose the vulnerability of the poor who are dependent on markets for food. A country dependent on imports combined with a falling exchange rate could mean food disentitlement could happen on a national scale

3. **Food use**: Appropriate use based on knowledge of basic nutrition and care, as well as adequate water and sanitation

This definition of food security moved beyond production of food, to include consideration of access to food, equitable distribution, and healthy diets. As we are perhaps already beginning to see, climate change will disrupt production at a time of rapid population growth meaning now more than ever we need systems of distribution. Table 10.3 summarizes the current threats to food security.

History has shown that even when there is enough food to go around, there can be famines. Panic buying and hoarding make markets freeze even when there is plenty of food, and financial speculation adds to price volatility.

Recommendations for improved food security must navigate opposing approaches of market liberalization or local protectionism (Table 10.4). Tackling poverty is a priority that must never be overlooked, along with optimizing the current system

Table 10.4 Approaches to food security

Trade liberalization	Some proponents still argue trade will lead to much needed investment and increased increase yields. However, global markets increase price volatility and tend to remove local food market safeguards
Food sovereignty	Food sovereignty is when communities define their own means of production protected from the influence of international markets and multinational corporations
Food justice	Food justice is ensuring equitable distribution, observing there is already enough food to feed the world and the problem of distributing it fairly
Vegetarian food	Meat requires ten times as much land to produce the same amount of calories as through grain. Vegetarian diets can produce all the nutrients required for humans and reduce cardiovascular risk

where 25 % of crops are lost due to pests and diseases, and the developing world loses 37 % of food in storage and transportation [16].

Longer-term plans should avoid overreliance on mechanized agriculture as seen on large farms in the West, which may prove unsustainable, but optimize current farming practices such as using simple irrigation techniques. Land reform should take place but should focus on recognition of traditional land rights.

Box 10.2: Food Price Crisis 2007–2008

In 2007–2008, dramatic food price inflation led to political upheaval and riots in many countries around the world and restated the importance of food security. The UN called the High-Level Conference on World Food Security in 2008, and nations committed $1.2 billion in food aid to the 60 hardest hit countries.

It is thought droughts in producing nations combined with an oil price spike to trigger the initial rise and this was compounded by poorly thought through biofuel schemes. Other factors such as population growth, financial speculation, and increased demand for Western diets in Asia also contributed.

Bill Clinton summed it up "*we all blew it, including me as president… treating food crops as a commodity rather than a right of the poor…Food is not a commodity like others. We should go back to a policy of maximum food self-sufficiency. It is crazy for us to think we can develop countries around the world without increasing their ability to feed themselves.*"

Prompt 5: How Is Food Security Measured?

British colonial administrators created food security codes to predict the likelihood of famine in India in the 1880s. Nowadays, many different codes are in practice—often specific to the country they are predicting for. Variables like rainfall, livestock status,

Table 10.5 Devereux and Howe's famine intensity scale [17]

Level	Phrase	Lives	Livelihood
0	Food secure	Crude mortality rate (CMR) less than 0.2/10,000/day and wasting less than 2.3 % of population	Cohesive social system, food prices stable, coping strategies not utilized
1	Food insecure	CMR 0.2–0.5, wasting 2.3–10 %	Cohesive social system, food prices unstable, seasonal shortages, reversible coping strategies taken
2	Food crisis	CMR 0.5–1, wasting 10–20 %, and/or prevalence of edema	Social system stressed but largely cohesive, dramatic rise in food and basic items prices, adaptive mechanisms begin to fail, increase in irreversible coping strategies
3	Famine	CMR 1–5, wasting 20–40 %, and/or prevalence of edema	Clear signs of social breakdown, markets begin to collapse, coping strategies exhausted and survival strategies (migration in search of help, abandonment of weaker members of the community) adopted, affected population identifies food scarcity as the major societal problem
4	Severe famine	CMR 5–15, Wasting over 40 %, and/or prevalence of edema	Widespread social breakdown, markets close, survival strategies widespread, affected population identifies food scarcity as the major societal problem
5	Extreme famine	CMR > 15	Complete social breakdown, widespread mortality, affected identifies food scarcity as the major societal problem

Table 10.6 Famine magnitude scale

Category	Phrase	Mortality range
A	Minor famine	0–999
B	Moderate famine	1,000–9,999
C	Major famine	10,000–99,999
D	Great famine	100,000–999,999
E	Catastrophic famine	1,000,000 and over

market prices for cereals, and enrolment on food aid programs dictate the levels of alert. Devereux and Howe's measurement of famine with scales for both "intensity" and "magnitude" has been widely accepted (Tables 10.5 and 10.6).

Prompt 6: How Are Famines Created?

Famine is widespread scarcity of food, associated with regional malnutrition, starvation, disease epidemics, and increased mortality. The UN declares a famine when "at least 20 per cent of households in an area face extreme food shortages with a limited ability to cope; acute malnutrition rates exceed 30 per cent; and the death rate exceeds two persons per day per 10,000 persons" [18].

Traditionally, famine is portrayed as a freak occurrence due to natural events causing a failure of crops (e.g., drought, floods, or disease). However, this simplistic view overlooks the long-term events and wider problems that are causing famine. Since 1980, there have been three important conceptual developments in the understanding of famine:

1. Sen/Dreze 1981: Famine can occur in times of plenty due to "disentitlement." This is when food price inflation means rural workers can starve if their wages do not keep up with food prices [19].
2. Rangasami 1985: Famine is a long-term process taking years. Economic violence against people leads to destitution, loss of livelihoods, and mass movements of population. Media portrayals of starving people are the last step in an insidious process [20].
3. De Waal 1990: Most famine deaths are not directly from lack of food but from forced migration resulting in dangerous camp environments with unsafe water, poor sanitation, and overcrowding [21].

Failure to recognize the social causes of famine explains why famine relief efforts have failed many times in the past. Sometimes, famines may even be exploited by those not affected; labor becomes cheap as people become desperate for work and traders profit from inflated food prices. So-called famine economies have been observed and contribute to complex emergencies (Chap. 4) and may work against relief efforts.

Prompt 7: What Are Other Emerging Challenges for Global Health?

Many emerging risks threaten global health. Epidemics of new and resistant diseases (HIV, MDR-TB, SARS, pandemic flu) and an increasingly urban and mobile population. There are also now much greater numbers of people living in places vulnerable to natural disasters. Figure 10.3 shows the economic risks identified by the World Economic Forum which are also health risks due to their effects on food security. Growing inequalities in wealth, unsustainable use of critical resources (water, oil, minerals, and land), and social upheaval and conflict all impact health [22]. Many are interrelated and have the capacity to compound one another.

Further Information 2

You research Senegal on the CIA Factbook, the Human Development Index, and Relief Web and find that the country is experiencing high ***population growth*** *as it goes through* ***demographic transition****.*

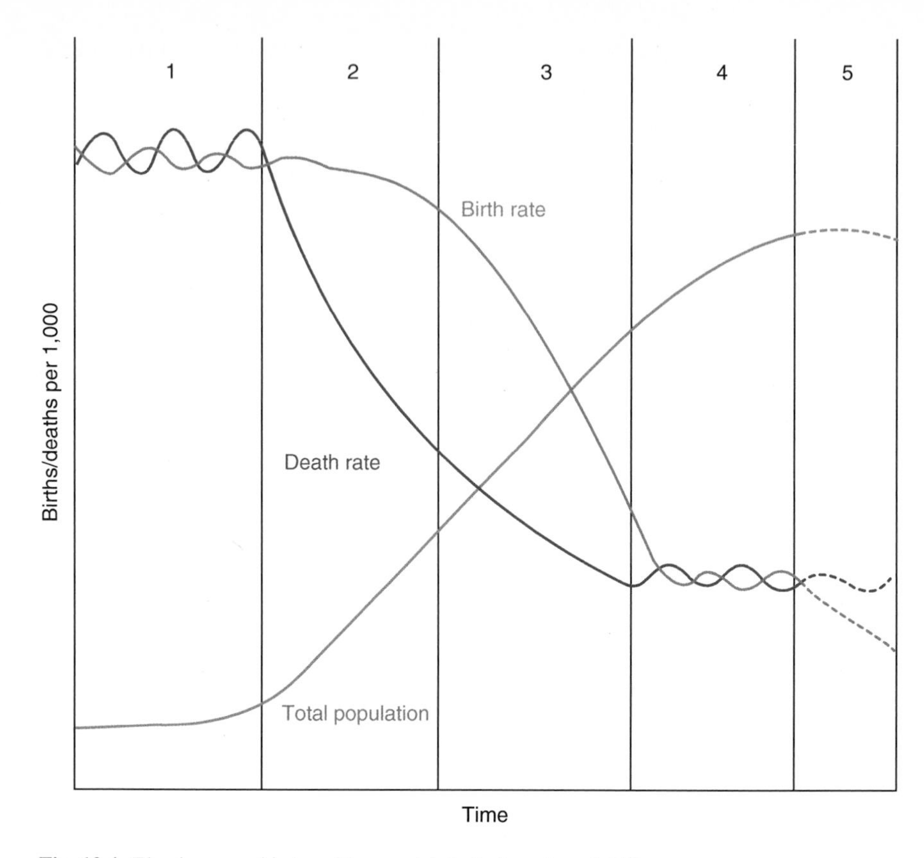

Fig. 10.4 The demographic transition model, including stage 5 [23]

Prompt 8: What Is Demographic Transition?

Demographic transition is the movement from high birth rate and high mortality to a low birth rate and low mortality. It a process that occurred in developed countries, leading to stable populations with longer life expectancy. One characteristic feature of entering the demographic transition is a large initial increase in the population.

Some countries, e.g., China and Brazil, passed through the transition rapidly. However, many countries, especially in sub-Saharan Africa, appear stuck in early stages with persistent high birth rate and relatively high death rate due to failures in development and the AIDs epidemic.

Stages of demographic transition (Fig. 10.4):

1. High birth rate, high death rate.
2. Death rate decreases due to increased food supply and better sanitation with population growth as a result.

3. Birth rate decreases due to contraception, and death rate decreases further, slowing population growth.
4. Birth and death rate stabilizes with low rates for both.

Demographic transition is seen as desirable as it provides a pathway to stable populations with low rates of mortality and morbidity through childhood and adult life. This brings economic benefits with a healthier workforce and equity between people across classes.

It has been seen to occur as a natural phenomenon with increasing wealth; however, approaches have been attempted to expedite the process:

1. Policies lowering birth: An extreme example is central planning as seen by China's one-child policy. Less controversially empowering women though education or access to family planning is very effective. It is estimated it would cost $17 billion annually to meet the global unmet demand for contraception, one of the most cost-effective interventions for global health.
2. Reducing overall mortality especially through better child survival (e.g., preventing disease, vaccination programs, nutrition, reducing accidents, MDG4).
3. Increasing wealth: Producing a skilled workforce through education, industrialization, and economic development. Allowing business and trade.

Note: GDP is a poor measure of productivity ignoring some major contributions to society, e.g., breastfeeding, subsistence farming, and preventative medicine. It also does not measure the damage of environmental degradation, pollution, or disability due to accidents. The Human Development Index (HDI) is a much better marker of true societal wealth [24].

Prompt 9: What Are the Critiques of the Demographic Transition Model?

Worldwide population growth now is very high: In the UK, the population growth never exceeded >1.7 % per year; in central Africa, it is 3–4 %.

Reversal of development: Population growth, conflict, and HIV have led to a reversal of development in many African countries perhaps preventing transition.

Historical differences: Many developed countries like the UK exported some of their population growth and had the economic benefit of food imports from empires.

Slow changes in birth rates: Rapidly declining mortality in many developing countries has failed to be matched by decreasing birth rates.

Lack of industrialization: Industrialization may not happen universally as industrialized countries export products to poor countries, and trade agreements work against industry in developing nations.

Inequalities: Increasing inequalities within countries will still leave billions in poverty as global wealth increases [25]. Some sections of society may go through demographic transition, while others may not, leaving a two-tiered society leading to social upheaval and conflict [8].

Demographic transition itself can lead to challenges. In developed countries such as the UK and USA, an ageing population is providing massive fiscal challenges for governments, decreasing funds for overseas development aid. In China, this is exacerbated by the four-two-one challenge where the one-child policy could make one grandchild responsible for supporting two parents and four grandparents if they survive past retirement age.

Further Information 3

Another famine savages the country, and conflict erupts with a neighboring country over use of water from a major river. Many people point to the growing developments in technology, and that this will solve climate change.

There is an uprising using the internet and mobile technology with hope that change will bring in more equitable times.

Prompt 10: Amid All These Disasters, Is There Any Hope?

At present, we are stealing the future, selling it in the present, and calling it GDP. [26]

Technological solutions are appearing, but it would be foolish to rely on something that does not yet exist for a problem as great as climate change. Nuclear fusion may be a possibility for limitless energy without the risks of nuclear proliferation; however, the earliest a commercial reactor could be available is estimated to be 2050. At the same time, new technologies like shale gas and underground coal gasification look set to make climate change worse.

Scientific developments are allowing better prediction of natural disasters (tsunamis, volcanoes, droughts) and are allowing vulnerable people to escape and respond, but these rely on the capacity of people to respond and may prove useless to those in extreme poverty.

The internet and mobile phones are perhaps the most exciting development, as a means for educating everyone and giving even the poorest a voice. The best people to respond to a disaster are often the people affected, and phones and internet may allow new developments in organization.

Taking a step back to look at the goals of society, interesting precedents have been set by Bhutan which in 1972 defined its economic progress to be gross national happiness, or Bolivia which has protected the environment by enshrining in law the rights of the mother earth [27].

Case Study: Drought in the Horn of Africa [28, 29]

In 2011, the worst drought of several decades affected Ethiopia, Kenya, and Somalia. By June 2011, staple foods had increased in price up to 180 % making them unaffordable by the poor. The famine was a catastrophic famine (affecting 15 million people with CMR of 0.6–2.8); the UN warned that 750,000 people could die as a result, mainly children [30].

It is important to realize while a drought was triggered by lack of rainfall, most of the famine was man-made due to poor governance and conflict. The hardest hit areas were ones with deep poverty following years of conflict and ethnic marginalization.

Misinformed agricultural reforms contributed, with farmers forced off their land by new farms among the affected, and still only 1 % of smallholder farmers in Ethiopia are using irrigation techniques.

Early warning systems also failed, and there was a delayed international response. Oxfam estimated that this delay costs thousands of lives and millions of pounds as donors waited for certainty that a famine was occurring [31].

The inequality of global trade can be seen in Ethiopia where simultaneously there was a Saudi investment of $100 million to grow and export grain on 99-year land lease, while the World Food Program still planned to spend $116 million over 5 years providing food aid [32].

It is unclear if this drought was due to man-made climate change, but it highlighted the vulnerability of people in East Africa to climate variability. It also shows the potential global consequences of climate change [16].

References

1. Mollica M. Informal horse garage on the sides of the new toll highway in construction in Dakar Senegal. Part of "En Route To Dakar" series by Mimi Mollica. Copyright Mimi Mollica. Available from http://www.mimimollica.com. Cited 20 Mar 2012.
2. Muller R, Curry J, Groom D, Jacobsen R, Perlmutter S, et al. Decadal variations in the global atmospheric land temperatures. Berkeley: University of California; 2011. Available from http://berkeleyearth.org/pdf/berkeley-earth-decadal-variations.pdf. Cited 20 Mar 2012.
3. Intergovernmental Panel on Climate Change [Internet]. Geneva: World Meteorological Organization. Available from http://www.ipcc.ch/. Cited 20 Mar 2012.
4. Costello A, et al. Managing the health effects of climate change: Lancet and University College London Institute for Global Health Commission. Lancet. 2009;373(9676):1693–733. ISSN 0140–6736. Available from http://www.thelancet.com/climate-change. Cited 20 Mar 2012.
5. Godlee F. How on earth do we combat climate change? BMJ 2011;343:bmj.d6789. Available from http://www.bmj.com/content/343/bmj.d6789?tab=full. Cited 20 Mar 2012.
6. Jarvis L, Montgomery H, Morisetti N, Gilmore I. Climate change, ill health, and conflict. BMJ. 2011;342:bmj.d1819.
7. Rapley C. The health impacts of climate change. BMJ. 2012;344:e1026. doi:10.1136/bmj.e1026.

8. World Economic Forum. Global risks 2011 sixth edition an initiative of the risk response network. 2011. Available from http://www.weforum.org/reports. Cited 20 Mar 2012.
9. McMichael T, Montgomery H, Costello A. Health risks, present and future, from global climate change. BMJ. 2012;344:e1359. doi:10.1136/bmj.e1359.
10. Treasury HM. Stern review executive summary. Cambridge: Cambridge University Press; 2006. Available from: http://www.hm-treasury.gov.uk/d/Executive_Summary.pdf. Cited 20 Mar 2012.
11. Treasury HM. Stern review on the economics of climate change. Cambridge: Cambridge University Press; 2006. Available from http://www.hm-treasury.gov.uk/sternreview_index.htm. Cited 20 Mar 2012.
12. Skepticalscience.com [Internet]. Brisbane. Available from http://www.skepticalscience.com/. Cited 20 Mar 2012.
13. Thölken H. Politics and policies: making change happen. BMJ. 2012;344. doi:10.1136/bmj.e1356.
14. The Government Office for Science. Foresight: migration and global environmental change. Final Project Report. 2011.
15. UN Food and Agriculture Orgnisation. Rome Declaration on World Food Security. 1996. Available from http://www.fao.org/docrep/003/w3613e/w3613e00.htm. Cited 20 Mar 2012.
16. Cochrane L. Food security or food sovereignty: the case of land grabs. J Humanit Assist. 2011. Available from http://sites.tufts.edu/jha/archives/1241. Cited 20 Mar 2012.
17. Howe P, Devereux S. Famine intensity and magnitude scales: a proposal for an instrumental definition of famine. Disasters. 2004;28:353–72. doi:10.1111/j.0361-3666.2004.00263.X.
18. UN News Centre. When a food security crisis becomes a famine. 2011. Available from http://www.un.org/apps/news/story.asp?NewsID=39113. Cited 20 Mar 2012.
19. Sen A. Poverty and famines: an essay on entitlement and deprivation. Oxford: Clarendon; 1981.
20. Rangasami A. "Failure of exchange entitlements" theory of famine: a response. Econ Pol Wkly. 1985;20:1747–52.
21. de Waal A. A re-assessment of entitlement theory in the light of the recent famines in Africa. Dev Change. 1990;21:469–90.
22. Department for International Development. Humanitarian Emergency Response Review. Chaired by Lord Ashdown. 2011. Available from http://www.dfid.gov.uk/Documents/publications1/HERR.pdf. Cited 20 Mar 2012.
23. Niknaks. The demographic transition model, including stage 5. Available from http://en.wikipedia.org/wiki/File:Stage5.svg. Cited 20 Mar 2012.
24. Human Development Reports [Internet]. New York: UNDP. Available from http://hdr.undp.org/en/humandev/. Cited 20 Mar 2012.
25. Wilkinson R, Marmot M, editors. Social determinants of health, the solid facts. 2nd ed. Copenhagen: WHO; 2003. Available from: http://www.euro.who.int/__data/assets/pdf_file/0005/98438/e81384.pdf. Cited 20 Mar 2012.
26. Hawkin P. Gross National Happiness [Internet]. Available from http://www.gnhusa.org/gnh-quotes/. Cited 20 Mar 2012.
27. Vidal J. Bolivia enshrines natural world's rights with equal status for Mother Earth. The Guardian. 2011. Available from http://www.guardian.co.uk/environment/2011/apr/10/bolivia-enshrines-natural-worlds-rights. Cited 20 Mar 2012.
28. Oxfam. Briefing on the Horn of Africa Drought: climate change and future impacts on food security. 2011. Available from http://www.oxfam.org/sites/www.oxfam.org/files/briefing-hornofafrica-drought-climatechange-foodsecurity-020811.pdf. Cited 20 Mar 2012.
29. Food and Agriculture Organisation of the United Nations. Drought-related food insecurity: a focus on the Horn of Africa. Rome. 2011. Available from http://www.fao.org/crisis/28402-0-f9dad42f33c6ad6ebda108ddc1009adf.pdf. Cited 20 Mar 2012.
30. Famine Early Warning System Network [Internet]. Washington: United States Agency for International Development (USAID). Available from http://www.fews.net/. Cited 20 Mar 2012.

31. Oxfam, save the Children. A dangerous delay. The cost of late response to early warnings in the 2011 drought in the Horn of Africa. Joint Agency Briefing Paper. 2012. Available from http://reliefweb.int/sites/reliefweb.int/files/resources/Dangerous-delay-UK-version.pdf. Cited 20 Mar 2012.
32. The economist. Outsourcing's third wave. 2009. Available from http://www.economist.com/node/13692889. Cited 20 Mar 2012.

Part III
Trauma and Surgery

Section reviewed by Jim Ryan

Physical trauma is encountered in almost every disaster and has the ability to kill patients quicker than any other condition. Adequate care needs to be timely but appropriate to the patient's need. Surgery may often be indicated but will likely be performed in sub-optimal conditions. Difficult decisions have to be made, where resource-poor environments can often be compounded by multiple severely injured casualties.

This section aims to provide an introduction to the clinical management of trauma in disaster scenarios. It also explores the wider role of surgery in such settings, focusing not just on acute care but also on the management of disease endemic to the tropics, and the practice of surgery in austere environments.

This section begins with the basic management of a single trauma casualty. The following cases attempt to extrapolate the common themes of such management to more complicated and challenging scenarios.

Disasters are by nature overwhelming, difficult, and dangerous. Before practicing, individuals should take note of their limitations. Moreover, successful patient outcomes depend not just on an individual's skill and experience but perhaps more on the organizations, processes, and logistics facilitating such care.

James Houston

Chapter 11
Prehospital Care

Will Barker

Learning Objectives

- Learn how to safely approach a trauma site
- Learn the principles underpinning the ABC trauma approach
- Learn how to conduct a primary survey
- Discuss some common forms of life-threatening injury and their management
- Understand the next steps including the secondary survey
- Discuss rescue and transport including C-spine management
- Discuss controversies around prehospital care, including the debate around "stay and play" and "scoop and run" philosophies
- Discuss the relevance of historical concepts in trauma such as the golden hour and trimodal distribution of death

Initial Scenario

You are a GP volunteering as a first responder doctor with BASICS to keep up your trauma skills [1]. *You get a call from a local ambulance dispatch center; there has been a road traffic collision between a lorry and a car on a motorway in your covering area.*

You arrive quickly on scene, and the ambulance crew have just unpacked their gear when you arrive. There is only one casualty, and she is trapped in the wreckage of her car and is breathing with difficulty. The driver of the lorry appears unhurt but is walking around, and several people have stopped and got out of their vehicles.

W. Barker, MBBS, MPhys
FY2 Doctor, St Thomas' Hospital, Westminster Bridge Road,
London, UK
e-mail: willbarker@doctors.org.uk

D. MacGarty, D. Nott (eds.), *Disaster Medicine*,
DOI 10.1007/978-1-4471-4423-6_11, © Springer-Verlag London 2013

Prompt 1: What Are the Problems Facing You as the First Responder?

Sites of trauma are hazardous, and your first priority is to prevent getting injured yourself and further casualties. Adequate time should be taken assessing personal safety, scene safety, and survivor safety (Box 11.1). This time very rarely negatively impacts on patient survival but prevents further casualties and helps extraction [2].

With multiple casualties, all efforts should be spent triaging patients (covered in Chap. 16). Remember, for each casualty there are a diverse number of possible injuries, many of which may not be present initially and many that could be fatal.

Box 11.1: 1, 2, 3 of Safety at Scenes of Trauma

1. Personal safety	Personal protective equipment, e.g., latex gloves, goggles, high-visibility clothing
	Avoiding dangerous areas, e.g., fuel leaks
2. Scene safety	Assessing the scene for hazards
	Being aware of fires, sources of explosions, or falling objects
	On roads, use two people to stop traffic in both directions
	Cover or make visible sharp pieces of metal
3. Survivor safety	Evacuating survivors from places of danger, e.g., falling vehicles, fires, explosions
	Preventing confused patients straying into danger

Further Information 1

You don your high-visibility jacket, goggles, and gloves. You ensure traffic is stopped in both directions and onlookers are safe. A minute after you arrive, you move on to attend the patient in the car with breathing difficulties.

Prompt 2: How Should You Approach Treatment of This Patient?

Trauma patients should always be treated using a rigidly structured "ABC" approach regardless of type of trauma (Table 11.1). Trauma kills on predictable timescales; an airway problem kills before a breathing problem, and breathing before a circulation problem.

Other injuries can be distracting but should never cause the airway and breathing to be overlooked. A few minutes of airway obstruction is all it takes for hypoxia to lead to secondary irreversible brain injury. Following any intervention, it is

Table 11.1 The "ABC" approach to trauma or "primary survey"

Airway	Maneuvers to ensure a patent airway, adjuncts, and C-spine immobilization
Breathing	Assessment for life-threatening thoracic injury; oxygen
Circulation	Assessment for signs of hemorrhage and shock; control external bleeding
Disability or neurological status	Best response, alert, responding to pain, voice or unresponsive (AVPU score), and assessment of pupil size, equality, and reactivity.
Extrication to definitive care,	Extrication by what means, where to, in what time frame.
Environmental control Exposure	Environmental control such as blankets to keep patient warm while remembering to expose the patient and check head to toe for injuries. Remember glucose and noninvasive monitoring of pulse, saturation, and blood pressure

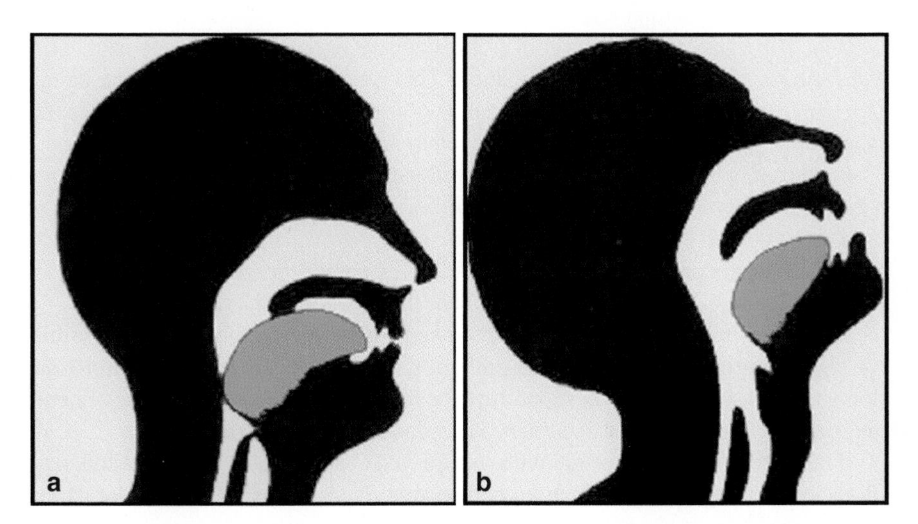

Fig. 11.1 Head tilt and jaw thrust to clear airway [3]. (**a**) in an unconscious patient the tongue can easily obstruct the airway (**b**) head tilt and jaw thrust move the tongue forward clearing the airway

important to reassess ABC for effect, returning to A if there is any deterioration in the patient's condition.

Prompt 3: How Do You Assess and Manage a Patient's Airway (A)?

Look and listen for signs of respiratory compromise. Observe for cyanosis, signs of respiratory distress, maxillofacial trauma, and use of accessory muscles. Hold your ear to patient's mouth and listen for breathing or any additional noises, stridor or gurgling.

If the patient has decreased consciousness, the tongue can easily fall backward in the mouth preventing the patient from being able to breathe (Fig. 11.1a).

If the airway is compromised, perform an airway maneuver; jaw thrust (use 2–3 fingers behind the jaw to move it forward) or chin lift if no neck injury (slightly extend the neck using fingers below the jaw). This clears the upper airway by preventing the tongue obstructing the back of the throat (Fig. 11.1b).

Check mouth for vomit or debris and clear anything that may obstruct breathing. Do not insert finger as you may risk pushing objects down further, but instead, use suction if available, and only suction what you can see since blind suction can trigger airway spasm.

Airway adjuncts can be used if the responder is trained: an oral pharyngeal airway (OPA), nasal pharyngeal airway (NPA), or laryngeal mask airway (LMA) all maintain pharynx patency. They can be inserted with less skill and sedation than full endotracheal (ET) intubation.

If the patient is falling into a coma (unresponsive or only responsive to pain, GCS < 8), she requires endotracheal intubation. This is usually by rapid sequence induction where the patient is given a combination of medicines to quickly sedate and paralyze them and cricothyroid pressure is given to reduce the risk of gastric aspiration.

In all trauma, the spine must be immobilized unless you can confidently exclude a C-spine injury (Box 11.2). An unstable bony or ligamentous injury risks spinal cord damage and total paralysis from the neck down, particularly if the head is moved in an uncontrolled way. Spinal fractures should be given a high index of suspicion in high impact collisions or where there is head injury.

Manual in-line immobilization can be used where one person takes responsibility for supporting the head. This is preferably not the doctor as it stops him from doing other tasks. The person supporting the head leads any log rolls or movements and can give jaw thrust at same time as C-spine immobilization.

If the patient is sitting upright with a suspected C-spine injury, forehead and nape of neck stabilization should be used before applying a semirigid neck collar. Note: A spinal board with straps and bolstering devices is the only way a C-spine is immobilized, it is not stable in a collar alone.

Box 11.2: Clearing a C-Spine Injury Clinically

In the UK, this is usually only done in the hospital setting by a registrar level or consultant. The criteria are as follows:

- No distracting injury, GCS 15/15, no alcohol
- No reported pain in neck or bruising
- Painless neck forward flexion/extension and rotation
- No point tenderness on palpation of spinal processes of C1–7

If the criteria are not met or are doubtful, the patient needs a CT head and neck or a neck X-ray series (AP, Lateral, and Peg). *Note*: The gold standard investigation for all polytrauma patients is whole-body CT, with the benefits far outweighing the radiation risks [4]

Further Information 2

The casualty is seated in the front seat of the car. You suspect a cervical spine fracture and so approach from in front, introduce yourself, and explain to her not to move her head, while you then approach from behind. The casualty does not respond and is breathing but with difficulty and you can hear a gurgling noise. You put a spinal collar on her and perform a careful jaw thrust. She appears to breathe a little easier but is still unconscious.

You attach high-flow oxygen through a nonrebreather mask and a saturation probe. You then perform a pinch of the trapezius. The casualty responds to the pain and opens her eyes. Due to decreased consciousness, you know she might not be protecting her airway and so insert an oropharyngeal airway and continue to assess her for potential need to fully intubate when further medical support arrives.

Prompt 4: How Do You Assess and Manage Breathing (B)?

Oxygen must be given to all trauma patients to support breathing in the form of high-flow oxygen (>12 l/min) through a tight-fitting "Hudson" nonrebreathing mask.

Look for external signs of trauma and count respiratory rate (RR). RR is a very sensitive marker of almost any physiological distress. Feel for tenderness, tracheal deviation, or rib fractures. Auscultate and percuss the chest to aid diagnosis and identify and treat common immediate life-threatening conditions in trauma (Table 11.2).

Pulse oximetry can be very useful for noninvasive recording of blood oxygenation and heart rate. If saturations >95 %, this is strong evidence of adequate peripheral oxygenation, but if the patient is cold or shivering, this may interfere with measurement. If following performing airway maneuvers the patient is still not adequately breathing (i.e., sats < 94 %), a bag valve mask may be used to give manual breaths.

Further Information 3

The patient's respiratory rate is 40 BPM; you notice the trachea is deviated to the right, and the left side of the chest is resonant to percussion with absent breath sounds. You diagnose a left-sided tension pneumothorax and insert a large needle (wide-bore cannula) into the second intercostal space, midclavicular line above the rib to avoid the neurovascular bundle. You hear a hiss of air as the pressure escapes, and the patient breathes easier; however, the patient soon appears cold and pale, and the saturation probe shows her heart rate has increased to 120 BPM.

Table 11.2 Life-threatening injuries in trauma [5]

Cause	Description	Symptoms/signs	Treatment
Tension pneumothorax	Air leaking into chest cavity.	Respiratory distress.	Narrow window from symptoms to cardiac arrest.
	Intrathoracic pressure increases obstructing blood flowing back to the heart	Hyperresonant percussion note and absent breath sounds on affected side.	Needle thoracostomy.
		Tracheal deviation away from affected side	Insertion of chest drain once stabilized
Massive hemothorax (>1,500 ml)	Blood leaking into pleural space due to hemorrhage.	Signs present late, typically >1 l blood loss.	Narrow window from symptoms to cardiac arrest.
	Intrathoracic pressure increases obstructing blood flowing back to the heart	Respiratory distress, hypotension.	Chest drain insertion once IV access established for circulatory support
		Dull percussion and decreased breath sounds on affected side	
Flail segment (one of the most common serious injury to the chest)	Two or more ribs broken in two places. Failure of chest wall movement	Respiratory distress. It may be possible to see the flail segment paradoxically move inward on inspiration	Analgesia. Mechanical ventilation is reserved for patients with pulmonary insufficiency despite adequate analgesia
Sucking chest wound	Hole in chest wall allowing air in on inspiration	Respiratory distress	Three-sided airtight dressing.
		Obvious open chest wall injury	Insertion of chest drain once stabilized
Aortic disruption	Tear/dissection of aorta or great vessels	Evidence of mediastinal trauma	If the patient is hemodynamically unstable, surgery to control hemorrhage is essential.
		Often rapid death	If hemodynamically stable, manage BP with adequate analgesia and antihypertensives
		However many patients asymptomatic	
Cardiac tamponade	Blood leaking into heart pericardium compromising venous return and heart filling	Muffled heart sounds	Subxiphoid cardiocentesis
		Raised JVP/distended neck veins	
		Hypotension	

Prompt 5: How Do You Assess and Manage Circulation (C)?

Shock is where cardiac output is insufficient to adequately perfuse organs. A good early marker is a capillary refill time (CRT) >3 s. Cold peripheries and increased heart rate (HR) are typically then seen, and it is important not to mistake this as a physiological response to pain and cold. Look for any obvious external bleeding and think about sites of concealed bleeding such pelvic fractures or hemothorax.

Low blood pressure gives a definitive diagnosis of shock; however, a drop in systolic blood pressure (SBP) is a very late sign in shock, only occurring after 30 % blood loss [6]. The early signs are a drop in consciousness level and RR/HR. Anxiety may be another early sign the patient is going into shock, giving way to agitation or confusion as the brain becomes underperfused.

If needed, systolic blood pressure (SBP) can be measured using noninvasive blood pressure monitoring with an automated cuff. If not available, palpable pulses provide a guide; a palpable radial pulse indicates SBP >80, femoral pulse indicates SBP>70, and the carotid pulse indicates SBP > 60.

Treat any obvious signs of bleeding with direct pressure, elevation above the level of the heart or pressure on artery upstream. Tourniquets can be considered if pressure is ineffective; this is of particular relevance to military trauma and is covered in Chap. 13.

Secure IV access ideally with two large-bore IV cannulas. New research indicates this should not be a reason to delay patient transport in many circumstances where urgent surgery is required as a delay in surgical referral costs lives [7]. Blood products can be considered; type of fluid is covered in more detail in Chap. 13.

Movement of a patient should be minimalized to reduce the risk of dislodging clots, and fractured limbs should be splinted. Permissive hypotension is now regularly employed, only giving fluids (crystalloid/colloid) if a radial pulse if not palpable. If hypotensive, 250-ml boluses should be administered until a radial pulse returns [8].

Note: Concealed bleeding can mask massive blood loss; a hemothorax only becomes clinically apparent when it reaches about 1 l. At this stage, 15–30 % of a patient's circulating blood volume has been lost into the chest, leaving little time from detection to arrest.

Further Information 4

The fire service informs you the extraction will take a further 20 min. You find the radial pulse is not palpable, but you manage to secure IV access in one arm and give boluses of 250 ml of 0.9 % saline. This does not improve so you give another crystalloid bolus.

The patient's radial pulse becomes palpable and the heart rate drops from 160 to 120 BPM. However, the casualty starts shivering and saying inappropriate words.

You decide that the patient is critically ill and inform the team that extrication is a priority and air ambulance will be useful. You conduct a secondary survey before the air ambulance arrives and try and prevent environmental exposure to the patient by wrapping her in a blanket.

Prompt 6: How Do You Assess Disability: Neurological Status (D)?

Look and feel for basal skull fractures. CSF otorrhoea/rhinorrhoea and severe tenderness of skull or boggy/depressed fractures can give a clinical diagnosis of a skull fracture. Periorbital ecchymosis and Battle's sign are late signs that will probably not be seen acutely.

AVPU provides a quick assessment of consciousness (awake/alert, voice response, pain response, unresponsive). Consider performing a full Glasgow coma score (GCS) if time, to monitor for neurological deterioration of patient. You can also consider testing pupils with a torch to test for blown pupil (raised ICP from head injury) or other pathology.

A full neurological exam would be impractical and time-consuming; however, the patient should be asked to wiggle her hands and feet to check for focal neurological deficit and asked about abnormal sensation. Remember that AB and C take priority and reassess them. Causes of decreased consciousness can be from hypotension, brain swelling, or pain.

Prompt 7: How Do You Plan Extrication (E)?

Once the patient has been stabilized and ready for transport, it is important to get her safely to definitive care, in a hospital equipped to deal with her injuries. Ideally, this should be planned at an early stage to give time for support to arrive. Consider the following:

- Who – will be required to safely extract and transport the patient
- How – will the patient be extracted
- Where – will the patient need to go to get definitive care
- When – do they need definitive care (how urgent)

Prompt 8: What Is the Secondary Survey (E-Exposure)?

Part of secondary survey is the AMPLE history (A – allergies, M – medication history, P – past med history, L – last meal, E – events leading to incident/mechanism).

The secondary survey requires the patient to be fully undressed (Exposure) and is a complete examination of the patient from head to toe, front and back. The aim is to identify any injuries missed by the primary survey of the head, neck, thorax, abdomen, pelvis, and upper and lower extremities. Ears, fingers, nose, and mouth should also be examined with gloved fingers. The patient should then be log rolled to check for bony spinal tenderness followed by a rectal exam to assess for neurological or abdominal injuries. If the patient is critically injured the secondary survey may be completed later in hospital when more stable.

Prompt 9: Why Is Environment Control Important (E-Environment)?

Hypothermia is a separate risk factor for major trauma as it leads to exhaustion and coagulopathy (covered in Chap. 13). Reducing heat loss through radiation, conduction, convection, and evaporation can prevent it. In practice, this is done by providing blankets for the patient, warmed IV fluids if possible; heated air blankets are useful if available. Note: In hot countries, hyperthermia, heat stroke, and dehydration can also be relevant to casualty management.

Prompt 10: How Do You Communicate the Patient's Condition to the Hospital?

MIST reporting is a standard trauma reporting system.

M – mechanism, e.g., RTC at 60 mph involving car and lorry
I – injuries sustained, e.g., pneumothorax
S – symptoms and signs, e.g., shock, CRT 4 s
T – treatment given, e.g., needle thoracostomy

Then give salient points from AMPLE history.

Further Information 5

You discover spinal tenderness at the C5 level and evidence of a fractured femur and major pelvic fracture. The fire brigade arrives to cut the patient from the vehicle. Another ambulance arrives on scene and informs you that the air ambulance is expected in 5 min. The patient becomes drowsy and starts vomiting.

Prompt 11: What Are the Possible Causes of Vomiting in Trauma and How Should It Be Managed?

There are many causes of vomiting in trauma (e.g., head injury, opiate reaction, abdominal injury, or pain), but it should always prompt a swift response to protect the airway and should heighten the suspicion of serious pathology.

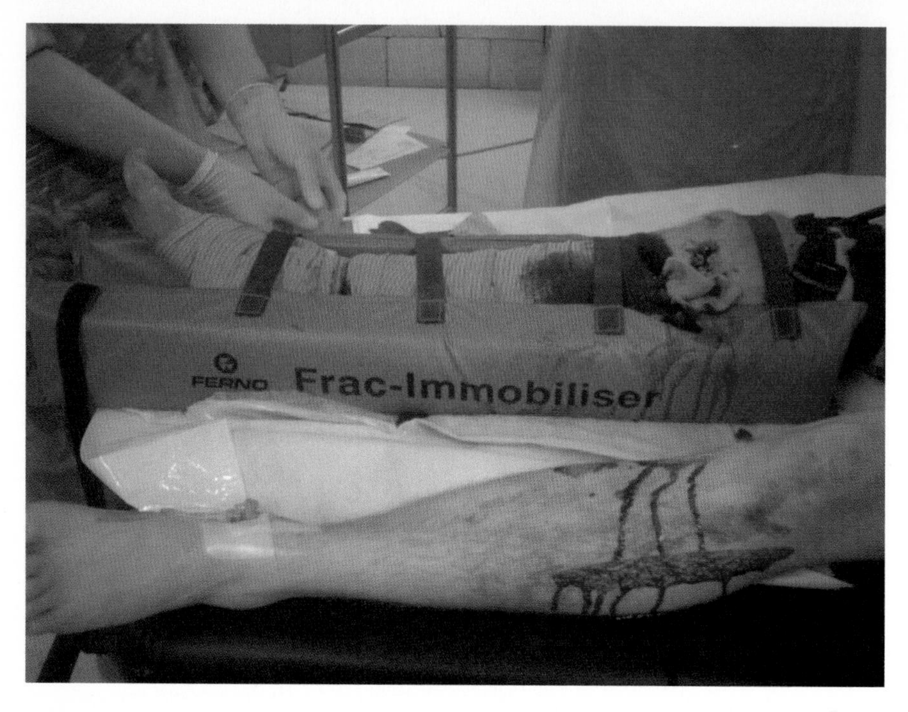

Fig. 11.2 Use of a split to stabilize a long bone fracture (Picture by David Nott)

Management involves returning to the ABCDE approach; airway management takes priority over immobilization if breathing is severely compromised. If the patient is immobilized, you can roll the stretcher to the side to avoid risk of aspiration. Suction is useful again if available and an antiemetic should be given where appropriate.

Prompt 12: How Do You Manage Major Orthopedic Fractures?

Major orthopedic fractures can conceal massive hemorrhage, and there is the possibility of lethal fat emboli progressing to the lung. The risks of this can be minimized through immobilization and traction.

Major pelvic fracture always presents a high risk of lethal hemorrhage, due to the energies required to fracture the pelvis and the proximity of major blood vessels. A splint should be applied to control bleeding; this could be done using a "SAM sling," or one can be improvised using a belt. The legs should be taped together. A femoral fracture can result in 1.5 l of blood loss. The limb should be immobilized in a traction splint. For other lower limb injuries, a stabilizing splint can be used (Fig. 11.2).

Table 11.3 The trimodal distribution of trauma deaths

Peak in mortality	Causes	Discussion
First peak Seconds to minutes 50 % of trauma deaths	Overwhelming injury, e.g., fatal head injury, rupture of the great vessels, or spinal cord	The first peak tends to be deaths that no matter what intervention or skill level is available would still occur. Very little has changed to this peak mortality, and little can be done in the disaster setting. It can still be reduced by public health measures such as road safety, seatbelts, and helmets
Second peak Minutes to hours 30 % of trauma deaths	Airway problems. Fatal hemorrhage	The second peak tends to be deaths that are preventable through early intervention as part of organized trauma system, e.g., early recognition in the field and subsequent early hospital care. Developments in the last 40 years have markedly reduced these deaths in developed countries, however they still contribute the largest proportion of preventable deaths and play a key role in disaster mortality
Third peak Over 4 h, days to weeks 20 % of trauma deaths	Infection Multi organ failure Blood clots	Almost all of these deaths can be potentially mitigated by good care in the prehospital environment followed by well-managed hospital care. However, they remain a major cause of death in disasters where health services are severely disrupted or overwhelmed

Further Information 5

The patient leaves by air ambulance and you debrief the team. There is discussion about whether the patient should have been transported earlier by standard ambulance.

Prompt 13: How Relevant Are Concepts Such as the Golden Hour of Trauma and Trimodal Distribution of Death?

Dr. R. Adams Cowley coined the term the “golden hour of trauma” in 1963 to persuade police helicopters to transport severely injured patients to trauma centers as soon possible for definitive surgery [9].

It was not based on evidence, and there is nothing magical about 60 min; however, in the early stages of trauma, rapid assessments, decisions, and managements are required to treat life-threatening injuries. The “golden hour” is therefore still a useful concept in that rapid treatment saves lives in trauma [10].

In 1983, another American surgeon Donald Trunkey analyzed trauma deaths in San Francisco and suggested they followed a trimodal distribution (Table 11.3, Fig. 11.3).

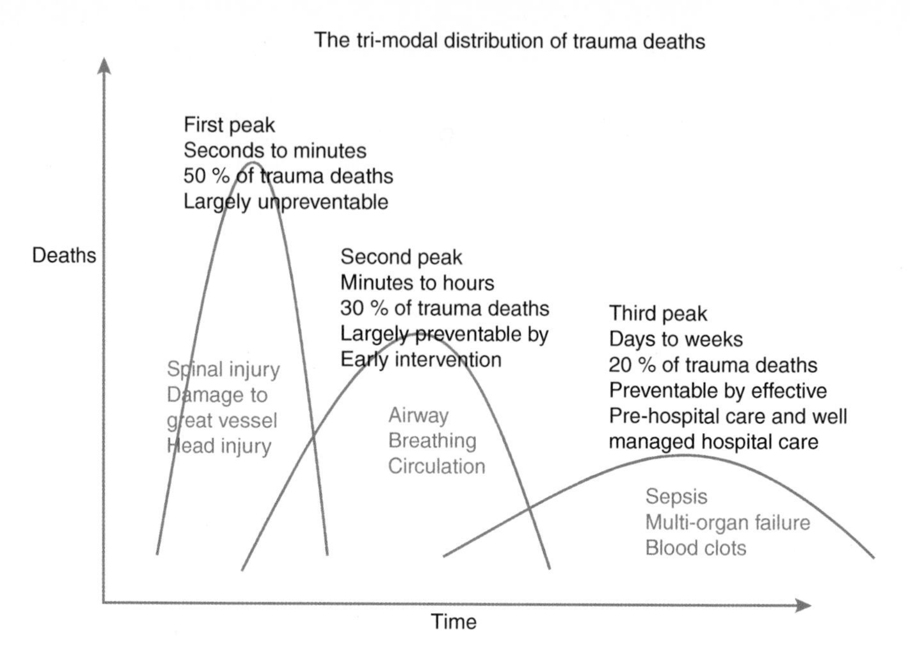

Fig. 11.3 The trimodal distribution of death

Subsequent studies in developed countries have failed to replicate this finding [11]. Moving beyond, both these concepts in developed countries are time-critical treatment considerations for various injuries or pathologies; head-injured patients must receive surgery within 4 h of injury, since hemorrhage and brain swelling can lead to lethal increases in cerebral pressure in this time. Those with severe hemorrhage require surgical intervention within 20 min, as it may be the only way of preventing further bleeding.

Prompt 14: Is a Preclinical Medical System Needed or Can It Be Replaced by a Speedy Transportation System?

There is much debate as to how much care should be given at the scene before transportation to the hospital setting. This depends on many variables such as type of trauma, skill of responder, and time to hospital setting. In this case where the patient is trapped in a vehicle, it is necessary to provide more care on scene. If early transport is available, should it be taken? Two opposing philosophies can be summarized by "stay and play" or "scoop and run."

Stay and play: The Doctor is brought to the patient resulting in longer prehospital time. In the case of a severely traumatized patient, administration of first aid, infusion therapy, early intubation, and ventilation are preformed to avoid/minimize secondary, shock-related organ damage. This is seen more in mainland Europe (France, Germany) where doctors attend a large proportion of prehospital trauma.

Scoop and run: To take the patient without primary treatment and hurry him to hospital and surgical services, typically by paramedics not doctors. This is seen more in the USA and UK.

As first responders become skilled in procedures, they are more likely to want to use those skills in stabilizing the patient before transport, delaying definitive surgery. Most recent evidence from the USA shows delayed transportation results in worse outcomes [12]. Reasons for this are as follows: there are dangers of increasing blood pressure by fluid resuscitation, with untreated bleeding sources as it can lead to increased bleeding, disturbance of clots, and dilution of coagulation factors [13].

Transport times to definitive care may be comparable to initial resuscitation. Insertion of a peripheral intravenous catheter takes an average of 8–10 min for the experienced rescuer. Transportation times in the USA are on average 8.5 min and take therefore less time than the insertion of a peripheral IV cannula [14].

In the case of severe hemorrhage, surgery may offer the only hope of survival, and speedy transportation to competent surgery is preferred. Ivatury et al. demonstrated that only 2 % of the victims with perforation injury of the chest survived preclinical treatment (oxygen administration, MAST, infusion therapy, and intubation) which took an average of 22 min. In the control group with no preclinical treatment with an average transportation time of 8.5 min, the survival rate was 18 % [7].

When to scoop and run:

- Suspicion of injury of the great vessels
- Shotgun and knife injuries of chest/abdomen
- Brain injury with GCS < 8
- Nonpenetrating abdominal trauma
- Polytrauma

Differences between the approaches of Europe and America may be partly attributable to the fact that in the USA the majority of trauma is caused by penetrating injuries from gunshot wounds and stabbings which tend to be singular and require urgent surgical intervention. In Europe most trauma is from blunt injuries, typically as the result of road traffic collisions, and patients have multiple injuries and extraction may be complicated.

A compromise has been suggested as "run and play" whereby patients are given immediate airway and breathing support and extricated to a trauma center in a vehicle equipped to provide intensive treatment with trained staff.

What these developments show is like the rest of medicine the field of prehospital care is continually evolving and seeks to build an evidence base for continual improvement based on studies rather than intuition.

Case Study: History of the ATLS® Program

Advanced Trauma Life Support (ATLS) has been a massive leap forward in the management of polytrauma patients but like many medical developments, comes from a situation managed badly.

In 1976, a light aircraft being piloted by an orthopedic surgeon Dr. Jim Styner crashed into a field. Dr. Styner's wife was killed instantly, three of his children received critical injuries, and Dr Styner himself was seriously injured. He managed to keep his children alive as he awaited the emergency services. Unfortunately, the care they received afterward was poor and uncoordinated failing to protect their airway or cervical spine, and they were lucky to survive the 10-h wait for definitive care.

This inspired him to campaign to improve trauma management and led to the development of ATLS. The course philosophy is to teach a simple approach to manage emergency situations. The founding principles being:

Trauma is a surgical disease.

Treat the greatest threat first.

Lack of history should not prevent assessment starting.

Lack of precise diagnosis should not prevent treatment starting.

The course teaches one safe system [15] applicable to manage any trauma situation.

ATLS has since become the core philosophy for trauma; however risks becoming the new dogma. Trauma is not purely a surgical disease since many trauma patients may benefit more from supportive medical and respiratory care. Unfortunately, studies have failed to capture better outcomes for patients after responders have completed the course [16].

There are alternatives such as Trauma Evaluation and Management (TEAM) [16] and Anaesthesia Trauma and Critical Care (ATACC) [17], which adopt a slightly different focus.

Despite these criticisms, the philosophy of treating the greatest threat first and treating before diagnosis is known remains as relevant today as when the course was started.

References

1. BASICS.org.uk [Internet]. Ipswich; British Association of Intermediate Care; c2008 [updated 2012 Feb 18; cited 2012 Feb 28]. Available from: http://www.basics.org.uk/.
2. Johnson C, Anderson S, Dallimore J, Winser S, Warrell D. Handbook of expedition and wilderness medicine (Oxford medical handbooks). Oxford: OUP; 2008.
3. Atanassova V [Internet]. Tongue-blocking-airways.png; c2008 [updated 2008 Apr 26; cited 2012 Feb 28]. Available from: http://en.wikipedia.org/wiki/File:Tongue-blocking-airways.png.
4. Huber-Wagner S, Lefering R, Qvick L, Körner M, Kay M, Pfeifer K. Effect of whole-body CT during trauma resuscitation on survival: a retrospective, multicentre study. Lancet. 2009;373(9673):1455–61. doi:10.1016/S0140-6736(09)60232-4.
5. Bjerke S, Geibel J. [Internet] Emedicine: Flail chest; c2011 [updated 2012 Jan 20; cited 2012 Feb 28]. Available from: http://emedicine.medscape.com/article/433779-overview.
6. Kolecki P, Brown D. [Internet] Emedicine: Hypovolemic Shock Clinical Presentation; c2011 [updated 2010 Mar 11; cited 2012 Feb 28]. Available from: http://emedicine.medscape.com/article/760145-clinical#a0217.

7. Ivatury R, Nallathambi M, Roberge R, Rohman M, Stahl W. Penetrating thoracic injuries: in-field stabilization vs. prompt transport. J Trauma. 1987;27:1066.
8. NICE. Pre-hospital initiation of fluid replacement therapy in trauma. c2004 [updated 2004 Jan; cited 2012 Feb 28]. Available from: http://www.nice.org.uk/nicemedia/live/11526/32820/32820.pdf.
9. Cowley R. The resuscitation and stabilization of major multiple trauma patients in a trauma center environment. Clin Med. 1976;83:14–22.
10. Lerner E, Moscati R. The golden hour: scientific fact or medical "urban legend"? Acad Emerg Med. 2001;8(7):758–60.
11. Demetriades D, Kimbrell B, Salim A, Velmahos G, Rhee P, Preston C, et al. Trauma deaths in a mature urban trauma system: is "trimodal" distribution a valid concept? J Am Coll Surg. 2005;201(3):343–8.
12. Pepe P, Mosesso V, Falk J. Prehospital fluid resuscitation of the patient with major trauma. Prehosp Emerg Care. 2002;6(1):81–91.
13. Bickell WH, Wall MJ, Pepe PE, et al. Immediate versus delayed fluid resuscitation for hypotensive patients with penetrating torso injuries. N Engl J Med. 1994;331(17):1105–9.
14. Apprahamion C, Darin J, Thompson B, Mateer J, Tucker J. Traumatic cardiac arrest: scope of paramedic services. Ann Emerg Med. 1985;14:583.
15. Driscoll P, Wardrope J. ATLS: past, present, and future. Emerg Med J. 2005;22:2–3. doi:10.1136/emj.2004.021212 l.
16. TEAM. [Internet]. Chicago; American College of Surgeons; c2008-11 [updated 2011 Jan 31; cited 2012 Feb 28]. Available from: http://www.facs.org/trauma/atls/team.html.
17. Anaesthesia, Trauma and Critical Care. [Internet]. Warrington; ATACC c2012 [cited 2012 Feb 28]. Available from: http://www.atacc.net/index.asp.

Chapter 12
Mass Casualty Incident

Shao Foong Chong

Learning Objectives

- Discuss how to assess and act as the first medical responder.
- Define and declare a mass casualty incident.
- Understand the importance of triage.
- Apply the principles of triage sieve and triage sort.
- Describe the organization of a major incident around bronze, silver, and gold areas.
- Outline the roles and responsibilities of the major multiagency emergency services.
- Describe the key aspects of a structured approach to a mass casualty incident.

Initial Scenario

You are an emergency medicine consultant on your way home from a busy night shift in the accident and emergency department, when you hear a huge explosion nearby that shatters the windows of the surrounding buildings. You smell pungent fumes and see people stumbling around the street covered in blood crying for help. You have attended a major incident medical management and support (MIMMS) training program where you acquired some familiarity with dealing with mass casualties in prehospital care and you begin to put your skills into action as a first responder.

S.F. Chong, MBBS, M.A. (Oxon)
FY2 Doctor, Department of Emergency Medicine,
St George's Hospital, Tooting, London, UK
e-mail: shaofoong@hotmail.com

D. MacGarty, D. Nott (eds.), *Disaster Medicine*,
DOI 10.1007/978-1-4471-4423-6_12, © Springer-Verlag London 2013

Prompt 1: What Can You Do as the First Medical Responder?

- The aim for any first responder in the prehospital environment is to optimize casualties' physiological status to a satisfactory level to be able to transport them to hospital for definitive treatment as soon as possible.
- The area must be assessed for any dangerous hazards. This may include fire, explosions, structural collapse, and terrorist attack. In recent years, there has been an increase in threat posed by a CBRN terrorist attack. This includes chemical, biological, radiological, and nuclear threats.
- Perform a quick but thorough initial assessment estimating the number of patients, hazard that requires specialist equipment, and number of emergency responders already present.
- Call the communications center early to declare a major incident. The key to an effective emergency response is to call for plenty of help as early as possible. It is better to call for too much help than too few [1].

Prompt 2: Define a Mass Casualty Incident

- Mass casualty incident (MCI) is a situation in which the number, severity, or type of live casualties are out of proportion to the available medical and logistical capabilities necessary for optimal care.
- The aim in these circumstances is to effectively utilize the limited resources to do the greatest good for the greatest number. The population as a whole, rather than the individual, is the management priority.

Prompt 3: How Do You Declare a Major Incident Effectively?

- You call the communications center via 999 and declare a mass casualty incident using the critical message structure METHANE as taught by MIMMS [2] to pass information from the scene to control:

  M: Major incident – standby or declared.
  E: Exact location – grid reference if possible.
  T: Type of incident – e.g., railway crash, terrorist bomb, mass gathering events, industrial spill.
  H: Hazards at scene, present, and potential – e.g., fire, hazardous materials, incoming traffic, security.
  A: Access and egress routes.
  N: Number, severity, and types of casualties involved.
  E: Emergency services present and required – e.g., police, fire brigade, ambulance service, and HM coastguard.

The communication center will then report the incident to the various emergency services on all frequencies to provide dispatch.

Further Information 1

From your initial assessment, you report 5 deaths and at least 20 critical injuries. People start screaming for your help. One walks to you bleeding from a big laceration to his arm, another is groaning in agony on the floor, and you notice one more slumped next to a fence in silence. While waiting for the emergency services to arrive, you perform primary triage. The casualties present with the following signs and symptoms:

1. *Female, 40s, walking, screaming, lacerated forearm*
2. *Male, 30s, lying with impaled object in abdomen, groaning, RR 34, P 136, CRT 4*
3. *Male, teens, unresponsive, you open the airway – does not breathe*
4. *Male, 10-year-old child crying, obvious open fracture of the left lower leg, RR 24, P 100, CRT 2*
5. *Female, 30s, mother of child, confused with superficial burns to the face and hands, but walking*
6. *Female, 20s, unconscious, bleeding from ears, no breath sounds after positioning airway*
7. *Male, teens, walking, complaining of severe abdominal pain*
8. *Male, 40s, lying on ground holding chest, gurgling breath sounds, RR 36, P 130, CRT 5*
9. *Female, 60s, holding left ankle, unable to walk, RR 18, P 92, CRT 4*
10. *Female, 30s, unconscious, breathing, RR 34, absent radial pulse, CRT 5*

(RR = respiratory rate, P = pulse, CRT = capillary refill time)

Prompt 4: What Is Triage?

- Triage is the prioritizing of patients according to injury severity and the need for immediate care. Triage comes from the French verb "trier," which means "to sort" or "to choose." Much is owed to the work of a French surgeon, Baron Dominique Jean Larrey, who in the Napoleonic Wars devised this method to rapidly assess and categorize the large numbers of wounded soldiers in battle and evacuate those requiring the most urgent medical attention. The concept is now in widespread use in military conflicts and civilian disasters.
- Triage must take into account various factors: the number of casualties, the severity of injuries, the availability of assets and resources, means and distances for transportation, and number of beds on standby in surrounding hospitals [3].

- There are many triage systems. "triage sieve" is used at the initial scene of a MCI to assess casualties who require immediate medical care to save their lives as opposed to patients who can wait for help. These patients are later reevaulated using "triage sort" to prioritize casualties for evacuation to hospital.
- Triage is important because time matters. Trauma patients in particular may require definitive treatment within the "golden hour." People requiring surgical care may be sent by helicopter or ambulances to dedicated trauma hospitals.

Prompt 5: Explain How You Would Prioritize Patients Using Triage Principles?

- Triage sieve allows for rapid categorization of patients for priority movement into the triage sector for further assessment, treatment, and transport. In the UK, Smart Incident Command System is taught as a triage system on the major incident medical management and support (MIMMS) training program [5].
- The systems of priorities in common use at MCIs are referred to as the treatment (T) system and the priority (P) system. The only difference is the additional expectant category included in the T system.
- Patients are usually labeled as red, yellow, green, or black for easy recognition by rescue services. A variety of methods may be used from simple colored tape or marker pens to more sophisticated triage tags with bar codes for patient tracking.

P1/T1 – Red

- Life-threatening injuries as determined by abnormal vital signs – e.g., compromised airway, respiratory distress, uncontrolled or severe accessible hemorrhage, severe burns, shock.
- Immediate treatment: Emergency life-saving resuscitation and/or surgery required within 1 h.

P2/T2 – Yellow

- Potentially life-threatening injuries with some abnormal vital signs – e.g., major fracture or joint injuries, burns without airway problems, lesser visceral injuries.
- Delayed treatment: Early resuscitation and/or surgery needed, but a delay of 2–4 h is permissible without endangering life.

P3/T3 – Green

- Minor injuries and ambulatory patients or "walking wounded" – e.g., minor soft tissue injuries, fractures, or burns.
- Minimal treatment: Relatively minor injuries and ambulatory patients where a longer delay of >4 h is acceptable. May be able to assist in own care.

P1 Hold/T4 – Blue

- Expectant category: Serious multiple injuries needing extensive treatment or with a poor chance of survival – e.g., severe head and spinal injuries, extensive burns, radiation exposure.
- Expectant treatment: Treating these casualties would divert resources from potentially salvageable casualties. Therefore, supportive treatment may be provided, such as analgesia.

Dead – Black or White

- Deceased or fatal injuries
- The dead should be transported to a temporary mortuary.

Prompt 6: How Do You Quickly Assess the Condition of Patients Using Triage Sieve?

- Triage sieve is a rapid, dynamic, and reproducible system that looks at the physiological systems that change as a consequence of injury. It involves an assessment of the casualty's mobility, then an assessment of their breathing, respiratory rate, and circulation. No treatment should be commenced during triage, with the exception of inserting simple airway adjuncts such as oropharyngeal or nasopharyngeal tubes or tourniquets [4], which take a matter of seconds. Assessment of each casualty should not take more than 30 s to complete.
- The triage algorithm (Fig. 12.1) is devised to prioritize the important physiological systems compatible with life. For example, it is essential to initially check for signs of breathing because an obstructed airway from burns or maxillofacial injury may cause irreversible brain injury if not managed immediately. Meanwhile, ambulatory casualties probably have sufficient cardiac output and respiratory reserve to not require immediate medical treatment and can take care of themselves.
- *Walking?* Upon initial triage, any patients who are already walking around the scene or are able to walk, regardless of injuries, are considered to be a lower priority 3 initially and are tagged (green). These patients are asked to move to "casualty collection points" [4], which help to clear the area and provide possible assistants to responders. Yelling or speaking through a loudspeaker "anyone requiring assistance should move to the designated casualty collection point" may help. Note that victims of large blast injuries who are rendered temporarily deaf may not be able to hear these instructions. Any patients unable to walk are then assessed further.
- *Breathing?* Assess whether the patient is breathing. If there are no signs of breathing, use simple airway opening procedures such as head tilt chin lift. Upon opening the airway, if there still is no respiratory effort, consider the patient dead. Do not start CPR as several other persons may die while you are trying to

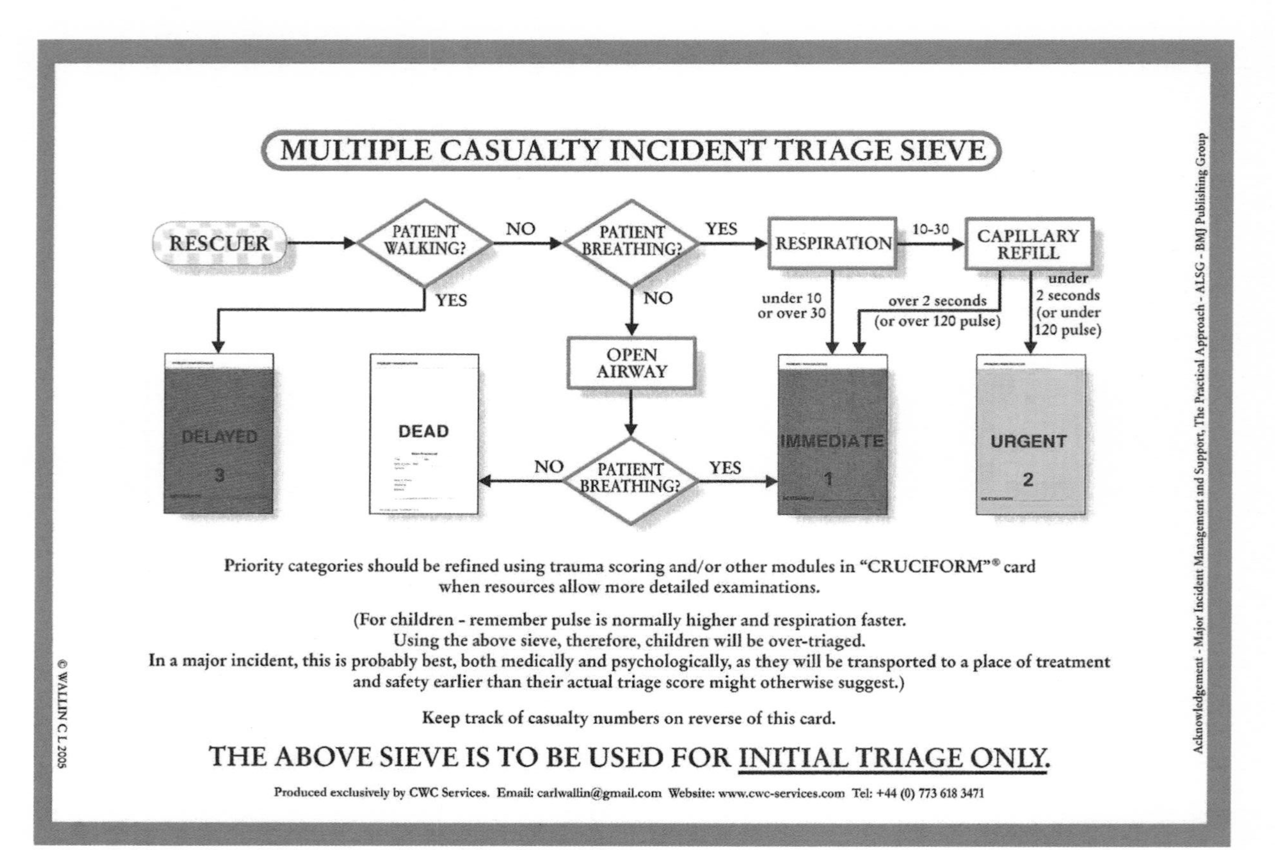

Fig. 12.1 Triage sieve flow chart (Courtesy of Carl Wallin; CWC Services [6])

save just one. If they do start breathing consider this a priority 1 (red), then move on to the next patient.

- *Respiratory rate?* If the respiratory rate is greater than 30 per minute or less than 10 per minute, tag red and move on. If it is within this range then move on to assess perfusion.
- *Capillary refill time or pulse rate?* Perfusion status is determined by assessing capillary refill or radial pulse. If pulse is <40 or >120 or capillary refill is prolonged more than 2 s, tag the patient priority 1 (red). If the pulse is between 40 and 120 or capillary refill is below 2 s, tag the patient priority 2 (yellow). Note that capillary refill may hard to assess in the dark, in cold environments, or wet conditions.

Prompt 7: In What Order Would You Care for These Patients? Briefly Outline Your Rationale for Prioritizing These Patients in the Manner You Did

1. *Despite her lacerated forearm, your first casualty is making a lot of noise screaming and walking, and you know she is noncritical = P/T 3.*
2. *This man lying on the ground with impaled object is tachypneic, tachycardic, and needs help urgently = P/T 1.*
3. *Unfortunately after a simple head tilt chin lift, there are still no signs of respiration = Dead*
4. *This child with a left lower leg fracture of the left lower leg has a raised RR, but is hemodynamically stable, therefore his treatment can be delayed temporarily = P/T 2.*
5. *This mother has superficial burns and is walking. You tell her to keep her child still as much as possible until help arrives = P/T 3.*
6. *No breath sounds after simple airway maneuvers = Dead.*
7. *Although this male is complaining of severe abdominal pain and may have a severe pathology underneath, he is walking. You tell him to talk to the casualty clearing station and be reassessed there = P/T 3.*
8. *This man is a priority patient with a RR 36 and breathing pattern that is very worrying = P/T 1.*
9. *This patient cannot walk with a broken ankle but is otherwise stable = P/T 2.*
10. *This unconscious female who is breathing quickly requires urgent treatment = P/T 1.*

Further Information 2

You feel you are doing your triage well, but around you, it is chaos. There has been very poor communication to casualties as many of the walking wounded (P/T 3's) are still on scene, although some are helping others to apply dressing to others in need. You need the P/T 1's to be stretchered off; however, ambulances seem to be deployed to the wrong area far away, so incoming paramedics need to run far distances to pick up casualties. You remain with the P/T 2's who wait for treatment and use makeshift material around you as splints for extremity injuries. You are then asked to move to the treatment sector, where your skills may be more useful in secondary triage. Patients are placed in rows according to their triage category, some of them you have seen before. You work closely with the triage officer, where you reassess the patients and categorize them for treatment and transport. You have the following new casualties:

1. *Female, 34, lying immobilized on a long board with head blocks and a leg split. RR 32, SBP 140. Eyes opening spontaneously, screaming for help and moving all hands and feet.*
2. *Male, 16, lying unconscious on the ground, gasping for air, RR 7, SBP 70. No eye opening, groaning, flexing toward painful stimuli.*
3. *Male, 45, sitting in the corner mumbling to himself, eyes open with tears streaming down his cheek, with a large shard of glass stuck in his upper arm. He can move all four limbs with encouragement. RR 18, SBP 100.*
4. *Female, 23, 2nd degree burns to 30% of her body surface area. Eyes open spontaneously, talking normally, and moving spontaneously. RR 32, SBP 60.*
5. *Male, 28, walking with blood streaming down from a scalp laceration, eyes staring at his blood soaked clothes, talking to himself. RR 22, SBP 110.*

(RR = respiratory rate, SBP = systolic blood pressure, GCS = Glasgow coma scale)

Prompt 8: What Type of Trauma Would You Expect From a Bomb Blast

- You suspect that the majority of injuries from this car bomb will be from blast explosion, which results in injuries at high pressures and high temperatures. There are different ways to categorize blast injuries [3]. You can expect primary blast injuries from overpressure effects associated with the shock wave, such as tympanic membrane rupture, blast lung causing hemorrhagic alveolar and pulmonary edema, and bowel injury. Secondary injuries resulting from shrapnel may lead to a range of problems: from superficial soft tissue wounds to fatal penetrating injuries. Tertiary injuries are those sustained by people being thrown through the air by the blast wind, causing head injuries, fractures, and amputations. Other injuries include toxic gas inhalation, crush injury, and burns.
- Trauma is a transfer of energy, leading to damage of tissues. Overall damage will depend on the amount of energy transferred and the characteristics of the tissue. [3] Injuries from physical trauma may result from penetrating, blunt, blast,

thermal or chemical causes. The timing of the onset of symptomatology is important to consider when performing triage for further management [4]. Bomb blasts will result in a large influx of casualties very quickly, so hospitals need to be well prepared for this. Exposure to chemical or biological agents may require personal protective equipment for emergency departments and a proper decontamination procedure to be in place.

Prompt 9: Describe Secondary Triage According to Triage Sort

- Secondary triage occurs at the casualty clearing station and is designed to detect any deterioration or improvement in the casualties' clinical conditions and refine triage sieve decisions. At this stage, a casualty's priority status may be upgraded or downgraded depending on his or her score.
- Triage sort, based on the revised the trauma score, is one method used for triage that has been shown to have a significant relationship from severity of injury to prognosis. This triage tool codes three physiological parameters – Glasgow coma score (GCS), systemic blood pressure (SBP), and the respiratory rate (RR) – each having a value of 4 (Fig. 12.2). These values are added together, and casualties are numerically scored from 0 (dead) to 12 (physiologically normal); this score provides an indication for priority evacuation and/or definitive treatment.
- Priorities are assigned as follows: P3 = 12, P2 = 11, P1 = 1–10, P1 Hold = 1–3, Dead = 0.

Calculate the Triage Sort Score					
Respiratory Rate		**Systolic Blood Pressure**		**Glasgow Coma Score**	
10 – 29	4	≥ 90	4	13 – 15	4
> 29	3	76 – 89	3	9 – 12	3
6 – 9	2	50 – 75	2	6 – 8	2
1 – 5	1	1 – 49	1	4 – 5	1
0	0	0	0	3	0

Assign a Triage Priority		
12	=	Priority 3
11	=	Priority 2
≤ 10	=	Priority 1
0	=	Dead

Fig. 12.2 Triage sort score

Table 12.1 Answers for triage sort

Casualty number	RR	SBP	GCS	Total score	Priority
1	3	4	4	11	2
2	2	2	2	6	1
3	4	4	4	12	3
4	3	2	4	9	1
5	4	4	4	12	3

Prompt 10: Use Triage Principles to Manage Your Evacuation of Casualties Effectively

- The accuracy of triage has a major effect on casualty outcome. Health care providers seldom practice true triage as mass casualty situations are rare to come by. Large amounts of overtriage, the assignment to immediate treatment, and evacuation of casualties who are not of high priority, may stretch limited resources so much that it prevents those who are critically ill from gaining the immediate care they require. A direct correlation of overtriage with the critical mortality rate has been demonstrated in 10 major bombing disasters [7]. Thus, it is essential that evacuation in an MCI be reserved for the most critically ill casualties.
- Assessing the new casualties at the treatment center, you prioritize them as illustrated in Table 12.1.

Further Information 3

Meanwhile, reports of a bomb in the city have alerted emergency medical services. Sirens come from every direction. Communications between emergency responders are initially wrought with problems, as there is a channel gridlock. Parked vehicles that have arrived at the beginning are now blocking access routes for incoming emergency services vehicles. The fire services arrive and ask you whom they should report to. Dead bodies on the ground need to be removed. You work with the incident commander to coordinate the emergency response.

Prompt 11: How Do Emergency Services Describe the Scene of a Major Incident?

- *Bronze area* – The actual scene of the incident, surrounded by a cordon demarcated with tape ideally. Managed under forward commanders, one for each of the emergency services. In a terrorist or firearms incident, the police control this area. Meanwhile, the fire services are appropriately in charge in the case of a fire or chemical hazard.
- *Silver area* – The outer cordon surrounds the entire incident side. Between the inner and the outer cordon is the bronze area where designated locations such as the casualty clearing station, treatment sector, and command and control post are

Table 12.2 Roles of emergency services at a MCI [8]

Medical	Scene assessment of personnel and equipment requirements
	Coordinate information to and from local hospitals
	Oversee treatment from medical and nursing personnel
Ambulance	Triage and patient transfer from the scene
	Health service communications
Fire	Eliminate fire and chemical hazards
	Rescue trapped casualties using specialist equipment
Police	Control traffic to aid evacuation
	Identify and move the dead
	Maintain law and order
	Liaise with the media
Armed forces	Explosive ordnance disposal
	Special forces

located. Silver (or incident) commanders are responsible for gathering incident scene information, coordinating emergency vehicles, and liaising with other emergency services.

- *Gold area* – Gold command is situated at a predesignated location away from the incident scene, responsible for the overall organization and flow of the mass casualty incident response. The greatest challenge in any MCI is the ability to effectively coordinate the all the different emergency services rapidly.

Prompt 12: What Are the Roles and Responsibilities of the Agencies? (Table 12.2)

Further Information 4

After 4 hours of being on scene, the most critically ill casualties have been transported to nearby trauma hospitals, and others are making their own way to the closest A&E department. This is been extremely stressful for you, and you are plagued with doubts about whether you made the right triage decision and the quality of your patient care. At the end of the day, you are asked to debrief. The whole event seemed like such a blur to you as you were on the front line. You realize at the meeting that there was an organized structure to the event.

Prompt 13: Describe the Phases of a MCI

The response to a mass casualty incident is considered under the following headings based on the CSCATTT mnemonic [2]:

- *Command* – Each emergency service will have a commander at the scene, each with his or her own responsibilities.

- *Control* – Enforced by inner and outer cordons surrounding the actual side of the incident with the wreckage and hazards and the entire incident site with various designated site, respectively.
- *Safety* – The "1-2-3 of safety" that should not be forgotten in the heat of the moment is 1-self, 2-scene, and 3-survivors in order of priority. You are no good to others if you become a casualty yourself because you have not assessed surrounding hazards.
- *Communications* – Effective communications must be established between incident commanders. Regular face-to-face communication permits constant updates, ongoing needs, and progress. The ambulance service is responsible for health service communications.
- *Assessment* – Assessment of the number, severity, and types of injury.
- *Triage* – Prioritizing of patients for treatment and evacuation according to their severity of injury using triage sieve and sort.
- *Treatment* – Designated area close to where ambulances arrive, a safe distance from the incident and clearly marked. Some treatment will be undertaken here but should be restricted to what is necessary to allow the patient to be evacuated safely to hospital for definitive care.
- *Transport* – A transportation officer coordinates casualty evacuation with the triage officer according to priority status, determines the capacity of local hospitals, and communicates an estimated time of arrival. The aim is the right patient to the right place at the right time and by the right method.

Case Study: 7/7 London Bombings (Fig. 12.3)
In the morning rush hour of 7 July 2005, there was a series of four coordinated suicide bombings, three on the London Underground and one on a double-decker bus. Fifty-six people were killed, and about 700 were injured, of whom about 100 required overnight hospital treatment or more.

Initial confusing reports suggested that a power surge had caused explosions in power circuits and that six explosions were reported. A couple of hours after the bombings, these rumors were corrected and the government confirmed the incidents were terrorist attacks. The Tavistock Square bus detonation took place near the British Medical Association, and a number of doctors in the building were able to provide immediate emergency medical assistance.

An enquiry into the 7/7 bombing found that overall the multiagency emergency response was very successful; however, there were some shortcomings. There were limited first aid emergency supplies at public transport stations. Rescuers phones and radios failed, meaning ambulances were delayed or sent to the wrong place, and medical equipment was insufficient. The police casualty bureau was overwhelmed with calls from the public trying to get further information. As a result, a number of recommendations have been proposed and incorporated into future MCI planning.

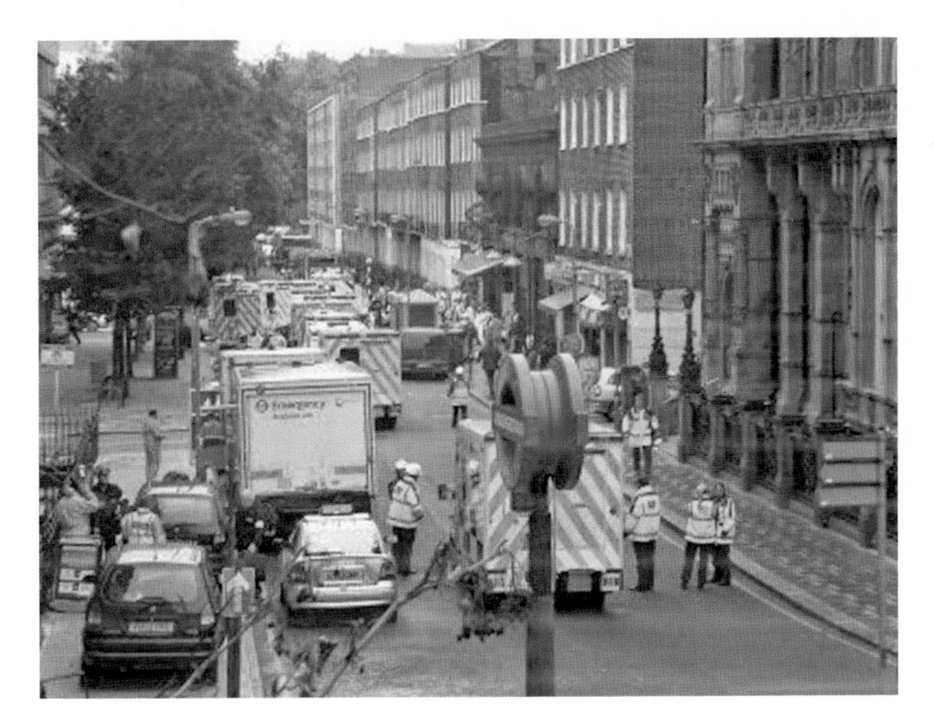

Fig. 12.3 Ambulances at Russell Square, London, after the 7th July bombings

References

1. Mistovich J, Hafen B, Karren K. Multiple-Casualty Incidents. In: Prehospital emergency care. 7th ed. Prentice-Hall; 2003. p. 937–51. Chapter 43.
2. Greaves I, Porter K. Major incident management and triage. In: Oxford handbook of pre-hospital care. Oxford University Press; 2007. p. 575–618. Chapter 10.
3. Henny W, Hopperus Buma A. Trauma and triage. In: Hopperus Buma A, Burris D, Hawley A, Ryan J, Mahoney P, editors. Conflict and catastrophe medicine: a practical guide. 2nd ed. London: Springer; 2009. p. 418–27. Chapter 29B.
4. Glarum J, Birou D, Cetaruk. Triage principles. In: Hospital emergency response teams: triage for optimal disaster response. Butterworth-Heinemann; Oxford; 2010. p. 147–156.
5. Hodgetts T, Kackway-Jones K. Major incident medical management and support (MIMMS). 2nd ed. London: BMA Books; 2002.
6. CWC Services. The cruciform system: The triage sieve. [cited 2012 March 09]. Available from: http://www.cwc-services.com/information/product-in-depth/triage-cruciform/in-the-box?start=1.
7. Born C. Disasters and mass casualties: I. General principles of response and management. J Am Acad Orthop Surg. 2007;15:388–96.
8. London Emergency Services Liaison Panel. Major incident procedure book. 7th ed. Norwich: TSO; 2007.

Chapter 13
Military Trauma

James Houston and Jim Ryan

Learning Objectives

- Describe injury in war and conflict
- Detail battlefield advanced trauma life support (BATLS) and its differences to civilian advanced trauma life support (ATLS)
- Explain echeloned care
- Discuss casualty evacuation
- Describe medical care of the injured in war and conflict
- Define shock, outline its classification, and discuss management principles
- Explain the triad of trauma death
- Briefly describe damage control resuscitation (DCR) and damage control surgery (DCS) (Fig. 13.1)

Initial Scenario

You are a military doctor working as part of a relief effort to a country in the midst of civil war. A strong foreign military presence is set up in the country, currently under a mandate to protect civilians from an oppressive regime that will stop at nothing to remain in power. You have been primarily tasked with providing medical care to civilians caught up in the conflict. While the majority of what you have seen has involved treating cases of malnutrition and chronic diseases endemic to the

J. Houston, MBBS, MEng (✉)
FY2 Doctor, Department of Surgery,
Chelsea and Westminster Hospital, London, UK
e-mail: jameshouston@doctors.org.uk

J. Ryan
Emeritus Professor of Conflict and Catastrophe Medicine,
Centre for Conflict and Catastrophe Medicine, St George's University of London,
London, UK

D. MacGarty, D. Nott (eds.), *Disaster Medicine*,
DOI 10.1007/978-1-4471-4423-6_13, © Springer-Verlag London 2013

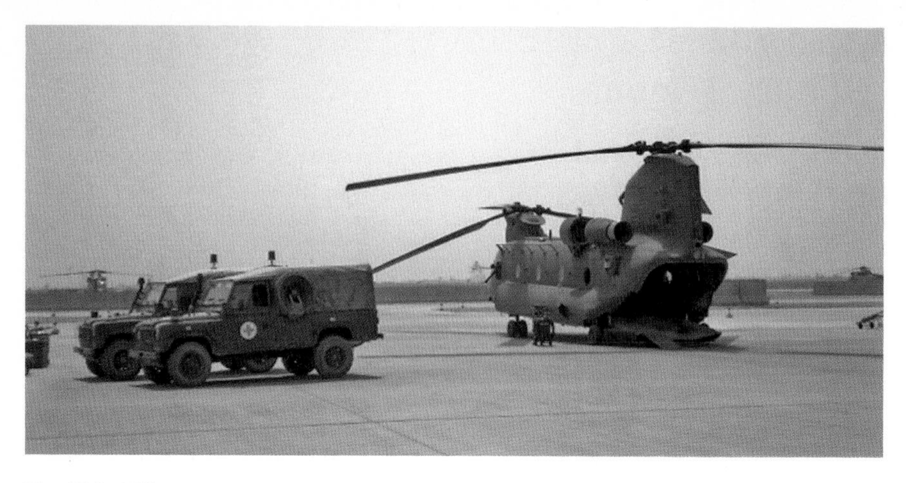

Fig. 13.1 Military helicopter used in casualty evacuation (Picture by David Nott)

area, you have also encountered a wide variety of trauma victims caught up in sporadic fighting. Troubles have been escalating for the last 6 months, and regime forces are now attacking peacekeeping forces and those seen to be providing aid. While much of the incumbent power base has been removed in the cities, many regime supporters have moved to isolated rural towns where they can stage guerrilla attacks on "foreign invaders" and those seen to sympathize. The story picks up as you are traveling in a convoy heading between two such rural towns. A column of four supply vehicles travels along the desert roads guarded front and back by military vehicles. Suddenly the convoy comes under fire. The convoy stops to investigate. Seconds later, further gunfire is heard. A call comes over the radio that one of the escorting soldiers has been shot. You are asked to assist in any way you can.

Prompt 1: What Is the First Priority When Coming Under Fire?

Personal Safety

Personal safety should be of primary concern. There is a possibility of an ambush or that other snipers could be planted in the area. Further casualties could seriously jeopardize the entire convoy.

Further action by you will depend on:

- Your current location and access to effective cover
- Personal protective equipment (PPE)
- The ability to defend your position
- The need for backup

Prompt 2: What Wound Patterns Are Likely in This Environment?

Injury patterns associated with battlefield trauma are primarily from penetrating projectiles, which include bullets and fragments from explosive weapons. The trend in recent conflicts is increasingly toward wounds caused by explosive devices compared to gunshot wounds [1]. Bullets and fragments are broadly classified into high and low velocity, and result in wounds associated with either high- or low-energy transfer to tissues. However, readers are not to be unduly concerned by the physics of wounding missiles – the most pertinent threat from such injuries is their propensity to cause life-threatening hemorrhage.

Likely injury mechanisms and patterns include:

- Bullets or fragments causing injury to soft tissue, bone, blood vessels, nerves, and body organs
- Significant phenomena associated with bombs and blast – these include:
  - High-pressure shock wave – associated with overpressure causing injury to structures with air/fluid interfaces such as lung and middle ear
  - Blast wind – dynamic pressure with disturbance of the environment causing whole-body displacement (Fig. 13.2)
  - Disruption of the environment with generation of fragments – including bits of people
  - Exothermic reactions – flash and ignition occur
  - Generation of toxic fumes and smoke
  - Collapse of buildings with potential for crush and entrapment

In war and conflict, urgent control of hemorrhage is a priority and is achieved by direct pressure or tourniquets. Wounds of war are always contaminated; blast phenomena may also cause dirty field clothing; soil and debris to be in driven into wound cavities as seen in Figs. 13.3 and 13.4.

Conserving limbs can be difficult if widespread debridement and extensive wound excision is necessary. To make matters worse, some improvised explosive devices (IEDs) have been deliberately contaminated with feces to maximize the threat of post-injury sepsis.

Most battlefield weaponry is specifically designed to kill, severely injure, or maim victims. It is their intention to make the injuries difficult to treat since such wounds will prevent any enemy from being able to continue to attack or defend a position. Likewise if a team member is injured but not killed, other members of the team may stop in their combat roles to attend to his wounds, giving the other side a strategic advantage.

Injury patterns in modern war may have a negative effect on unit morale, particularly where single or multiple amputations result. Mines that may permanently disable but not kill may well cause more anxiety about carrying out duties than the threat of being shot.

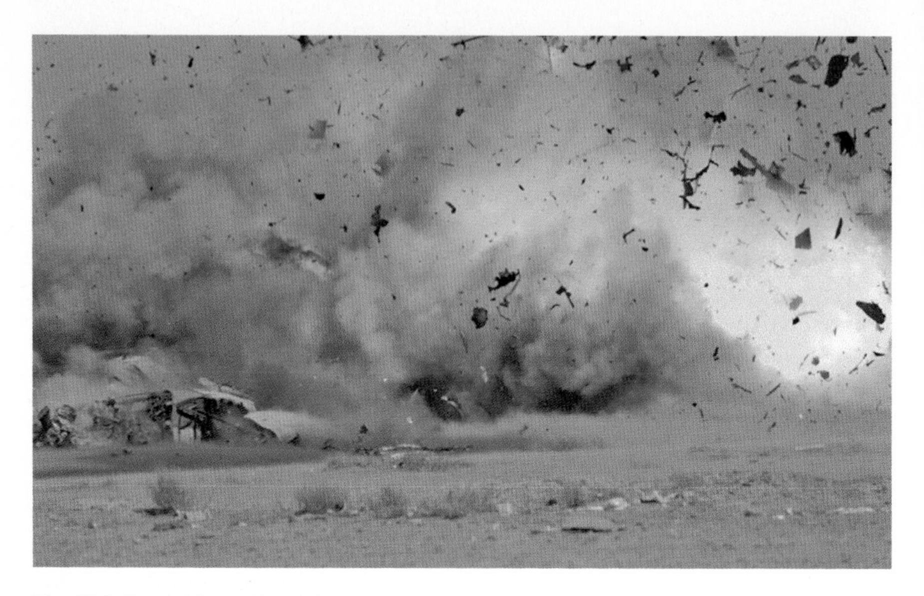

Fig. 13.2 Bomb blast with debris

Champion [2] describes the features of combat trauma associated with significant morbidity and mortality. These are:

- High energy and high potential lethality of wounding agents
- Multiple causes of wounding and multiple wounds, often involving more than one body region
- Preponderance of penetrating injury
- Persistence of threat in tactical settings
- Austere resource-constrained environment
- Delayed access to definitive care

Prompt 3: What Is Roled or Echeloned Care?

The nature of war and conflict imposes unique difficulties in providing medical care. Medical care is shared over time and place. Care requires constant backward evacuation from front line to more secure areas in the rear where more sophisticated care can be given. Four levels, termed roles or echelons, are described, each progressively more sophisticated in terms of capability or capacity.

Role 1 provides care at or near the front line and is discussed further below. Role 2 care is further back in a more secure area, allowing advanced resuscitation and possible emergency lifesaving surgery. Role 3 care is centered on field hospital well to the rear.

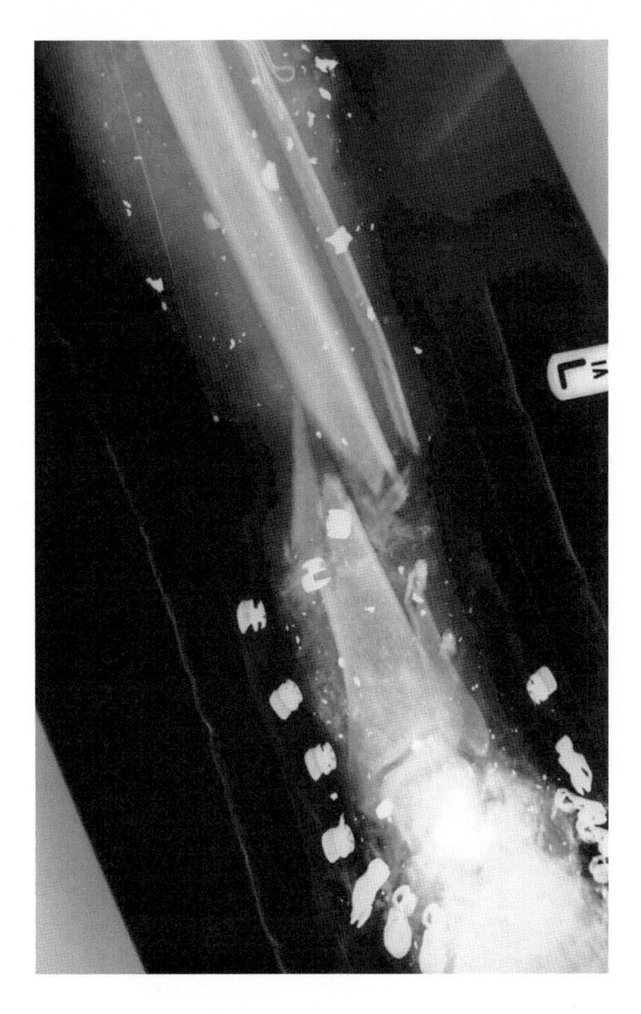

Fig. 13.3 X-ray of fracture showing shrapnel contamination (Picture by David Nott)

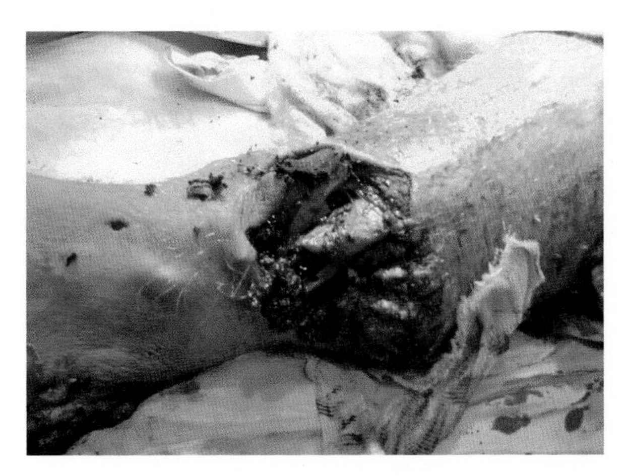

Fig. 13.4 Open fracture as result of blast with soil contamination

Role 4 care is centered on static hospitals with full capability which may be hundreds or thousands of miles away.

Care at role 1 is most problematic and has undergone dramatic reorganization in recent years. Butler [3] describes an approach to trauma care depending on environment and is divided into:

- Care under fire at the forward edge of the battlefield (the firefight is still going on).
  - Here treating the casualty may be secondary to defeating the enemy, and little can be done, apart from perhaps positioning the airway or rapid application of a field dressing for major hemorrhage. The most effective approach is to win the firefight and move the injured person back to a safe place.
- Tactical field care – still very far forward; no firefight but resources are constrained.
  - The complex injury patterns associated with military trauma may make effective treatment difficult on the battlefield, but airway care and effective control of hemorrhage is usually possible.
- Combat casualty evacuation care (casualty is being extracted from the incident).
  - The casualty needs to be taken to a point for advanced resuscitation in a sophisticated field medical facility.
  - A secondary transfer may then be made to a place where definitive care can be provided. In the case of military trauma, this may be an evacuation to a field hospital or back to the casualty's home country.

The approaches outlined above takes into account that more complex treatment is better done at places that have the facilities to deliver it. Thus complex surgery is best performed in a hospital in a country at peace with permanent facilities; resuscitation is better performed in a semipermanent facility where blood and central lines can be used. Echeloned care also takes note that while extraction to adequately resourced and stable facilities is useful, extraction must also be timely. Thus minimal interventions necessary to the patient's care can be performed at each step to enable the best possible outcome.

Further Information 1

The soldiers perform a thorough search of the building and surrounding area. Further gunshots are heard in the resulting chaos. A report comes in that an enemy sniper has been killed in the firefight although there is no other sign of any contact. One soldier has been shot in the leg. He is currently lying prone and screaming for help. Blood can be seen visibly darkening his combat trousers although it is not currently clear where the wound is situated. His compatriots form a protective cordon and shout anxiously for your help. The military medic traveling in the convoy starts using a "BATLS" approach toward the casualty, and you go over to assist. The medic exposes the wound, and a gush of blood squirts up from his upper thigh. You suspect an arterial injury.

Prompt 4: What Is BATLS and How Is It Different from ATLS?

BATLS (battlefield advanced trauma life support) is a derivation of ATLS used in the military. While ATLS focuses on an ABC approach in a hospital A&E environment, BATLS modifies this to a<C>ABC [4] (adding catastrophic hemorrhage) to take into account the significant mortality associated with acute hemorrhage in military contexts. Using a combination of field dressings, tourniquets, and topical hemostatic agents, life-threatening hemorrhage can be brought under control, after which standard ABC should be instigated.

ATLS (advanced trauma life support) was designed to give medical professionals a systematic approach to treating trauma victims in the setting of an A&E/ED resuscitation room. It involves primary and secondary surveys as detailed in previous chapters.

Prompt 5: How Should Hemorrhage Be Managed Acutely?

Focusing on the catastrophic hemorrhage emphasis from BATLS, immediate pressure should be applied over the wound using a bulky field dressing. Should traumatic amputation have occurred or bleeding cannot be stopped, a tourniquet can be applied to stop bleeding.

The above Figs. 13.5 and 13.6 show pictures of standard issue battle tourniquets. Its advantages over other tourniquets are that it is easily applied to limbs and has a simple tightening mechanism. The pressure is applied over a sufficiently wide area to reduce the incidence of localized limb ischemia. Research [6] has shown that their use has been successful in saving lives and that the earlier they have been used, the more effective they have been. Anecdotal stories have arisen of soldiers actually wearing the tourniquets into combat zones. Tourniquets must only be used in life-threatening situations. Their overuse can cause more harm than good, and after a couple of hours, limbs can be lost due to irreversible ischemia.

Other options are the use of topical agents such as hemostat or quick-clot gauze. Some of these products contain a substance called chitosan, which causes rapid clotting of both arterial and venous bleeding.

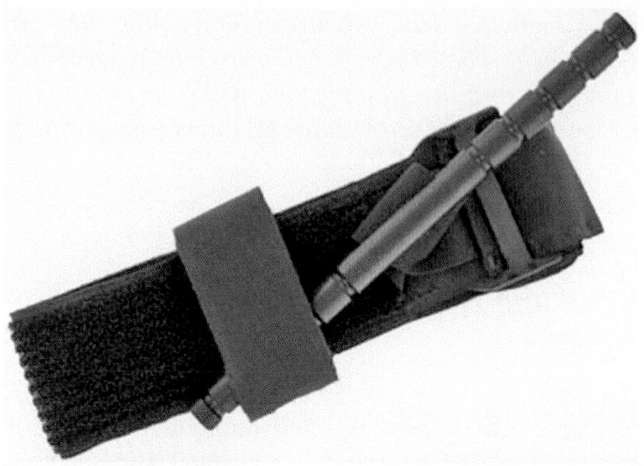

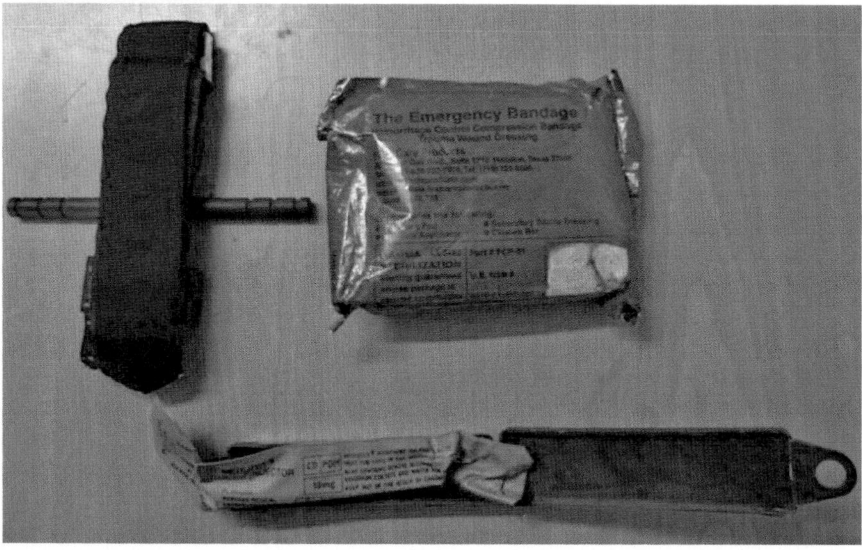

Figs. 13.5 and 13.6 Combat tourniquets (Fig. 13.5 Source: US Government National Archives, accessed online from www.olive-drab.com [5], Fig. 13.6 Reproduced with permission of D. Nott)

Further Information 2

Fortunately a battlefield tourniquet is available. This is placed upon the patient's limb while the medic calls for a MERT (Medical Emergency Response Team) helicopter. The casualty is described as male, 25-year old with gunshot wound to leg with massive hemorrhage. Airway is self-maintained. Breathing is increased in rate but not compromised. Circulation is compromised. There are no other injuries. The request is accepted, and a helicopter dispatched with a flight time of 20 min. You set up a drip of a liter of crystalloid solution. Small incremental doses of morphine are given for pain control. While the tourniquet seems to control most of the bleeding, the casualty is becoming increasingly drowsy and pale. After a 20-min delay, the helicopter arrives and picks up the casualty to return to a nearby base. As you are an experienced medic and have prior knowledge of the situation, you are asked to accompany the patient during the evacuation. During the flight, further fluids are given, and basic monitoring started. You arrive at the military base within another 25 min where a stretcher awaits to carry the patient inside to the emergency room. Although you are not strictly part of the emergency team, you are given permission to come inside and provide any help that is requested.

Prompt 6: What Is a MERT Team and How Does It Operate?

The patient needs evacuation to a definitive point of care. This means a place where advanced resuscitation and surgical procedures can be carried out to repair the blood vessels and stop the bleeding. In most civilian cases, the patient would be taken by vehicle to the nearest hospital.

Military evacuation to definitive care in remote settings often demands the use of a helicopter. The British military currently uses the MERT system (Medical Emergency Response Team) consisting of a multidisciplinary trauma team such as that based out of camp Bastion in Afghanistan.

- The medical team consists of four personnel including a doctor, two paramedics, and an emergency nurse.
- Armed soldiers will accompany the helicopter to secure the landing area, and Apache attack helicopters provide air support.
- The flight team itself consists of a pilot and copilot flying a Chinook helicopter.
- Other helicopters such as the Merlin have also been used in Iraq.

The American evacuation system uses Blackhawk helicopters, which are able to land in hotter zones than the vulnerable large Chinooks. While this may help get to casualties sooner, there is only basic medical support able to be given to casualties until they reach the hospital. The MERT on the other hand are fully equipped medical flying ambulances carrying much equipment used in prehospital care. They also carry blood and blood products that can be transfused as soon as the patient is in the helicopter.

Prompt 7: How Does a Military Emergency Room (ER) Differ from a Normal ER?

The military has led the way in advances in trauma in recent years. Research learned from Afghanistan and Iraq has made a real difference to the way complex cases are managed. Due to the nature of military engagement, their ERs are set up for trauma scenarios as seen in Fig. 13.7. It is likely that clinicians will have a high degree of

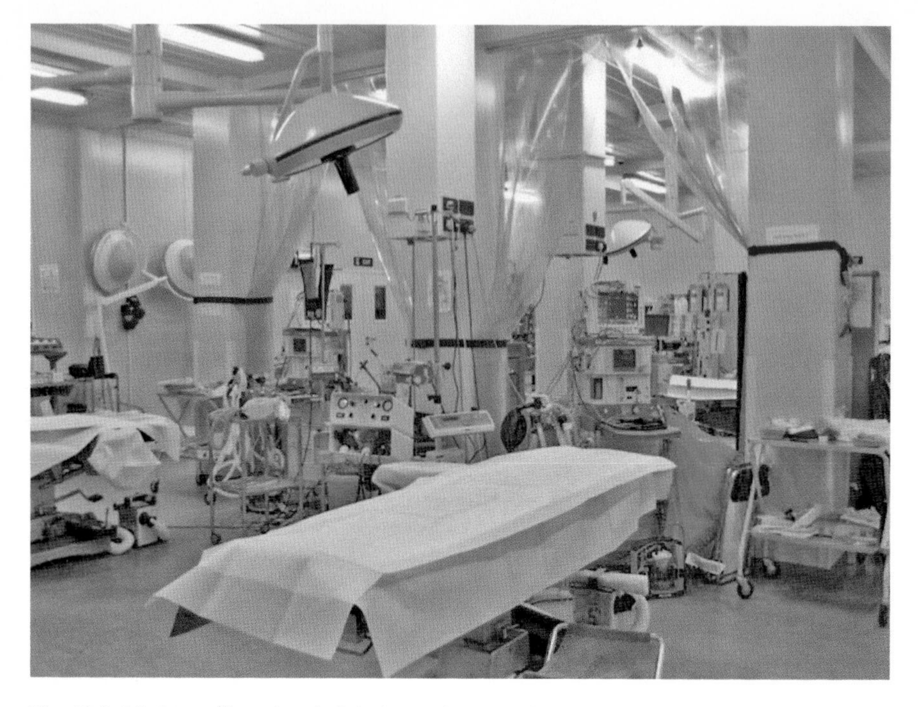

Fig. 13.7 Modern military hospital dual capacity operating room (Picture by David Nott)

trauma experience and rapid access to investigations such as cross-sectional imaging (CT). Adequate funding and resources, when compared to most NGO field hospitals in disaster settings, mean that improved outcomes are more likely.

Prompt 8: Detail Initial Management and Investigations in a Gunshot Victim

- A full CABC reassessment should be made in line with BATLS guideline.
- Any suspected C-spine fracture must be ruled out, and until then the patient must be kept immobilized using a well-fitting semirigid collar.
- 12–15L of oxygen should be administered via a "non-rebreathing" trauma mask.
- IV fluid resuscitation should continue to counter blood loss. As the blood loss is severe, emergency blood transfusions will likely be required.
- Investigations should include FBC, U&E, baseline CRP, LFT alongside a G&S, and crossmatch.
- An ABG is required.
- Fractures must be ruled out through X-rays and a likely CT – some trauma centers make use of a Lodox scanner that can provide a low-resolution X-ray of the entire body to assess quickly for any long bone fractures.

Prompt 9: How Should a Shocked Patient Be Managed?

Shock is defined as a failure in the circulatory system that results in inadequate end-tissue oxygenation.

Hypovolemic shock refers to inadequate circulatory volume. Causes include blood loss, plasma loss in burns, and dehydration.

The body compensates to this by increasing heart and breathing rate. Other signs of shock include cool, clammy skin due to vasoconstriction. Reduction in end-organ perfusion such as the brain, kidneys, and heart can cause confusion, acute renal failure, and cardiac arrest, respectively.

By convention, shock is graded into classes clinically – see Box 13.1 below.

Box 13.1: Grades of Shock

Class I: Up to 15 % loss of blood volume (750 ml), mild tachycardia.
Class II: 15–30 % loss of blood volume (750–1,500 ml), moderate tachycardia, coolness and pallor of the skin, decreased pulse pressure.
Class III: 40 % blood loss (1,500–2,000 ml), increased pallor and sympathetic response, some confusion, and decompensation leads to a drop in blood pressure.
Class IV: Over 40 % blood loss (>2,000 ml), profound hypotension leading to life-threatening end-organ damage.

Hypovolemic shock from hemorrhage may also cause abnormal blood gas readings such as lowered pO_2, lowered pH, lowered bicarbonate, an increased ion gap and base deficit, and an increased lactate. Thus a metabolic acidosis is likely to be taking place. This will reflect the patient's oxygen debt, where anaerobic glycolysis now takes place, producing lactate and a resulting acidosis. It has been shown that the more severe the base excess, the greater the mortality risk [7]. The hemoglobin may not drop immediately since the absorption of diluting extravascular fluid to compensate may not have yet occurred.

Adequate management of hypovolemic shock due to hemorrhage is crucial in military trauma. The patient requires enough fluid replacement to allow perfusion in end organs. Correct fluids are important both in terms of quantity and components; while volume must be replaced, so must also the contents of the blood.

Prompt 10: What Fluids Can Be Used in Resuscitation?

- Crystalloids

These fluids can pass through any cell membrane, and the extent of their diffusion is determined by their osmolality.

- Normal Saline: Contains 0.9 % NaCl (9 g in 1 l of H_2O). Since this fluid is isotonic, it will stay briefly in the extracellular fluid and the circulatory system.
- Dextrose Solution: Most often 5 % glucose, this is hypotonic and will be distributed throughout all the body compartments. It should thus not be used for resuscitation.
- Hartmann's or Ringer's Lactate: This fluid is designed to be almost isotonically identical to blood. It is therefore a common choice in initial resuscitation scenarios with blood loss.

• Colloids

These fluids have molecules in them, which are too large to pass through semipermeable membranes and will thus stay longer in the intravascular volume. They theoretically have a more lasting effect in maintaining blood pressure.

- Examples of colloids include gelofusin and Voluplex.

• Blood Transfusion

Blood carries a greater risk to the patient than fluids due to the risk of transfusion reactions and the possibility of blood-borne viruses. While its use can certainly be lifesaving, the benefits to the specific person must be weighed up against the risk of complications. There are four different types of blood products that can be offered in the resuscitation setting:

- Packed Red Cells: A product containing primarily red cells from blood with some leucocytes and a small amount of plasma and additive. Each unit will normally correct the Hb by 1 g.
- Plasma (Fresh Frozen Plasma so-called FFP): This contains all the coagulation factors and proteins that maintain oncotic pressure. An adult dose is normally four units.
- Platelets: This is transfused as a platelet concentrate and is used in severe thrombocytopenia often less than 50. One pack is given per 10 kg mass of patient.
- Cryoprecipitate (Cryo): This contains factors VIII and XIII and fibrinogen and should be used in fibrinogen deficiency (<0.8)

Further Information 3

A more thorough primary and secondary survey is performed on arrival by the trauma team.

Airway – Patent
Breathing – Tachypneic, trachea central, RR=, good air entry bilaterally, Sa 90 %,
Circulation – BP 85/60, HR 120, CRT = 5
Disability – GCS 13/15 PEARL, moving all limbs, BM = 6

An ABG shows pO_2 8 kPa, pH 7.30, BE −3, Hb 9.5, and HCO_3^- 20.

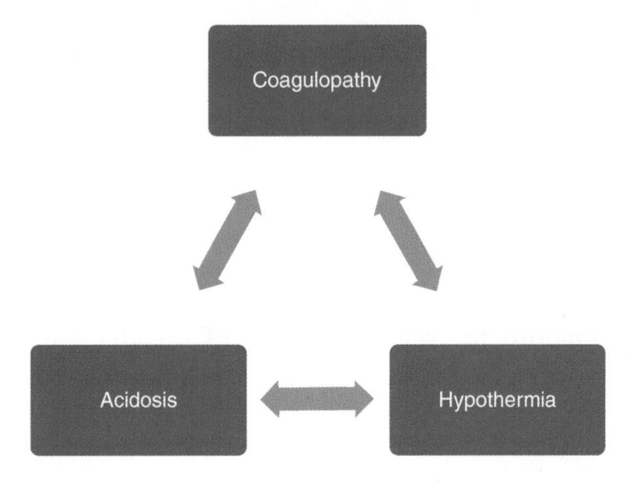

Fig. 13.8 The lethal triad in trauma

The patient looks pale and clinically unwell. He is estimated to be in class III shock. There are no other injuries seen on examination of the rest of his body during the secondary survey.

The patient had initially responded initially to crystalloid infusion during the helicopter transfer, but his blood pressure became unstable and dropped again, and the bleeding is ongoing. Crash blood products are requested, and the nurse asks the team what blood pressure the team should titrate to.

Prompt 11: What Is the Lethal Triad in Trauma?

The lethal triad refers to acidosis, hypothermia, and coagulopathy and is illustrated in Fig. 13.8. The pathophysiology of these complications of trauma has been described by Holcomb et al [8]. Likewise, one part of the triad can also make the others worse, and thus when these occur together, outcomes are poor. Much of recent trauma management has taken into account that complications from metabolic failure are more likely to kill patients than from failure to fully complete any required operation.

Prompt 12: How Actively Should Blood Pressure Be Managed in Hemorrhage?

- Massive bleeding stands second only to central nervous injuries in terms of the leading cause of death from trauma [9]. While little can be done to correct central nervous injury in the acute setting, much can be done to correct bleeding.

- While much has been said earlier about restoring fluids, a compromise must be made between providing perfusion of end organs and not raising the pressure too much, which might then disrupt previous clots.
- The concept of "permissive hypotension [10]" was coined bearing in mind such a balance, and a systolic figure of 90 with a palpable radial pulse is often quoted as optimal.

Prompt 13: What Important Considerations Should Be Made When Contemplating Blood Transfusion?

- There is debate about the ratios of FFP to RBC. Traditionally RBC was the only product given as the focus was on correcting the oxygen-carrying capacity of the blood. This however fails to take into account the coagulopathic state of trauma victims as described in the trauma triad. Traditionally FFP was given once clotting factors were diminished or at best in a ratio of 3:1. However, more recent research suggests giving the RBC in equal components to FFP, mimicking whole blood, and pre-anticipating any loss [11] of coagulation factors.
- Platelets have suggested to be added in a similar way as FFP, resulting in a 1:1:1 ratio in massive transfusions [12, 13].
- Antifibrinolytics such as tranexamic acid have been shown in trauma patients to reduce the risk of death [14].
- One dose of cryoprecipitate can be given which will provide sufficient fibrinogen for hemostasis although evidence is still not concrete. Likewise another additive recombinant factor VIIa has been suggested in trauma victims to correct coagulopathy but remains controversial.
- In the emergency setting, hospitals often have a "crash blood call" often known as a code blue. Calls refer to an urgent request for blood, which normally means 4 units of O negative blood with immediate crossmatching for another 4 units of red blood cells. In the military setting, a call is sent for one or more "shock packs," each consisting of 4 units blood, 4 FFP, and platelets.
- Massive transfusion is defined as replacing more than half a patient's entire blood volume in less than 24 h. Such large transfusions bring an extra set of complications when considering replacing all components of blood including clotting factors. See Fig. 13.9 for an illustration of the sheer number of products that may need to be used in a resuscitation setting.
- An important consideration of massive transfusion is hypothermia. Thus where possible, all fluids should be warmed to body temperature before infusion. Care should be made to keep the patients warm with blankets where possible or to keep the hospital environments at a warm enough temperature to prevent hypothermia.
- Assessing coagulopathy is a vital and very early consideration. Conventional use of INR, fibrinogen, or APTTr for the assessment of coagulation profile provides

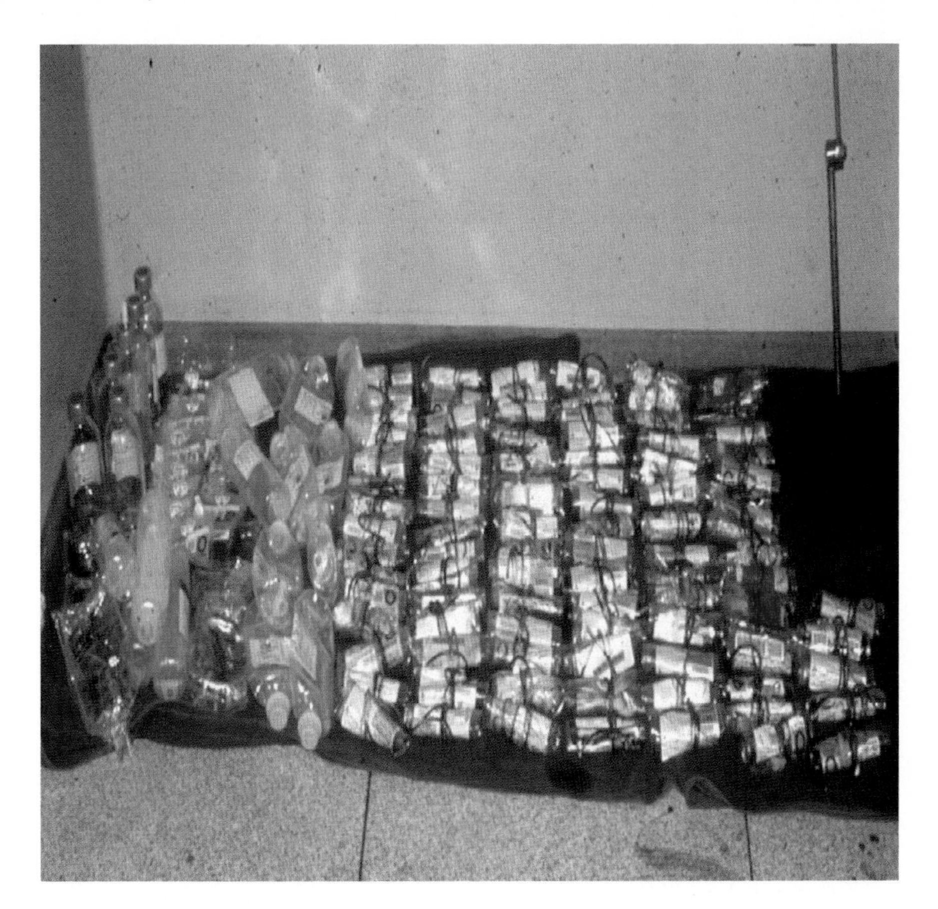

Fig. 13.9 Resuscitation products used in a trauma setting (Picture by David Nott)

a picture that is unidimensional and is often several steps behind where the patient is, clinically speaking, by the time results get back. Thromboelastography and more currently ROTEM™ measures the speed and strength of clot formation and can provide a more rapid and timely measurement of coagulopathy. These measurements have now been used in wartime settings for the management of massive hemorrhage.

Further Information 4

The patient is started on oxygen and given warmed fluids. He is resuscitated to a systolic of 90 with blood replacement products before being taken to the operating theater. A 2-h operation then takes place to repair the arterial supply to his leg and to control the bleeding. The time in the field hospital is short; however, 10 h later, the soldier is put on another ITU-equipped plane and flown back to the UK. On arrival back home, he then spends three days in an ITU bed before returning to the operating theater for a further operation to assess and repair the torn artery. The patient begins almost immediate physiotherapy, and 2 weeks later, the patient is fit enough to be transferred to a rehabilitation hospital. While the patient now has a limp and will not be able to return to front line duties that he craves, he is given the support required to start a new career in teaching.

Prompt 14: Describe Damage Control Surgery

Damage control surgery as described by Rotondo [15] reduces the emphasis on definitive surgical procedures in the first instance but instead provides lifesaving interventions before a stay in ITU. This is then followed by a longer, definitive surgical procedure once the lethal triad has been corrected [16]. Although in this case the injury is reasonably simple, a better example could be demonstrated in a bomb explosion where surgery may be performed to stop any immediate bleeding, with limb reconstruction taking place at a later date.

Prompt 15: Describe Damage Control Resuscitation

A balance must be made between the need for surgical care and the time taken for resuscitation. While surgical care may provide a definitive solution to the bleeding, weakened reserves through inadequate resuscitation may reduce the patient's chances of surviving the operation. A new concept called damage control resuscitation (DCR) [17] aims to add as an adjunct to damage control surgery. It aims to address the lethal triad earlier in the patient's management not only in the intensive care phase post-damage control surgery but also in the initial resuscitation. Key parts of DCR include previously mentioned topics such as keeping the patient within a permissive hypotension, using hemostatic resuscitation in a 1:1:1 ratio, and early correction of coagulopathy. Damage control surgery can then be used after this form of resuscitation.

Case Study: Afghanistan and Trauma Services in the UK
Recent military conflicts in Afghanistan and Iraq have provided a wealth of research into new ways of dealing with complex trauma. Soldiers are now surviving injuries that would have previously been fatal. Emphasis has particularly been made on controlling hemorrhage and addressing the triad of trauma death. In practice, this has come through using combat tourniquets,

rapid evacuation using MERT, use of 1:1:1 blood products, damage control resuscitation, and damage control surgery. Years of conflict have made trauma teams well experienced to deal with the daily trauma cases coming into Camp Bastion. Echelons or roles of care have been established to get the casualties to the trauma center and then stabilized before being flown back in the UK – often to the Queen Elizabeth Hospital in Birmingham. Many of the military advances, such as use of dedicated trauma teams, ratios of blood products, rapid imaging, and damage control resuscitation have now been adopted in civilian settings. This type of service is heavily resource intensive, and funding is often debated when bearing in mind the amount of serious trauma a hospital will encounter. Thus in London, specific trauma centers have been set up where trauma casualties will be referred to as opposed to their local hospital. However, improvements in trauma mortality do not paint the whole picture. Soldiers although surviving may well have great incapacity due to loss of limb, neurological, or cognitive function. Trauma's success has begun to rear the most difficult of questions: bearing in mind the likely outcome, are we now going too far to save a life?

References

1. Owens BD, Kragh Jr JF, Wenke JC, Macaitis J, Wade CE, Holcomb JB. Combat wounds in operation Iraqi Freedom and operation Enduring Freedom. J Trauma. 2008;64(2):295–9. PubMed PMID: 18301189.
2. Champion HR, Bellamy RF, Roberts CP, Leppaniemi A. A profile of combat injury. J Trauma. 2003;54(5 Suppl):S13–9. Review. PubMed PMID: 12768096.
3. Butler Jr FK, Hagmann J, Butler EG. Tactical combat casualty care in special operations. Mil Med. 1996;161(Suppl):3–16. PubMed PMID: 8772308.
4. Hodgetts TJ, Mahoney PF, Russell MQ, Byers M. ABC to<C>ABC: redefining the military trauma paradigm. Emerg Med J. 2006;23(10):745–6. PubMed PMID:16988297; PubMed Central PMCID: PMC2579588.
5. U.S. Government National Archives. Available from: www.olive-drab.com. Accessed on Mar 2012.
6. Kragh Jr JF, Littrel ML, Jones JA, Walters TJ, Baer DG, Wade CE, Holcomb JB. Battle casualty survival with emergency tourniquet use to stop limb bleeding. J Emerg Med. 2011;41(6):590–7. Epub 2009 Aug 31. PubMed PMID: 19717268.
7. Davis JW, Parks SN, Kaups KL, Gladen HE, O'Donnell-Nicol S. Admission base deficit predicts transfusion requirements and risk of complications. J Trauma. 1996;41(5):769–74. PubMed PMID: 8913202.
8. Holcomb JB, Jenkins D, Rhee P, Johannigman J, Mahoney P, Mehta S, Cox ED, Gehrke MJ, Beilman GJ, Schreiber M, Flaherty SF, Grathwohl KW, Spinella PC, Perkins JG, Beekley AC, McMullin NR, Park MS, Gonzalez EA, Wade CE, Dubick MA, Schwab CW, Moore FA, Champion HR, Hoyt DB, Hess JR. Damage control resuscitation. J Trauma. 2007;62(2): 307–10. PubMed PMID: 17297317.
9. Søreide K. Epidemiology of major trauma. Br J Surg. 2009;96(7):697–8. PubMed PMID: 19526611.
10. Kreimeier U, Prueckner S, Peter K. Permissive hypotension. Anaesthesist. 2002;51(10): 787–99.

11. Ramaiah R, Grabinsky A, Williamson K, Bhanankar SM. Trauma care today, what's new? Int J Crit Illn Inj Sci. 2011;1:22–6.
12. Borgman MA, Spinella PC, Perkins JG, Grathwohl KW, Repine T, Beekley AC, et al. The ratio of blood products transfused affects mortality in patients receiving massive transfusions at a combat support hospital. J Trauma. 2007;63:805–13.
13. Holcomb JB, Wade CE, Michalek JE, Chisholm GB, Zarzabal LA, Schreiber MA. Increased plasma and platelet to red blood cell ratios improves outcome in 466 massively transfused civilian trauma patients. Ann Surg. 2008;248:447–58.
14. Shakur H, Roberts I, Bautista R, Caballero J, Coats T, et al. Effects of tranexamic acid on death, vascular occlusive events, and blood transfusion in trauma patients with significant haemorrhage (CRASH-2): a randomised, placebo-controlled trial. Lancet. 2010;376:23–32.
15. Rotondo MF, Schwab CW, McGonigal MD, et al. "Damage control": an approach for improved survival in exsanguinating penetrating abdominal injury. J Trauma. 1993;35:375–83.
16. Rotondo MF, Zonies DH. The damage control sequence and underlying logic. Surg Clin North Am. 1997;77:761–77.
17. Jansen J, Thomas R, Loudon MA, Brooks A. Damage control resuscitation for patients with major trauma. BMJ. 2009;338:b1778.

Chapter 14
Tropical Surgery

Ed Mew

Learning Objectives

- Understand how clinical practice might be complicated when working in tropical settings
- Explore how a doctor's approach to patient assessment may differ in tropical settings
- Explain how tropical presentations of disease may differ from the nontropical
- Formulate a differential diagnosis and management plan for acute peritonitis in the tropics
- Understand surgical and anesthetic considerations in tropical surgery
- Explain how to perform a midline laparotomy
- Outline the clinical presentation, pathophysiology, and management of typhoid fever
- Explore postoperative considerations in the surgical patient in the tropics (Fig. 14.1)

Initial Scenario

You are a surgical trainee nearing the end of your training. You decide to take a break from surgical training and volunteer your services for 6 months in a rural hospital in southern Uganda. Your role initially concerns training local clinical

E. Mew, MBBS
FY2 Doctor, Trauma, Emergency and Acute Medicine (TEAM),
King's College Hospital, Denmark Hill, London, UK
e-mail: eau.mew@gmail.com

D. MacGarty, D. Nott (eds.), *Disaster Medicine*,
DOI 10.1007/978-1-4471-4423-6_14,

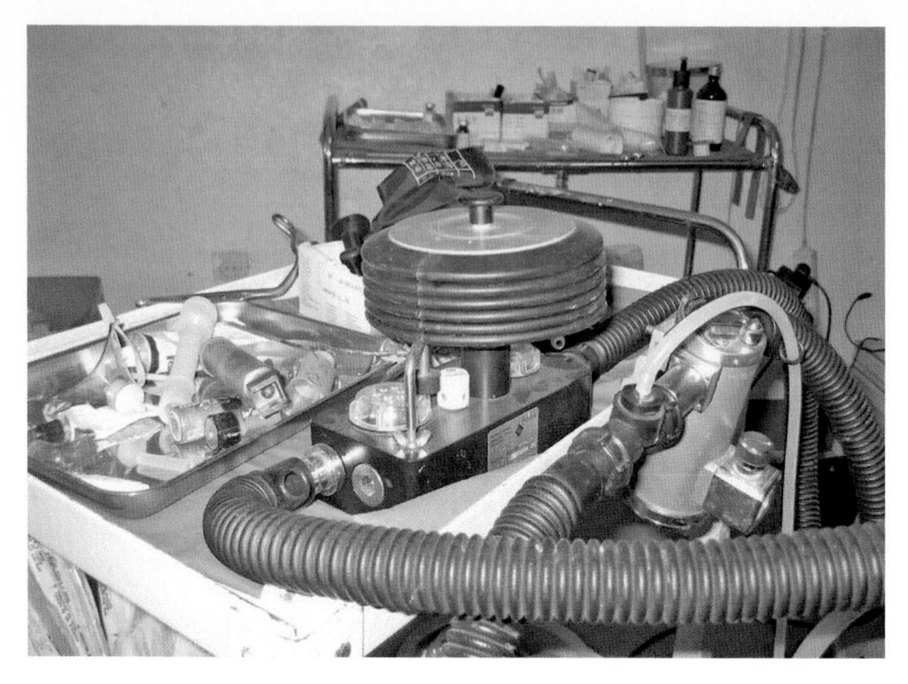

Fig. 14.1 Miscellaneous equipment in operating theater (Picture by David Nott [10])

officers in surgical techniques, while you adapt to the change in environment before taking on service provision. However, 3 days after your arrival, you are told that the senior surgeon has had to leave the hospital temporarily to care for a family member, and so you are left on your own. As you are digesting this information, a nurse walks into the ward bringing a message from the outpatient department which acts as an emergency department. There is someone with severe abdominal pain that the clinical officers are concerned about and have requested a surgical opinion.

Prompt 1: How Might Your Clinical Practice Be Complicated When Working in Tropical Countries?

Cultural Issues

You should ideally have talked to your new colleagues in the hospital or returning practitioners back in the UK about local customs. It is important to have ascertained the limits of local acceptability concerning the following areas of practice:

Examinations by male health professionals
Abortion and fertility questions
End of life and palliative care issues

Blood products and organ transplant
Use of animal products
Plastic surgery [1]

Endemic Conditions

You should definitely have thought about the conditions that are endemic in this part of the world as this will obviously shape your differential. Is there seasonal, socio-economic, or gender variability in distribution? Again, this information is best gleaned before practicing and from individuals with good local knowledge.

Local Resources

You must know the limitations of the hospital you are working in. Working in developing countries is often characterized by lack of resources. If possible, undertake an informal tour of the hospital, considering the following:

Laboratory Tests: What tests done, time period for tests, and out-of-hour services, techniques, and accuracy of testing
Radiology: Facilities, location, method of patient transportation to facilities (sometimes patients are told to make their own way there!)
Critical Care Units: Presence of, facilities contained, and criteria for admission
Equipment: Equipment commonly used on the wards, alternatives, drugs available, antibiotic protocols, and other protocols

Payment

The UK has a system of nationalized health care that is mostly free on point of delivery. In other countries, patients may have to pay for admission, tests, and treatment. This will influence the willingness of your patients to be admitted, have tests, and accept treatment. Some rural areas may have an operating insurance scheme that pays for their treatment. There may also be a "Good Samaritan" fund that provides financial assistance to those in abject poverty although criteria may be specific.

Work Circumstances

The work load that you will be expected to handle may differ markedly from what you are used to in the UK. How many patients are you expected to assess today?

How long is your operating list? Are there any other commitments that doctors in your position are expected to attend to? Other issues to consider include:

Contractual issues – what is your remit?

Cover for professional liability insurance (arranged either by host country or home country)

Legal permission to work in country: You may need to join a national association to practice medicine or allied health sciences.

Personal Protection

HIV and hepatitis B are the norm rather than the exception in many parts of Africa, and operating theaters may be underequipped without personal protective equipment.

Prompt 2: How Can a Doctor's Approach to Assessing Patients Differ in Tropical Conditions?

History

What language/dialect does your patient speak? You will need an appropriate translator. Your history may be limited by the language barrier, despite the best wishes of your interpreter.

You should take a focused surgical history for acute abdominal pain, templates for which are in all good books on clinical skills. The presenting complaint, relevant past medical history including HIV status, medications, and allergies are important features.

In regional settings, patients may come from far and wide to access health care. Does your patient have dependents or a livelihood that precludes a prolonged inpatient stay? How far has he come from and who is accompanying him? He and those that brought him may need accommodation. Discharging him to a tent 30 miles away for convalescence may spell death [2].

Examination

Examination should follow as per normal physical examination. Learning a few commands in the local dialect may help. You may have to rely more than usual on general impression – is the patient well or unwell? Basic observations like pulse rate (PR), respiratory rate (RR), blood pressure (BP), temperature (T) and, if possible, oxygen saturations (SaO_2) provide important information but may well not be done – necessitating the application of clinical acumen.

For example, blood pressure measurement may not be available, but you can estimate a blood pressure from palpation of the peripheral pulses: very roughly, a radial pulse → systolic blood pressure of above 70 mmHg, a femoral pulse → above 60 mmHg, carotid pulse → above 50 mmHg.

The fullness of the pulse will give you a measure of the pulse pressure – thin and thread suggests low pulse pressure in conditions like hypovolemic shock and advanced peritonitis; bounding pulse occurs in conditions like sepsis and hypercapnia.

Pallor of the conjunctiva, palmar creases, or tongue suggests anemia. Jaundice can be elicited in dark skin by blanching it with pressure and observing.

An important feature of surgical examination is the ability to elicit features of peritonitis (see Box 14.1 below):

Box 14.1: Peritonitis

Peritonitis means inflammation of the peritoneum – a membranous covering of abdominal viscera and the abdominal walls.

Localized peritonitis refers to local inflammation and may occur with minor pathologies or as a precursor to more serious generalized peritonitis. It manifests as abdominal tenderness that is localized to a specific area on palpation of the abdomen.

Generalized peritonitis, widespread inflammation of the abdominal wall, is generally recognized as:

Signs of shock + abdominal tenderness/percussion tenderness + rigidity + absent bowel sounds

A patient may not show obvious rigidity if having large habitus and weak abdominal muscles and is very toxemic, ill, old, immunosuppressed, or pregnant (abdominal muscles pushed laterally by uterus) [3].

World Health Organization – endorsed priorities for assessing surgical patients should be:

Sick or well?
Stable or needs resuscitation?
What is your differential diagnosis?
Needs surgery? [4]

Further Information 1

You have ascertained some key facts concerning the area from the Internet and testimonies of others who have previously worked in the hospital. Local endemic

conditions include malaria, diarrheal disease, typhoid fever, ascariasis, tuberculosis, and HIV/AIDS. There are no services for radiography. You have seen doctors ordering hemoglobins, blood slides for malaria, HIV tests, Widal tests for enteric fever, and urine dipsticks. Equipment is scarce. You have checked with the clinical officers, and you have a full operating list this afternoon and a ward round to do. You are expected to be quick. You hurry down to outpatients and turn your attention to the young man who you are told is called Gabriel.

Gabriel speaks a local dialect – a nurse translates. Gabriel describes a two-week history of moderate central abdominal pain with fever. It has suddenly got much worse two days ago, and he has started to vomit his food up, prompting him to come in. His bowels last opened yesterday. No urinary symptoms. He has never been to hospital before. He takes no medications and has no known drug allergies. He has come from a remote village two days travel away.

On examination:

Lying, he keeps still, and looks unwell.
Pallid conjunctiva, sclera not jaundiced. No abdominal scars.
RR: 24/min, PR: 126/min, radial artery palpable – normal volume.
Lungs clear to auscultation.
Abdomen rigid with generalized tenderness and percussion tenderness. Bowel sounds not heard. Non-tender mass in left hypochondrium, dull to percussion.
PR – feces on glove, no blood.

Prompt 3: How Do Tropical Presentations of Disease Differ from the Nontropical?

Tropical presentations may be confusing in a number of ways:

Disease-specific:

Tendency to affect multiple body systems.
Often nonspecific presenting features – e.g., fever and shortness of breath.
Late presentations give signs and symptoms unfamiliar to Western health-care professionals [3].

Context-specific:

Often multiple undiagnosed comorbidities.
Largely unknown past medical histories.
Lack of investigations able to perform.
Often empirical treatment is started before investigations, further confusing findings.

Therefore, local epidemiology and clinical acumen will have to determine your working diagnosis. In tropical surgery, the surgeon often has to think outside the

Table 14.1 Contrasting "traditional" and "tropical" surgical etiologies

Condition	"Traditional" common cause	"Tropical" cause
Large bowel obstruction	Tumour	Tumour, sigmoid volvulus
Small bowel obstruction	Hernia, adhesions	Hernia, adhesions, ascariasis
Bowel perforation	Diverticulitis, appendicitis, inflammatory colitis	Appendicitis, trauma, Salmonella typhi
Fracture	Accidental trauma, osteoporosis	Violent trauma, osteomyelitis
Pregnancy complications	Hemorrhage, thromboembolism	Hemorrhage, thromboembolism, infection, obstructed labor, complications of abortion, fistula
Common comorbidities	Cardiovascular, respiratory	Anemia, vitamin deficiency, malnutrition, ascariasis, malaria, TB, HIV/AIDS [2]

"box" of traditional medicine as taught in Western medical schools, as shown in Table 14.1:

Patients often present when complications have made their lives unbearable. Late presentations occur due to lack of money for treatment, lack of transport, reliance on local remedies and traditional healers, or even reluctance to leave jobs (and therefore livelihood) [3].

Expect patients to have comorbidities due to lack of primary health care.

Anemia may be relatively common in resource-poor settings due to parasitic infestations, malaria, etc.

In tropical areas with endemic malaria, a palpable spleen is a common occurrence (although splenomegaly may have other causes).

Prompt 4: What Is the Differential Diagnosis and Management Plan for a Patient with Peritonitis in the Tropics?

Differential Diagnosis

Gabriel is sick as he has features of peritonitis (tachycardia, tachypnea, rigid abdomen with percussion tenderness, absent bowel sounds). He may need resuscitative treatment. His symptoms and signs point toward an abdominal pathology. On balance, you can come up with the following differentials (see Box 14.2 below):

Box 14.2: Differential Diagnosis of Peritonitis in the Tropics

- *Appendicitis*: Very common cause of peritonitis throughout the world, especially in the young. Vague central abdominal pain with anorexia that becomes localized in right iliac fossa. Pain precedes the fever [3].

- *Perforated Peptic Ulcer*: Sudden onset of severe abdominal pain with board-like rigidity and guarding. Patient may have history of ulcer or melena [3].
- *Typhoid Perforation*: Infection with Salmonella typhi, via feco-oral route. Variable presentations, normally with preceding malaise, pyrexia, cough, and constipation. Perforation manifests as superimposed peritonitis.
- *TB Peritonitis*: Chronic abdominal pain, associated weight loss, ascites and night sweats, may be HIV positive.
- *Amoebic Colitis*: Infection with Entamoeba histolytica, spread by feco-oral route. 10 % are symptomatic (especially pregnant, young, malnourished) [5] with associated bloody/mucoid diarrhea [5]. Look for trophozoites in stool [4].
- *Pelvic Inflammatory Disease*: For females only – added for completeness! May have history of chronic pelvic pain or discharge. Risk factors for sexually transmitted infection include age<21, unmarried, new partner last 3/12, >1 partner last 3/12, and symptomatic partner [5].

- Acute appendicitis is a very common cause of acute abdomen throughout the world and is a reasonable first diagnosis to make.
- Perforation secondary to typhoid fever is a good differential given Gabriel's symptoms, signs, and the fact that enteric fever is endemic here.
- Another common cause of perforation is peptic ulceration, but Gabriel had no previous dyspeptic symptoms.
- Incomplete obstruction could cause Gabriel's symptoms, but his bowels are loose, and we would expect constipation. Also, it would not explain his fever or how unwell he is at present. Ileus/pseudo-obstruction from systemic disease is an unlikely option. The presence of tenderness suggests abdominal pathology.
- Malaria is also endemic here and can cause a wide range of symptoms. Although unlikely, it should be kept at the back of your mind as a possible differential. Other infective causes like abdominal tuberculosis should be considered.

Management

- Ideally you would want blood tests like amylase and full blood count plus an erect chest radiograph to exclude perforation and a CT scan or ultrasound. Obviously, these tests are impossible in this environment.
- If your patient shows signs of generalized peritonitis, but is not moribund, proceed to laparotomy.
- If localized peritonitis only, with local abdominal tenderness and generally "'well," consider nonoperative treatment.
- If your patient is moribund with a distended or board-like abdomen, a thready pulse, and a very low blood pressure, prognosis is poor. Operative treatment may not alter the outcome.
- Resuscitation is critical, especially fluid rehydration if dehydrated [3].

Further Information 2

Gabriel is admitted. He is started on fluids – you can only find 1 liter of normal saline that is in date. You have prescribed antibiotics which you give yourself as the nurses have gone home. You order a hemoglobin and Widal test for typhoid fever but are not hopeful that these will be done today. You want to explain to Gabriel that he is very sick and needs an operation, but there are no translators.

You send a text message to a colleague to discuss the case. Your main suspicion is appendicitis, as Gabriel is young and appendicitis is common. You feel he has separate comorbidities that explain his long-term abdominal pain, splenomegaly, and pallor. However, you are persuaded to operate on Gabriel with a midline laparotomy incision as the diagnosis is equivocal. Gabriel's hemoglobin test is back; Hb: 6 g/dL.

Prompt 5: Outline Surgical Considerations in Tropical Surgery

Surgery in resource-poor environments deserves unique considerations:

General Considerations

What is the indication for surgery? What will happen if you do not operate – is your patient likely to die? When life is in danger, risky surgery can be rationalized – although with consideration toward prospects for life after the surgery including rehabilitation and social impacts. When a patient is very sick, be alert to the fact that surgery with inadequate postoperative care may not alter a poor prognosis.
How difficult is the operation? It is determine by technical knowledge, experience, skill, and resources. Be wary of undertaking difficult elective surgery, especially if limited/intangible benefit to the patient.
How safe is the operation? Ensure you have an experienced individual delivering the anesthetic. WHO recommends that the vast majority of acute surgical abdominal presentations can be managed with knowledge of three key incisions, midline laparotomy, gridiron, and groin incision for hernia [4].
What is the known or probable HIV status of the patient [3]?

Staff and Equipment

Essential Equipment: Dedicated operating room with table, washing area, lights, anesthetic equipment, necessary drugs, etc. [4]
Surgical Equipment: Forceps, scalpels, needle holders, retractors,and drapes
Layout and Function: Equipment to guarantee sterility, waste and sharps disposal [4]

Sterility

Sterility of equipment is crucial to avoid causing more harm than good to your patient. There are three commonly used methods for sterilizing reusable surgical equipment: autoclaving, dry heat, and chemical sterilization.

If routine methods of sterilization fail, WHO recommends the following:

Immerse towels and drapes for 1 h in antiseptic such as chlorhexidine/formaldehyde/glutaraldehyde, wring them out, and lay on patient's skin.
Treat gauze packs and swabs similarly but rinse them in diluted (1:1,000) chlorhexidine solution before using them in the wound. Rinse the gauze in this solution occasionally during the operation.
Hand wash instruments, needles, and natural suture materials, then immerse in strong antiseptic (chlorhexidine) for 1 h, and rinse them in weak antiseptic before use [4].

Ethical

The situation may seem desperate for the patient with little hope besides operation. However, you are not working abroad to practice and hone skills. For every operation that you conduct, you must be able to defend your choice on the grounds that it was a decision a reasonable doctor in your position would have taken.
Appreciation of local health infrastructures and attitudes toward disability are important. You should consider structures of rehabilitation and the prospects of your patient living a normal life post-op. There may be a heavy burden of social degradation associated with certain operations like amputations.
Informed, patient-led decisions should, whenever possible, be positively encouraged [2]. Consent should be obtained if possible.

Prompt 6: Outline Anesthetic Considerations in Tropical Surgery

Physiology

- Normal fluid requirements for an adult are 70 mL/kg/24 h or roughly 3 L/24 h (1.5 L urine, 1 L sweat, breath 0.5 L) [2]. In hot climates, an adult can lose up to 1 L of sweat per h, a significant loss that is exacerbated by febrile illness. Maintaining adequate fluid balance is therefore of utmost importance in the perisurgical period. Patients may need fluid resuscitation before they are ready for surgery.
- Blood loss is always a significant problem in surgery. In austere environments, anemia is common due to malaria, iron deficiency, hookworm or hemoglobinopathies. It may be hard to replace blood due to shortage of blood products or social mores. Consider a policy of a donation of a unit of blood from relatives of those to be admitted. Blood donated may be at high risk of passing on blood-borne infections like HIV, hepatitis B, and malaria. If syphilis or yaws is

common, blood may contain spirochetes, but these will die in 24 h storage. You must also take into account the nutritional status of the donor. No one under the age of 18 can donate blood products.

- Oxygen is often a scarce resource in tropical surgery. It should, if possible, be considered for those at extremes of age, the sick, or those with comorbidities like anemia. Oxygen concentrators are useful machines that run off main electricity and can produce fairly pure oxygen at a limited flow rate – 4 L/min maximum. Addition of 1 L/min of oxygen into the inspired gas can increase its oxygen concentration to circa 40 %, while 5 L/min can achieve a concentration of 80 % [4]. If there is a power failure, the oxygen supply will continue for about 1 further minute.

Anesthesia

Anesthesia in remote settings, like surgery, is subject to compromise. It is important to gauge level of anesthetic input required in a particular setting. If working in a remote health center with few available resources, you may be limited to local anesthetic techniques. Once you have the facilities for IV lines, resuscitation, and ventilation support equipment, then your arsenal can include inhalation, IV ketamine, and regional (e.g., spinal) techniques [4].

A popular anesthetic machine used in tropical countries and the military is the "draw over" apparatus. This comprises a vaporizer that atomizes liquid anesthetic into a gas (e.g., ether), with a delivery device like a self-inflating bag or Oxford inflating bellows. An alternative is a continuous flow system (Boyle's machine). This relies on compressed gases, commonly oxygen and nitrous oxide, which enter via flow-controlled valves, pick up vaporized anesthetic gas, and are delivered to the patient.

IV anesthetics are potentially very useful in tropical settings. Bonanno notes the utility of ketamine as it does not cause cardiovascular depression and can be used to sedate patients without the need for ventilation [6]. The use of regional anesthesia also avoids general anesthetic and reduces need for narcotics – with attendant side effects.

Prompt 7: How Do You Perform a Midline Laparotomy?

Midline laparotomy is a commonly used surgical incision.

- Incision: Make a midline incision through the linea alba big enough to allow access to the organs you want to operate on. Midline incisions enable good exposure of abdominal contents. Details can be found in reputable surgical textbooks.

As you incise the peritoneum, a puff of gas indicates perforated viscus. Insert your hand and gently break up any adhesions [3, 4].

- Observe: If the peritoneum is red with flakes of fibrinous exudate, suspect peritonitis. Fluid in the abdominal cavity may be:
  - Blood (e.g., ectopic pregnancy, trauma)
  - Small bowel contents (e.g., perforated peptic ulcer/typhoid ulcer)
  - Large bowel contents (e.g., ruptured appendix)
  - Ascites (e.g., hepatic cirrhosis, cardiac failure) [3, 4]

- Examine the Rest of the Abdomen: Limit your exploration to what is easily practicable [3]. Handle gut gently to avoid damage or ileus. Start at the ileocecal junction and work your way proximally until you reach the ileojejunal junction, looking for ileal ulcers/perforations (the jejunum does not perforate in typhoid). Tag each perforation you find. There is usually only one, and there are rarely more than three.
- Peritoneal Toilet: If localized peritonitis, do a local toilet only. If generalized peritonitis, wash out the entire peritoneal cavity. Pour in a liter of warm 0.9 % saline, mix it around with your hands, and then aspirate. Repeat up to four times.
- Close Abdomen: Completely without drains. Sometimes it is not possible to close the abdomen. Do not be afraid to leave the abdomen open – you may use an opened-out IV fluid bag to cover the wound and tack it to the wound edges – a "Bogota bag" closure. If you do not find any pathology, the peritonitis may be primary or related to a medical condition. Primary peritonitis without an established cause is common in Africa [3].

Further Information 3

Gabriel is anesthetized with ketamine induction and ether maintenance from a draw over apparatus that is driven by oxygen from an oxygen concentrator delivering 4 L/min due to his anemia. Your incision goes as planned with minimal blood loss. Gabriel's appendix is normal by eye – you remove it anyway. Moving to the small bowel, you notice that it is hemorrhagic and ulcerated with a small perforation, consistent with typhoid perforation (see Fig. 14.2):

You remove a section of Gabriel's distal small bowel with end-to-end anastomosis. You plan to continue his antibiotics for 2 weeks to cover Salmonella typhi. After 3 days of looking unwell, he makes a recovery. You also start him empirically on anti-roundworm medication. You discharge him with advice to tell family members to come to hospital if they experience similar symptoms and instructions to come back to hospital for reassessment in 6–8 weeks. He disappears and is lost to follow-up.

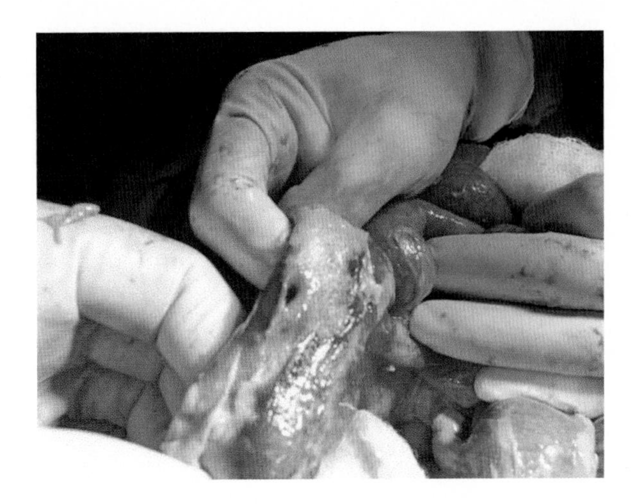

Fig. 14.2 Surgical view of typhoid perforation (Picture by David Nott [11])

Prompt 8: What Is *Salmonella typhi* and Typhoid Fever?

Typhoid (enteric) fever is infection by *Salmonella typhi*, a gram-negative bacteria. It is spread by feco-oral route to the gut where it infects mesenteric lymph nodes. From there, it spreads to reticuloendothelial tissue like other lymph nodes, spleen, and liver, thus causing a secondary bacteremia.

Classically, typhoid fever is a 4-week illness:

- Week 1: Malaise, pyrexia, cough, and constipation
- Week 2: Toxic, high temperature with relative bradycardia, rose spots (pink blanching papulae), hepatosplenomegaly
- Week 3: Very toxic with high fever, prostration, thread pulse, basal crackles on lung exam, and pea soup diarrhea
- Week 4: Convalescence [5]

Treatment is with early antibiotics, depending on local protocol – e.g., IV cefotaxime.

Complications include GI hemorrhage with per rectum bleeding and, most seriously, GI perforation which often necessitates surgery [5].

Further notes on typhoid perforation

- In areas where typhoid perforation is common (e.g., Ghana, West Africa), it is one of the commonest causes of an acute abdomen. Most patients perforate outside hospital.
- A typhoid perforation is seldom dramatic. Loops of gut stick together, preventing leaking gut contents from spreading widely. A patient can rarely identify the moment it happened. Tenderness usually starts in the right lower quadrant, spreads quickly, and eventually becomes generalized with guarding but rarely the board-like rigidity characteristic of chemical peritonitis.

- Percuss patient's lower ribs anteriorly; if there is gas between them and his liver, the percussion note will be resonant (absence of normal liver dullness).
- Hypotension, oliguria, and bradycardia are terminal signs [3].

Prompt 9: What Postoperative Considerations Must Be Made for Patients in a Tropical Environment?

In austere environments, one cannot take for granted that staff or equipment for routine postoperative management will be available. Follow-up should therefore include a careful examination and enquiry into postoperative symptoms.

Complications

- In sick postsurgical patients in poor-resource settings, be prepared for surgical complications: ileus, wound infection, wound dehiscence, intra-abdominal abscesses, fistulae, incisional hernia, and respiratory infections.
- Wound infection is more likely to occur in operations that:
  - Are lengthy.
  - Are for infective conditions.
  - Leave dead tissue/dirt/foreign bodies in the wound.
  - Involved inappropriate immediate primary closure when delayed primary closure may have been more appropriate.
  - Are carried out on immune-suppressed patients. If wounds fail to heal, think HIV [3].
- Do not forget the primary pathology. Renewed abdominal pain and peritonitis may signify another typhoid perforation. Sudden temperature spike may indicate wound infection, subphrenic abscess, or a fistula. Patients with typhoid fever may develop severe postoperative diarrhea that is difficult to treat [3].

Treatments

- It may be unreasonable to expect nursing staff to perform observations as regularly as in the UK.
- Check local attitudes toward oxygen therapy as it is often viewed as a palliative measure signifying that a patient is moribund, and so relatives may try to remove it.
- Analgesia can also be a problematic issue. In some sub-Saharan African cultures, the pain threshold is significantly higher than in the UK, and women give birth in silence! Furthermore, you should steel yourself for the reality that patients may often be left postoperatively with minimal analgesia.

Follow-Up

- Never count on being able to see your patients again! You should try and mold your plan for follow-up around the possibility of limitations of access to continual treatment for your patients.

- Alternatives are to provide community outreach clinics in which you can give limited treatment directly and follow up discharged cases.

Case Study: Future Tropical Surgery in Africa?

On paper at least, surgery began in Africa. Since its inception, it has been characterized by innovation, heterogeneity, and the challenge of few providers for bottomless wells of medical need. Indeed, surgical practice has arguably been blighted by the lack of trained surgical personnel, problems of maintaining equipment and sterility, and high infection rates with blood-borne viruses in blood transfusions [7]. This century, the world is turning, with more emphasis on developing countries finding locally devised solutions to their medical problems. Damien et al. note the need for increased accountability of surgical practice and greater involvement of mid-level practitioners for certain surgical procedures in Ghana [8]. This would spread the management of the surgical work load effectively. Similarly locally minded, Mungadi argues that most rurally presenting surgical cases are noncomplex and could be successfully treated by outreach surgical teams in the remote health centers that they presented to [9]. Precautions to be aware of limitations were crucial as a few adverse incidents were enough to scare communities away from health visitors [9]. The concept of health visitors introduces another pervasive issue in tropical surgery – access to skilled health-care workers. Problems surrounding lack of access to hospital or health clinic are multifactorial and penetrate to the infrastructural level.

References

1. Gill G, Beeching N. Tropical medicine. 6th ed. Chichester: Blackwell Press; 2009.
2. Nott D. Association of Surgeons in Training Yearbook, 2009-2010'. The Rowan Group, London 2010. Accessible online at http://www.asit.org/assets/documents/ASiT_Yearbook_2010.pdf. Accessed on 5 Jan, 2012.
3. Primary surgery. Accessible from: http://www.primary-surgery.org/. Accessed on 5 Jan, 2012.
4. WHO manual, surgery at the district hospital. Accessible from: http://www.who.int/surgery/publications/en/SCDH.pdf. Accessed on 5 Jan, 2012.
5. Eddleston M, Davidson R, Brent A, Wilkinson R. Oxford handbook of tropical medicine. 3rd ed. Oxford: Oxford University Press; 2008.
6. Bonanno F. Ketamine in war/tropical surgery (a final tribute to the racemic mixture). Injury. 2002;33(4):323–7.
7. Umolu PI, et al. Human immunodeficiency virus (HIV) seropositivity and hepatitis B surface antigenemia (HBSAG) among blood donors in Benin city, Edo state, Nigeria. Afr Health Sci. 2005;5(1):55–8.
8. Damien P, et al. How are surgical theatres in Africa utilized? A review of five years of services at a district hospital in Ghana. Trop Doct. 2011;41:91–5.
9. Mungandi I. Quality surgical care for rural dwellers: the visiting option. Trop Doct. 2005;35:151–3.
10. Photo courtesy of D. Nott.
11. Photo courtesy of D. Nott.

Chapter 15
Surgery in Austere Environments

David MacGarty

Learning Objectives

- Describe the process of surgical deployment to international disasters
- Understand the importance of planning before departure
- Determine the priorities in postdisaster surgical management
- Describe the pattern and treatment of traumatic injury following an earthquake
- Investigate the burden of amputation on populations emerging from disasters
- Discuss criticism of short-term surgical intervention
- Outline the importance of clinical governance and audit to surgical aid

D. MacGarty, MBBS, BSc
FY2 Doctor, Department of Obstetrics and Gynaecology, St Peter's Hospital,
Chertsey, Surrey, UK
e-mail: dmacgarty@hotmail.com

D. MacGarty, D. Nott (eds.), *Disaster Medicine*,
DOI 10.1007/978-1-4471-4423-6_15, © Springer-Verlag London 2013

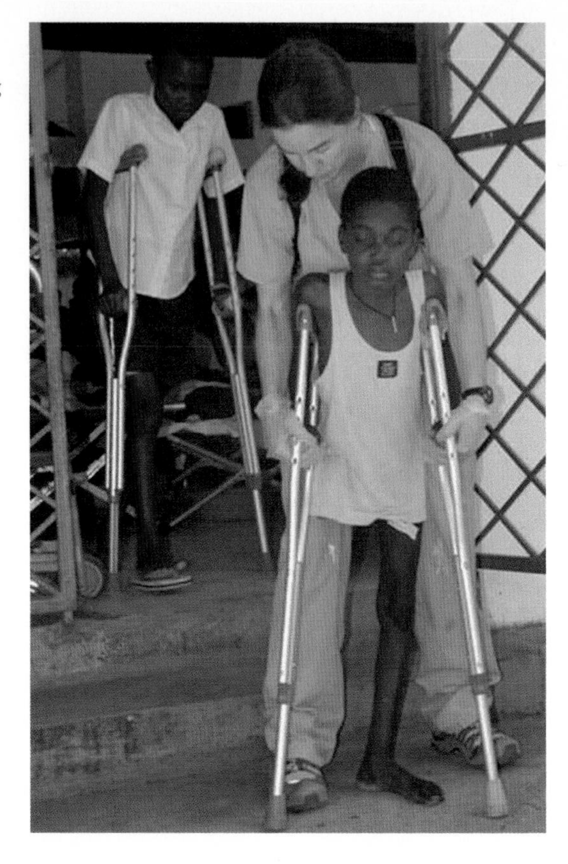

Fig. 15.1 A Haitian boy takes the first steps on his crutches with the support of a nurse after having a leg amputated at the Milot Hospital (Photo taken by Robert J. Fluegel - US Navy).

Initial Scenario

As you take a break during Monday's orthopedic list, you sit in the doctor's mess to eat your lunch. Your attention is snatched by a news report showing live footage of an earthquake on a Caribbean island. The footage shows devastated streets and buildings and panic-stricken locals wandering in shock. Initial reports predict a catastrophe with unprecedented casualties. Having previously deployed on two postdisaster missions, you contact your NGO and tell them you are ready to deploy. You complete your surgical list and go home.

You are woken early the next morning by a call from the NGO. They want you to prepare for departure. A hospital in a northern region of the island has been severely damaged. The hospital is inundated with the patient swell, and surgical trauma support is needed.

You will deploy with a team of 11 surgical staff on Tuesday evening and your team will be met at the airport with basic supplies and equipment. Reinforcements and further supplies will be flown in 48 h after your arrival.

Prompt 1: How Do You Make Yourself Available for Deployment?

The UK International Emergency Trauma Register was launched on 14th May 2011 at University Hospital of South Manchester NHS Foundation Trust [1]. It is a formal register of UK surgeons, anesthetists, emergency physicians, nurses, and other supporting medical and paramedical staff who are committed to deploying to international emergencies:

- The Trauma Register liaises with Trust executives to ensure volunteer deployments are fairly spread between Trusts and that Trusts are adequately compensated. It is hoped that colleagues who are not dispatched will cover for those who deploy and that each Trust understands the importance of the work.
- Registration with the Trauma Register allows deployment at very short notice, typically within 24–48 h of notifying the Trust. It is envisaged that each volunteer will be deployed for between 2 and 4 weeks per mission.

Prompt 2: What Must Be Considered Before You Deploy?

- Have you been invited by the host country? The WHO strongly advises humanitarian teams to avoid deploying until they are invited [2]. In many cases, NGOs will be present prior to disaster in the affected country and will invite personnel directly. Invites from the host nation will follow an initial postdisaster needs assessment and will come through official channels.
- Do you have access to information on the ground? Accurate, up-to-date information ensures you are directed to where you are needed while raising awareness of danger in the area. Again, this will be lead by organizations present on the ground.
- Do you have a clear mandate? The purpose and requirements of the deploying team must be clear to ensure the correct personnel, equipment, and supplies are provided for the correct amount of time.
- Humanitarian teams who turn up without invitation, local information, or a clear mandate are most likely to be a burden to the relief effort [2].

Prompt 3: Who Should Be Deployed in the Team?

- Experience: Deployed staff must be clinically experienced and have adequate preparation and training for disaster zones. Medical personnel unfamiliar with the environment have proven to be not only of limited utility but often have turned out to be a burden and a source of contention for the host community [2].

- Suitability: The deploying team must be familiar with the recipient Ministry of Health's or WHO's treatment guidelines. The team must be able to communicate and collaborate with patients, the local authorities, and colleagues in the health services. Dissimilarities in culture and language have resulted in misunderstandings between the external helpers and the local staff [2]. Some of the staff should speak the language, and interpreters should be provided.
- Team Structure: McIntyre et al. (2011) describe postdisaster surgical teams working in Haiti: "The common basic structure of each surgical team included varying numbers of orthopaedic, plastic and general surgeons as well as anaesthetists, operating room technicians and nurses. The average team size was 9 people" [3]. There are now very few general surgeons capable of managing all the surgical presentation following disasters. This has necessitated the deployment of groups of surgeons "hunting in teams," where several disciplines work together [4]. The composition of the team should reflect the location, the injury profile, and the time of arrival post disaster.

Further Information 1

After a long journey, you arrive at the hospital 48 h following the earthquake. It is early morning, and a sea of people surround the hospital with many families camped in the grounds and long queues seen outside tents.

The hospital director greets you. He explains hospital staff have been working nonstop since the earthquake and are exhausted. They have moved existing patients into makeshift wards outside the hospital, and tents have been set up for casualties of the earthquake. Both surgical theaters are ruined, and there is no trauma surgeon on-site. No major surgery has been attempted.

The director asks if your team could proceed with helping local staff treat and manage casualties, and he asks for surgical intervention to begin immediately. A quick tour reveals more patients than you anticipated, a third of whom are children. There is no salvageable anesthetic equipment, no pressurized oxygen, and very few drugs. The X-ray and biochemistry departments are ruined.

Prompt 4: What Are Your Initial Priorities?

As time passes following a sudden-impact disaster, the emphasis of casualty management changes:

- The priority in the first 48 h (phase 1) is early emergency medical care involving effective triage and application of ATLS skills [4]. The vast swell of initial casualties must be provided with immediate life-saving resuscitative and supportive care (including resuscitative or damage control surgery for those who are unable to tolerate delay – see "Military Trauma").

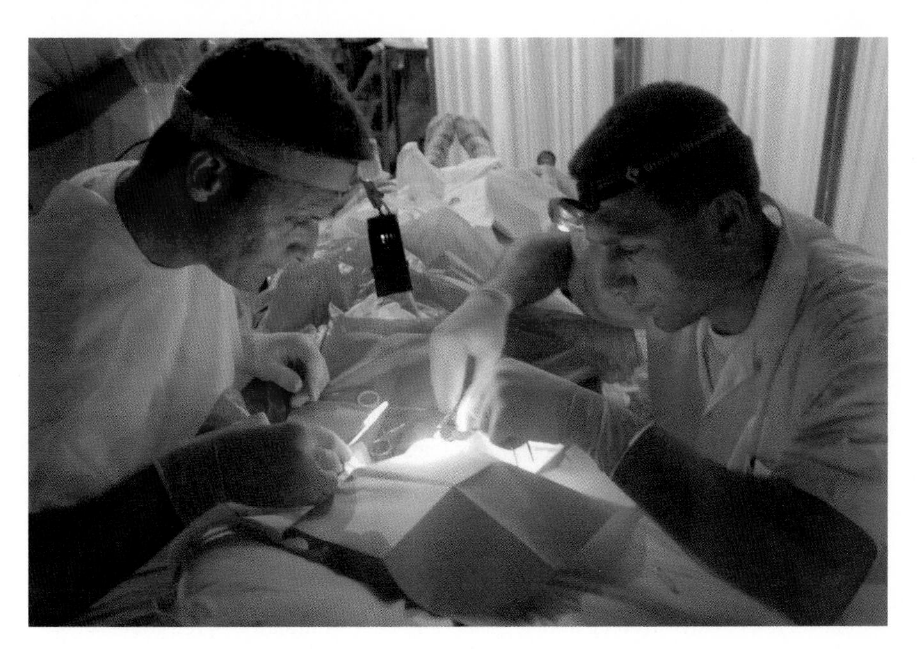

Fig. 15.2 Improvised surgical unit. (Photo taken by the Israel Defence Force)

- In phase 2 (48 h onward), the emphasis shifts toward elective surgery and follow-up care for trauma cases, new emergencies, and routine health care [2].

Given that the disaster response is entering phase 2, the priority is shifting toward trauma care. The WHO-PAHO guidelines for the use of foreign field hospitals in the aftermath of a sudden-impact disaster recommend [2]:

1. Set up an operating theater and an ICU:
   An enclosed environment is required for surgery so a new tent should be set up with a partition down the middle, one side for the operating theater, the other for an ICU. The operating theater must have adequate lighting and ventilation. The operating table and instrument counters may have to be improvised and all should be regularly cleaned with disinfectant. The ICU department is important for the postoperative care of major surgery cases (see Fig. 15.2).

2. Formulate a plan:
   A rotation should be established which gives each team member time to rest and ensures each member moves around and takes on different tasks.

   Collaboration with the local medical team should be planned to improve working efficiency. A team member who speaks the local language should be appointed to liaise with local staff and help coordinate care between teams.

3. Triage – prioritize patients for surgical treatment:
   A priority list of patients based on surgical need should be established. This will be used to form a surgical list. Life-threatening cases should be treated first.

4. Improvise medical record keeping:
   Adequate patient records are rarely kept during the first 48 h. A system for record keeping should be initiated to document patient identity, the procedure performed, operating staff, and any complications encountered. This will help the planning of follow-up care and will allow audit of case types and case load.

Prompt 5: Describe the Pattern and Treatment of Traumatic Injury Following an Earthquake

Without specialist, medical, and surgical help, patients with severe crush injury to the head, chest, and abdomen are likely to die in the first 48 h [5]. The most common injury presentations following earthquakes are lacerations, extremity fractures, and crush injuries [5–7]. Guidelines for the treatment of these injuries have been reproduced with permission from WHO's "Surgical Care at the District Hospital" [8].

Laceration wounds:

- Lacerations are most common on the face and scalp. These wounds may be associated with neurovascular injury, so a complete examination is required.
- Clean wounds should be sutured immediately and allowed to heal by primary intention.
- Clean contaminated wounds with normal but colonized tissue should be irrigated and packed open with saline gauze. The wound should be closed after 2 days (delayed primary closure).
- Infected wounds containing pus should be left to heal by secondary intention following wound toilet and debridement (see Box 15.1).
- All patients should receive antibiotics, e.g., ceftriaxone IV or oral amoxicillin, and should be immunized for tetanus.

Fractures of the extremity:

- Fractures during earthquakes are most frequently caused by collapsing structures.
- Closed fractures of the extremity do not require emergency treatment. Closed upper extremity fractures should be reduced under anesthesia and immobilized. Closed displaced fractures of the femur should be treated with skeletal traction.
- Open fractures should be urgently treated with wound toilet, debridement, wound excision, and fracture immobilization. The fracture should be stabilized after wound debridement with a padded posterior plaster slab, a complete plaster cast (split to avoid compartment syndrome) and traction or external fixation. Definitive fracture management should be performed at a later time.
- Infected open fractures require urgent toilet and debridement. If the wound is gangrenous and/or there are systemic signs of sepsis, amputation may be indicated (see Box 15.2 and Fig. 15.3). Early amputation is also indicated if vascular supply and sensation are lost or there is severe damage to three of the five major tissues (artery, nerve, skin, muscle, and bone). Amputations in children should, when possible, preserve the growth plate.

Box 15.1: Wound Debridement Procedure

Wound debridement is by far the most common surgical procedure following earthquakes [6, 7]. The WHO-approved technique is as follows:

1. Scrub the skin with soap and irrigate the wound with saline. Then prep the skin with antiseptic (do not use antiseptic within the wound).
2. Debride (clear) the wound meticulously to remove any loose foreign material such as dirt, grass, wood, glass, or clothing.
3. With a scalpel or dissecting scissors, remove all adherent foreign material along with a thin margin of underlying tissue and then irrigate the wound again.
4. Continue the cycle of surgical excision and saline irrigation until the wound is completely clean.
5. Leave the wound open after debridement and wound excision to allow healing by secondary intention.
6. Dress the wound lightly with damp saline gauze and cover the wound with a dry dressing (do not pack the wound).
7. Change the dressings daily [8].

Box 15.2: Guillotine Amputation [7]

Amputation refers to the surgical or traumatic removal of the terminal portion of the upper or lower extremity. Following an earthquake, amputation is performed to treat severe infection and to remove a limb following irreparable trauma to the extremity. Guillotine amputation is rarely necessary on modern deployments. However, in the face of mass casualties where resources are limited, it may be necessary to resort to this technique for limbs that are beyond salvage and nonviable and where time precludes creation of conventional muscle-covered flaps. It is the least desirable amputation approach as further definitive surgery is very difficult.

Crush injury:

- The longer a person is trapped under rubble or does not otherwise receive treatment following a crush injury, the more likely they are to suffer from crush syndrome. This is a serious condition resulting from damage to large areas of muscle which subsequently releases toxic muscle cell components and electrolytes into the circulation. It is associated with reperfusion syndrome which causes acute hypovolemia and metabolic abnormalities, lethal cardiac arrhythmias, and renal failure. In a postdisaster situation, crush syndrome is difficult to treat, and attempts should be made to prevent the crushed body part from abruptly releasing toxins. Amputation is frequently used to prevent crush syndrome.

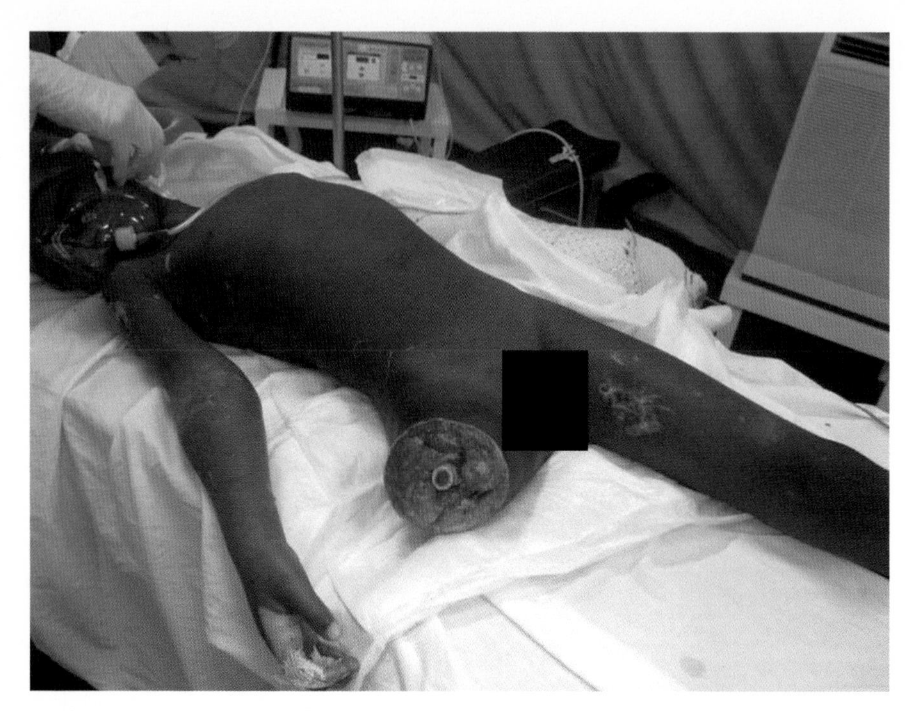

Fig. 15.3 Postguillotine amputation (Picture by David Nott)

Further Information 2

Thirty-six hours later, the swell of patients is unabated, and a high proportion of them require surgical intervention. The makeshift surgical theater has been operating nonstop, and staff are fatigued. Supplies of local anesthetic and ketamine are running low. Many amputations have been performed, and many more are needed, but continuing without ketamine would be unethical. You decide to suspend major surgery until supplies and reinforcements arrive.

The paramedic calls you to see a young patient named Luc who has an open compound fracture of the left tibia and fibula. Despite the injury, Luc lies motionless and quiet. He is tachypneic, sweating, and febrile, and he looks very pale. The soft tissue around the wound is deep purple in color, and it oozes pus and smells putrid. You decide not to amputate. It would be inhumane to operate without an anesthetic, and so you will manage Luc conservatively with antibiotics and analgesia until supplies arrive.

As red sunlight illuminates the lower tent edges, you hear the distant roar of a convoy. You are relieved from your post and take some rest. The last 48 h have been draining; there were many difficult surgical decisions to make. Luc died during the night of septic shock.

Prompt 6: What Factors Lead to the High Number of Amputees?

- Many late presentations: During the initial emergency response, only the most serious trauma cases are admitted for treatment. Lack of access to medical and surgical treatment results in many patients presenting late with complications [3]. In a warm environment with no medicine or antibiotics, infection spreads fast and may develop gangrene before the patient receives medical attention.
- Triage: Where urgent intervention is needed but there is an undersupply of surgical staff and supplies to cope with the patient load, early definitive treatment is favored over slow, intricate salvage procedures.
- Human factors: Limb amputation requires careful preoperative thought and consultation between surgeons and informed consent from the patient. The patient surge following a disaster puts extreme pressure on surgical teams and may compromise usual management processes [8].

Prompt 7: What Handicap Do Amputees Face?

- In 1980, the World Health Organization defined handicap as "the consequence of disability for the patient" [9].
- Handicap is the disadvantage in the fulfillment of an individual's role within society resulting from impairment and disability. Handicap results in a change in an individual's status within society and is thus as much a social problem as a physical one.
- In many countries, amputees suffer marginalization in society and are less able to access aid and resources following disasters [10].

Prompt 8: What Follow-up Care Must Be Provided for Amputees?

Handicap International works all over the world to reduce the handicap of injured people following disaster. They recommend the following [10]:

- Rehabilitation centers: Physiotherapy should be provided to help amputees adapt and to reduce their handicap (see Fig. 15.1). Centers should provide orthopedic device fitting and mobile fitting teams to supply emergency temporary orthopedic devices and fit permanent prostheses, orthoses, and walking aids. Long-term follow-up is needed as the lifespan of a fitted prosthesis is 3 years, and children must be refitted every 6 months.

- Assistance with basic needs: Amputees and other disabled are at a disadvantage in the scramble for resources post disaster. Amputees require targeted support including the provision of accommodation, resources for cooking, and the opportunity to earn money.
- Psychosocial support: The psychological trauma caused by the earthquake and the amputation should be addressed. A platform should be provided where amputees can share experiences and receive support. There must also be an attempt to raise awareness within local communities to prevent stigma and stop amputees becoming marginalized.
- Training: Intensive training should be given to local staff in both rehabilitation activities and fitting of orthotic devices. This will help build local capacity and allow local management of amputees in the long term.

Further Information 3

Two weeks after the disaster, a field hospital is operational on the site of the original tents. The field hospital will remain for up to 2 years until the original hospital is repaired and operational. The emergency patient load is reduced, and medical attention has shifted to chronic and ongoing medical care, though many patients continue to present with infected wounds, some requiring amputation. It is unlikely that you will see any of these patients again, and you hope they will be followed up.

Two days before you leave for home, you read a newspaper report criticizing the surgical response following the earthquake. They argue too many amputations were done, and the country has been left with a disabled generation who will be unable to cope in the deprived circumstances following the disaster.

Prompt 9: List and Explain Some Common Criticisms of Short-Term Surgery Projects?

The seven sins of humanitarian medicine give a clear summary of common faults with postdisaster surgical projects [11]:

- Sin 1: Leaving a mess behind.
- Sin 2: Failure to match technology to local needs and abilities. High technology care raises patient expectations and places unfair pressure on native resources when foreign teams withdraw.
- Sin 3: Failure of NGOs to cooperate and help each other and to cooperate and accept help from military organizations.
- Sin 4: Failure to have a follow-up plan.

- Sin 5: Allowing politics, training, or other distractive goals to trump service while representing the mission as "service."
- Sin 6: Going where you are not wanted or needed and being poor guests.
- Sin 7: Doing the right thing for the wrong reasons.

Surgery in the immediate postdisaster phase sits uncomfortably with many of the seven sins above. In the case of amputation alone:

- A mess is left behind in terms of the long-term human and economic consequences of limb loss.
- There is a lack of technology for reducing handicap following surgery (such as orthoses).
- Often, surgeons in the postdisaster phase never see their patients again and require others to follow them up.

Given the severe disability associated with amputation in developing countries (where rehabilitation and prosthetic services are not widely available), a high priority should be given to preserving injured limbs.

Prompt 10: How Could the Amputation Rate Following Future Earthquakes Be Reduced?

In the age of evidence-based medicine, effective clinical governance and audit are essential in justifying new approaches to humanitarian aid. Hence, the research carried out by surgical teams operating after an earthquake can provide evidence required for better surgical care for survivors of future earthquakes.

- Surgical caseloads: Analysis of surgical caseload over time allows for more efficient planning for similar future disaster. In an interview with the BBC, Susan Wright (director of Medecins du Monde UK) said, "You always have a big wave of amputations from around the third day, for about a week afterwards. Then the demand for such surgery becomes less intense" [12].
- Success of surgical teams: Tailoring the composition of future surgical teams depends on analysis of the success of teams in recent disasters. A surgical team from Ireland composed of rotating personnel of five orthopedic surgeons, five plastic surgeons, and five anesthetists reported lower amputation rates than other equivalent surgical teams following the earthquake in Haiti. They argue "changes in workload over time (post disaster) demonstrate the benefit that an ortho-plastic limb salvage team can provide in the early stage of disaster relief." They emphasize the need for a quick response following disasters to ensure surgical expertise in the management of the initial influx of acute injuries. The organizers of this orthoplastic team are creating lists of equipment and supplies, as well as surgeons and other medical professionals needed for response to future disasters [13].

Case Study: Haiti

At 16.53 on Tuesday, 12th January 2010, a magnitude 7 earthquake destroyed much of Haiti's capital Port-au-Prince and the surrounding area. There was huge demand for emergency surgical care in the aftermath, yet health care infrastructure around Port-au-Prince was devastated. The subsequent efflux of survivors into the surrounding regions placed enormous strain on district hospitals.

"Partners In Health" run a number of hospitals in Haiti, and they documented the delivery of emergency surgical care across all their medical facilities during the aftermath. They found that 9.7% of all the emergency surgery cases resulted in amputation [3].

Handicap International estimates the total number of amputations since the disaster at between 2000 and 4000. Fitting centers for orthopedic devices have been set up with mobile fitting teams visiting rural communities. By January 2011, 426 prostheses and 465 orthoses had been fitted. Training initiatives have increased local capacity to provide rehabilitative care and to allow the management of disability within communities [10].

References:

1. Redmond AD, O'Dempsey TJ, Taithe B. Disasters and a register for foreign medical teams. Lancet. 2011;377:1054–5.
2. WHO-PAHO Guidelines for the use of Foreign Field Hospitals in the aftermath of sudden-impact disasters, 2003, International Meeting: Hospitals in Disasters – Handle with care, Published in Washington, D.C.
3. McIntyre T, Hughes CD, Pauyo T, Sullivan SR, Rogers SO, Raymonville M, Meara JG. Emergency surgical care delivery in post-earthquake Haiti: partners in Health and Zanmi Lasante experience. World J Surg. 2011;35(4):745–50.
4. Ryan JM. Natural disasters: the surgeon's role. Scand J Surg. 2005;94:311–8.
5. Missair A, Gebhard R, Pierre E, Cooper L, Lubarsky D, Frohock J, Pretto A. Surgery under extreme conditions in the aftermath of the 2010 Haiti earthquake: the importance of regional anaesthesia. Prehosp Disaster Med. 2010;25(6):487–93.
6. Mulvey JM, Awan SU, Qadri AA, Maqsood MA. Profile of injuries arising from the 2005 Kashmir earthquake: the first 72 hours. Int J Care Injured. 2005;39:554–60.
7. Centres for Disease Control and Prevention. Post-earthquake injuries treated at a field hospital Haiti – 2010. JAMA. 2010;305:664–6.
8. Surgical Care at the District Hospital (WHO guidelines http://www.who.int/surgery/publications/scdh_manual/en/index.html).
9. International Classification of Impairments, Disabilities and Handicaps (ICIDH), WHO, 1980 (http://www.who.int/classifications/icf/en/).
10. Handicap International Report, 2011, A Year of Action in Haiti, 4th January update (http://www.handicap-international.org.uk).
11. Welling DR, Ryan JM, Burris DG, Rich NM. Seven sins of humanitarian medicine. World J Surg. 2010;34:466.
12. Susan Wright (director of Medicine du Monde UK), quotation from BBC interview quoted in article 'Haiti medics braced for wave of amputations.' (http://news.bbc.co.uk/1/hi/world/americas/8469206.stm).
13. Clover AJ, Rannan-Eliya S, Saeed W, Buxton R, Majumder S, Hettiaratchy SP, Jemec B. Experience of an orthoplastic limb salvage team after the Haiti earthquake: analysis of caseload and early outcomes. Plast Reconstr Surg. 2011;127(6):2373–80.

Part IV
Tropical Medicine

Tropical medicine as a discipline is focused on health problems that are either unique to tropical regions or are more difficult to manage in tropical regions. Although the hot climate in the tropics is an important factor in the prevalence of certain diseases (e.g., through sustaining vectors for disease transmission), climate in itself is not the sole reason for disease prevalence in tropical regions. Other factors such as deficiencies in medication provision, disease prevention measures, housing, diet, sanitation and personal hygiene also contribute to difficulties. As such tropical medicine encompasses the study and practice of medicine in the resource poor setting.

There are too many specific diseases to mention in a book with this format. The aim here is to discuss and work through the management of several key problematic tropical diseases. Disease outbreaks may result in a disaster when resources are insufficient and/or there is poor local and regional knowledge for disease management. In considering difficult decisions and situations, it is hoped the reader will garner an understanding of the reality of disease control in the resource poor setting.

David MacGarty

Chapter 16
Polio and Vaccination Campaigns

Will Barker

With thanks to Professor Kim Mulholland.

Learning Objectives

- Recognize polio as a persistent global challenge despite eradication attempts
- Outline important global vaccine-preventable diseases
- Discuss the role of childhood immunization in reducing childhood mortality (Millennium Development Goal 4)
- Outline key elements of a immunization campaign
- Discuss public health interventions associated with immunization campaigns
- Explore the concepts of vaccine acceptability and vaccine misinformation
- Outline the role of epidemiology and surveillance in immunization campaigns
- Discuss the role of WHO and UNICEF in global immunization
- Understand the role of public-private partnerships in immunization such as GAVI Alliance
- Discuss challenges of public-private partnerships against the benefits of new technology and investment

Initial Scenario

You are a doctor in rural India working with a children's charity. There has been an outbreak of polio in one of your regions, and the Ministry of Health asks if your charity can help respond.

With thanks to Professor Kim Mulholland.

W. Barker, MBBS, MPhys
FY2 Doctor, St Thomas' Hospital, Westminster Bridge Road,
London, UK
e-mail: willbarker@doctors.org.uk

D. MacGarty, D. Nott (eds.), *Disaster Medicine*,
DOI 10.1007/978-1-4471-4423-6_16, © Springer-Verlag London 2013

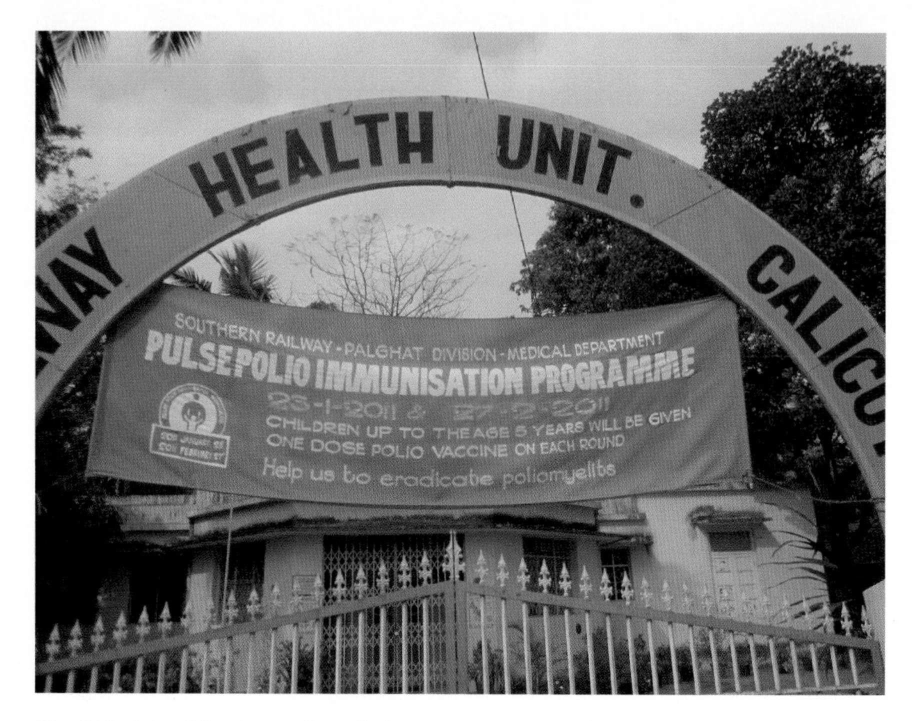

Fig. 16.1 Advertising for a pulse polio immunization program in southern India

So far, there are 23 confirmed cases of paralytic poliomyelitis, and the disease is in danger of spreading. The entire healthcare community is shocked as polio ceased to be endemic in India in 2011 after national polio eradication initiatives (Fig. 16.1).

Prompt 1: How Much Benefit Is Gained Through Childhood Vaccinations?

- In 1980, the WHO confirmed that smallpox had been eradicated from the world, making it the first and still the only human disease to be eradicated. This was a remarkable achievement considering that in the 1950s, 50 million cases occurred annually with mortality of 30–50 %. Eradication now saves an estimated 20 million lives a year.
- Building on the success of immunizing against smallpox, the Expanded Programme on Immunization (EPI) against polio, diphtheria, tetanus, pertussis, measles, and TB began in 1974. By 1990, the goal of universal childhood immunization to over 80 % of children in the world was achieved.
- Current vaccination programmes save about 2.5 million lives annually, although 1.5 million still die annually from vaccine-preventable diseases. Closing this gap

Table 16.1 Vaccines targeted by the Expanded Programme on Immunization (EPI) in 1974

Polio	Virus spread feco-orally causes permanent paralysis in some of those infected. Polio is close to being eradicated but remaining stubborn
Diphtheria	Bacteria transmitted by respiratory droplets causing serious respiratory illness. Mortality is 5–20 % of those affected
Tuberculosis	Bacteria commonly infecting the lung causing chronic infection that can disseminate throughout the body. Increasing in global importance due to multidrug resistance/total drug resistance and coinfection in people with HIV/AIDS
Pertussis	Bacteria causing whooping cough which can lead to serious respiratory complications such as bronchiectasis. It has a low case fatality rate but can lead to long-term lung disease
Measles	A very infective virus that infects the respiratory system. Mortality is low in developed countries but much higher among the immunosuppressed and vitamin A deficient and is particularly high when large epidemics occur in nonimmune populations. Despite good control in recent years, measles still claims over 100,000 lives every year [3]
Tetanus	Bacteria that produce a toxin that causes involuntary contraction of muscles and eventually paralysis and death. Transmitted by burns, cuts, and unskilled childbirth. Mortality is up to 80 % in developing countries, and it remains a major cause of neonatal mortality in the developing world [3]

is essential to meet the 2015 Millennium Development Goal of reducing child mortality by two-thirds relative to 1990 mortality levels.

- Vaccines are important players in reducing childhood mortality: UNICEF is the world's largest purchaser of vaccines, purchasing 40 % of vaccines used in the developing world. They also use supply chains to supply micronutrients such as vitamin A that reduces measles mortality further [1].
- The original EPI covered six diseases (Table 16.1). Before it started in 1974, less than 5 % of children worldwide were vaccinated in their first year; now, that figure is 79 % [2]. It is estimated this costs roughly $20 dollars per fully immunized child and saves one in ten making the cost per death averted only $200. Recently, the EPI has been further expanded to incorporate vaccines against hepatitis B and Hib and, most recently, against pneumococcus and rotavirus.
- The cost per disability-adjusted life year (DALY – see Box 25.1) saved may be as low as $7 in addition to other economic benefits such as parents able to work instead of caring for sick children [3].

Prompt 2: What Are Other Important Global Vaccine-Preventable Diseases?

- The WHO's highest-priority new immunizations available currently or potentially in the next 5 years are rotavirus and pneumococcal vaccines with malaria and dengue fever next.

Table 16.2 New and underused vaccines [4]

Meningitis A	A bacterial infection that is an important cause of septicemia and meningitis. Mortality untreated of >90% [4]. A breakthrough has been a new affordable meningitis A conjugate vaccine which was rolled out in 25 developing countries last year [5]
Pneumococcal	Protects against infections with Streptococcus pneumoniae, an important cause of pneumonia and meningitis and a wide range of other infections
Malaria	A disease caused by a blood parasite transmitted by mosquitos. It currently kills almost a million children under 5 each year but could be targeted by new vaccines currently in development
Hepatitis B	A highly infective virus endemic across Africa and Asia transmitted via blood and through vertical transmission. It causes massive morbidity from cirrhosis and liver cancer later in life
HiB	Effective against the most dangerous serotype of *Haemophilus influenzae*, which can cause meningitis and pneumonia especially in children. The vaccine is recommended for all countries. 27 million DALYs are lost each year in Asia as a result of infections with this organism [4]
Yellow fever	A viral infection transmitted by mosquitos, with a case fatality rate (CFR) of up to 20 % [4]. The vaccine is recommended in countries endemic for the disease, and proof of vaccination is required by some countries for those entering the country especially for travelers from endemic areas
Measles second dose	Increases immunity to measles and gives a second chance for children to be immunized. Of all the vaccines, it is likely to be most effective with lowest cost per death averted [4]
Rotavirus	Globally, over 500,000 children die each year from diarrhea caused by rotavirus, and two million are hospitalized. Many countries in Europe, Australasia, and Latin America are already using one of the two vaccines available [6]
HPV	A very common virus that is implicated in most cases of cervical cancer. New vaccines have become part of childhood immunizations in developed countries over the last decade, and several developing countries are using already them, including Fiji

- There is a "vaccine gap" whereby children in developed countries receive 10–12 antigens, whereas children in developing countries receive a maximum of 8 antigens if any at all [3]. The gap also exists for more modern vaccines with fewer side effects (e.g., the acellular pertussis vaccine) or simpler administration vaccines (e.g., MMR and other multivalent vaccines).
- There are also "neglected" vaccine-preventable diseases that primarily affect children in developing countries and hence receive little research. Table 16.2 shows some key new and underused vaccines in global health.

Prompt 3: What Is Polio?

- Polio is an acute viral illness spread through the fecal-oral route. Ninety percent of infections are asymptomatic. Sometimes, it infects the spinal cord causing meningitis with symptoms of an abrupt headache, fever, vomiting, and

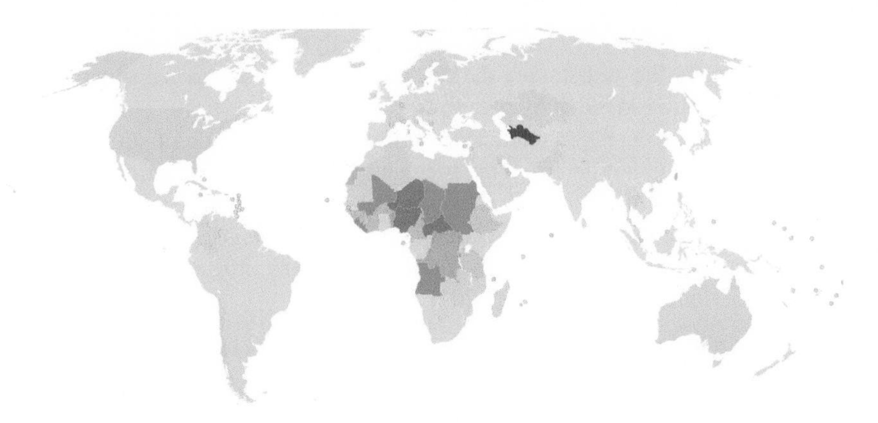

Fig. 16.2 Age-standardized disability-adjusted life year (DALY) rates from poliomyelitis by country (per 100,000 inhabitants) using WHO data from 2004 [8]. *DALY is disability-adjusted life year, a measure of health burden of a disease (see Chap. 25)

meningism. Normally, it resolves in about a week, but tragically, in 1 % of cases, lasting paralysis occurs.

- Polio outbreaks occur in countries with low rates of immunization, either when it is endemic in the population or following importation from endemic regions (Fig. 16.2). In tropical countries with poor hygiene and sanitation, it spreads rapidly through nonimmune populations. The incubation period is usually 7–14 days after which large numbers of virions are shed in feces for 2–3 weeks.
- Immunizations against polio were developed in the 1950s and have had a huge effect on controlling the disease. Two vaccine options are available, the oral (Sabin) vaccine and the injectable (Salk) vaccine.
- The oral polio vaccine is a live virus. It produces longer immunity, is cheap, can be delivered by untrained staff, and is transmitted to others in the community passing on immunity. As a live virus, it is contraindicated in immunodeficiency and pregnancy and has the capacity to mutate to cause vaccine-associated paralytic poliomyelitis (VAPP) in one in 750,000 vaccine doses [7]. In contrast, the injectable vaccine is more expensive but does not carry the risk of paralytic polio.

Prompt 4: What Is the Global Polio Eradication Initiative (GPEI)?

- The Global Polio Eradication Initiative (GPEI) began in earnest in 1988 with the goal to eradicate polio by 2000. GPEI aimed to maintain high levels of polio vaccination in infants, delivered both by routine immunization and by vaccination campaigns [9]. The eradication required huge effort as illustrated by the logistics required to immunize 200 million children in India (Box 16.1).

- In 1988, more than 350,000 children were paralyzed by polio in over 125 endemic countries. In the years since the eradication initiative was launched, the incidence of polio has fallen by over 99 %.
- Since 2000, progress to eradication stalled with "a decade of stalemate." This was due to failures in reaching adequate levels of immunization in the three remaining endemic countries (Nigeria, Pakistan, and Afghanistan*) and inadequate response to outbreaks in other nonendemic countries (Angola, Chad, and DR Congo) [9]. **Note*: Recently, India made strong progress against polio, and transmission was interrupted in 2011.

Box 16.1: The Equipment Needed for the National Polio Immunization in India [10]

- 225,000,000 doses of polio vaccine
- 2,000,000 vaccine carriers
- 6,300,000 ice packs
- 2,500,000 vaccinators
- 1,170,000 vaccination teams
- 155,000 supervisors in 155,000 vehicles
- 709,000 vaccination booths
- 174,000,000 children immunized

Further Information 1

You are asked to coordinate a vaccination program in response to the outbreak. You get funding approval for the campaign and start planning the logistics. Local staff inform you that outbreaks are occurring in areas with low vaccine coverage due to perceived harmful effects of the vaccination. The recorded national level of immunization is 70 %, although in rural areas you suspect it is lower.

To assess the severity of the outbreak, the ministry asks you to find the current immunization rates. You also investigate the capability of the Ministry of Health to respond and whether outside help is needed.

Prompt 5: What Are the Key Elements of a Vaccination Campaign?

- Vaccination campaigns can either target high-risk groups (e.g., Hep B for health workers) or follow a population strategy (e.g., the Expanded Programme on Immunization).

- Vaccination campaigns are exercises in logistics. They involve procuring large quantities of vaccine that must be safe and effective. Vaccines must be stored then distributed to the target population while keeping the vaccine and other important components (such as dilutants) refrigerated. Some vaccines are as sensitive to freezing or heating, and this requires careful control of the "cold chain."
- Where the immunizations are to take place, there must be facilities to store the vaccine and qualified staff to give the injections. An existing hospital or health center is ideal; otherwise, mobile immunization units are necessary. Parents must be encouraged to bring their children to the immunization center, and immunization must be done correctly with safe disposal of needles. Campaigns using fixed facilities instead of mobile units typically have half the cost per fully immunized child [4].
- Accurate records must be kept to measure the success of the campaign and prevent duplication of work; however, migration and low levels of literacy often complicate this. Overseeing the operation should be quality control: ensuring the quality of the cold chain, that vaccines are given correctly, and checking whether accurate records are made.
- There also must be disease surveillance at regional and national level involving both clinical and laboratory input.
- Part of a campaign may also be to introduce other effective public health measures such as hand washing, education, insecticide-treated mosquito nets, vitamin A, and other micronutrients.

Prompt 6: What Is Meant by Herd Immunity?

- For an infectious disease to spread through a population, a minimum proportion of susceptible individuals is required. If vaccination levels are high enough, chains of infection can be disrupted, protecting even nonimmune persons from the disease. The herd immunity threshold is the proportion of immunity in a population required to interrupt the spread of disease.
- The herd immunity threshold depends on the pathogen (mode of transmission, infectivity, etc.), population (general health, nutrition status, previous exposure to the pathogen or related organisms), and environmental factors (overcrowding, sanitation). For polio, immunity levels need to be about 80–86 %, and for measles, it is 83–94 %. Social factors such as overcrowding can increase infectivity and therefore increase the herd immunity threshold, as can factors that make people more susceptible to disease like malnutrition. A good example of herd immunity is Hib conjugate vaccines which have not only reduced the rate of invasive disease but the much more common rate of asymptomatic carriage [11].

- The ultimate goal of population vaccination is to get immunity levels over this threshold to prevent epidemics from happening. It also explains why, if vaccination levels are high enough, transmission can be halted. *Note*: Vaccination-based eradication campaigns will only work on pathogens for which there is no environmental (especially animal) reservoir.

Prompt 7: What Makes a Vaccine Acceptable and What Are the Complications of Vaccinations?

- For a vaccine to be acceptable, the disease must present a sufficient burden to justify the effort. The efficacy of a vaccine must then be demonstrated and tested in clinical trials before being introduced.
- Vaccinations carry very low risks, compared to the risk of the diseases they prevent. There are risks of minor reactions, usually a small rash, transient fever, or edema at injection site. In many fewer cases, there is the risk of anaphylaxis. Very low but important are the risks of serious side effects such as neurological impairment.
- Contraindications to vaccination are previous severe reaction to a vaccination and giving live vaccines to pregnant women or the immunosuppressed. Vaccination should also be postponed if the recipient has a severe febrile illness, but in general, WHO recommends vaccinating children with minor illnesses.
- As diseases become less prevalent, people may start to worry more about vaccinations than the illness. The MMR scandal in the UK has illustrated that even in developed countries where overwhelming evidence exists, conspiracy theories can seriously undermine vaccination efforts [12]. This is true in developing countries too; one discredited theory suggested polio vaccination was the source of the HIV epidemic [13]. Rumors are easily propagated and are hard to quell. For this reason, public health information campaigns form an integral part of effective vaccination programs.
- Vaccines must also be considered in the light of other disease management priorities (e.g., malaria, HIV/AIDS, and infectious diseases), balancing resources for existing and desired health programs. Campaigns must be sustainable for a national health service, but in practice, many require external financing support.

Further Information 2

As you strengthen disease-reporting capabilities, you find lack of information about the early stages of the epidemic allowed it to spread unnoticed.

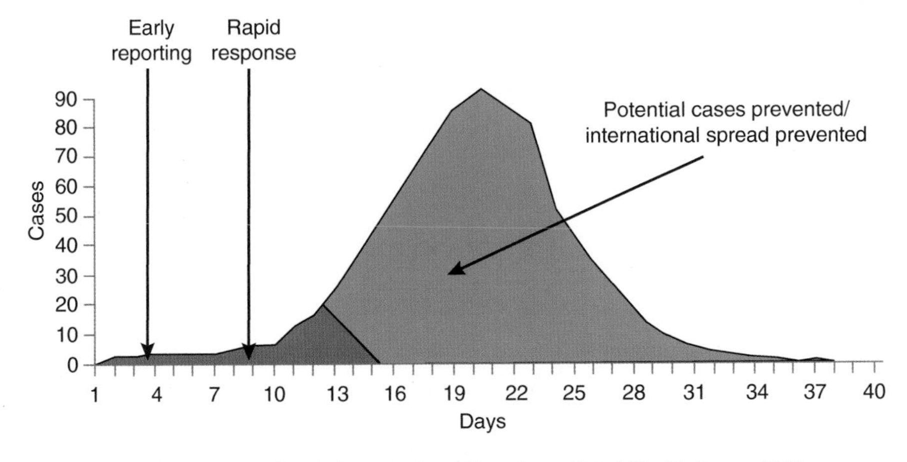

Fig. 16.3 The importance of early intervention (Taken from Global Health Report [15])

You discuss with your colleagues that better reporting would have allowed a quicker response containing the outbreak before it spread beyond the original villages. You also discuss other measures apart from vaccination which could have arrested the outbreak.

Prompt 8: What Is the Role of Epidemiology and Surveillance in Immunization Campaigns?

- WHO defines epidemiology as "the study of the distribution and determinants of health-related states or events (including disease), and the application of this study to the control of diseases and other health problems" [14; See Box 16.2 for definitions].
- Surveillance allows for rapid detection of and hence rapid responses to disease outbreaks, facilitating early containment (Fig. 16.3). Surveillance can either be clinical, microbiological, or both. For clinically based surveillance, there needs to be a good case definition to ensure uniformity of reporting.
- Serological epidemiology looks at previous exposure to a pathogen by testing for antibodies. With some diseases such as polio there is widespread subclinical infection significant in disease transmission since asymptomatic people may be highly contagious. However, serological date can be hard to interpret when there is widespread vaccine use.
- Developed countries manage disease surveillance by having notifiable diseases (based on clinical criteria and suitable case definitions) and reporting procedures and/or by a system of reporting from diagnostic laboratories.

- In developing countries, limitations come from lack of personnel, laboratories, communication technology, and infrastructure as well as fragmented health services. Development of suitable low-cost surveillance and reporting mechanisms are needed in areas where they are absent if there is to be sufficient information to assess the need for and effectiveness of disease control activities. Air travel now means people can travel the world in less time than the incubation period of most diseases meaning developed countries must also now have surveillance for exotic diseases.
- Targeted surveillance becomes more important in eradication campaigns as the disease approaches eradication, which adds to the expense. This is compounded by the fact that when the disease becomes rare, laboratories are particularly important to support clinical diagnosis.

Box 16.2: Definitions in Epidemiology [16]

Term	Definition
Case definition	A set of diagnostic criteria (either clinical or laboratory based or both) that must be fulfilled in order to identify an individual as a case of that particular disease
Prevalence	Number of cases at a particular time in a defined population
Incidence	Number of new cases during a particular period in a defined population
Endemic	Constantly present at a significant level in the community
Outbreak	Localized epidemic
Epidemic	An unusual increase in the number of cases in a community
Pandemic	Epidemic involving several continents at the same time
Primary index case	First case or group of cases
Secondary cases	People infected from the primary case[s]
Incubation period	Time from infection to onset of symptoms

Prompt 9: How Else Can Infective Disease Be Prevented? [17]

- The transmission of pathogens in analogous to the interaction of seed, soil, and climate [15]. In this analogy, the seed corresponds to pathogen factors such as survivability outside host, alternative hosts, mode of transmission, and pathogenesis; the soil corresponds to human factors such as number of susceptibles, demographics, nutrition, and immunity; the climate corresponds to environmental factors such as urban environment, animal vectors, overcrowding, and hygiene. To interrupt transmission, any step can be targeted.
- Actions on the individual level: Personal hygiene especially hand washing is usually the most important and simplest step. Personal behavior is also very important, e.g., safe sex against STIs.
- In addition to immunization, immunoprophylaxis or chemoprophylaxis can be used. Immunoprophylaxis is passive immunization and is performed by giving

preformed antibody for short-term protection, e.g., VZIG for nonimmune pregnant women exposed to chicken pox. Chemoprophylaxis is the giving of antibiotic or antiviral medication, e.g., rifampicin for people exposed to bacterial meningitis or antiretrovirals for people exposed to HIV.

- Actions on the community level: The most important is usually monitoring of safe water and food supplies. Longer-term town or camp planning can avoid slums and overcrowding and facilitate hygiene. Vectors such as mosquitos and flies should be controlled and information on safe behaviors shared.
- Isolation of those with dangerous infections can limit propagation of disease (e.g., limiting flows of people, implementing quarantines); social distancing works in a similar way (e.g., school closure, reducing workplace numbers, reducing social contacts, home isolation). Interventions targeted at those most likely to spread the disease can also be efficient use of resources (e.g., travelers or healthcare workers and surveillance of blood products).
- Quarantine gets its name from the seventeenth-century Italian word "quarantena" meaning 40 days – the time ships from plague-stricken countries had to wait off port. Since it involves the restriction of individual rights for the benefit of others, there is an inherent ethical conflict between the rights of the individual against that of society.
- Challenges to the battle against infective disease are immunosuppression (caused by AIDs and malnutrition), population movements (following drought, floods and conflict), and increasing amounts of international travel. Rapid global urbanization has led to the highest population densities in human history, which favor propagation of disease. Political or financial upheaval, insecurity, and decreased health funding all reduce the speed and effectiveness of response to new epidemics. It is no coincidence countries where polio eradication has been least successful are the world's most insecure.

Further Information 3

The campaign is successful, and you vaccinate 300,000 children in the affected area and neighboring provinces, achieving 90 % vaccination rates. The epidemic peaks and thankfully does not spread to other parts of the country or beyond India's borders.

In 6 months time, with no new cases, the epidemic is classified as arrested. You are pleased with the success of the campaign but know that you were lucky to contain the outbreak and ponder what can be done to improve vaccination rates.

Your campaign was only funded for one year, and so you are forced to lay off your trained staff and transfer responsibility to the health service. You worry if it can maintain sufficient vaccination rates and surveillance. You think about the role of WHO, public-private partnerships including GAVI Alliance, and new technology in facilitating vaccination.

Prompt 10: What Is the WHO Global Immunization Vision and Strategy?

Global Immunization Vision and Strategy (GIVS) is the framework developed by UNICEF and WHO to protect children from preventable diseases such as measles, tetanus, and whooping cough. Its delivery strategy has five objectives [18]:

1. To uphold immunization as a human right
2. To achieve equity in the use of vaccines
3. To seek synergies with other programs and reestablish immunization as a core component of primary health care
4. To develop immunization systems able to meet the challenges posed by the ambitious new goals
5. To bolster national self-reliance and partnerships

It aims for >90 % core vaccination coverage in every country over the coming 5 years and to reduce measles mortality by 90 % from rates in 2000 [19, Box 16.3]. It also hopes to ensure capacity for surveillance and monitoring, strengthen health systems, and make vaccinations sustainable.

The costs of implementing the GIVS goals in the 72 poorest countries were estimated to be $11–$15 billion over 2006–2015 [20]. To put it in perspective, this is the same cost as 8 B52 stealth bombers or 30 days of war in Iraq and Afghanistan.

Box 16.3: The Importance of Measles

Twenty years ago, there were over 1 million childhood deaths due to measles, and measles was a leading cause of blindness. Achievement of universal immunization goals in 1990 has controlled measles, bringing measles-related deaths down to 164,000 in 1998 [21]. However, its infectivity, high herd immunity threshold, and complacency mean current levels of vaccination still permit outbreaks in developed countries and epidemics in countries with low levels of vaccination. This is especially true in refugee camps created by disasters, highlighted by the Sphere Project as being the most important immunization in the disaster setting (Chap. 3). It remains a target for new vaccine deployment to increase the immunization rates above the herd threshold which may one day lead to it being targeted for eradication [21].

Prompt 11: What Is the Role of Public-Private Partnerships such as GAVI Alliance?

- By the end of the 1990s, immunization rates were stagnating or falling in the poorest parts of world. GAVI Alliance (formerly the Global Alliance for Vaccines and Immunisation) was launched in 2000 as a global health partnership to increase

vaccination development, uptake, and support vaccination campaigns in the poorest nations.
- GAVI Alliance's stakeholders include governments (developing world and donor); private sector philanthropists, e.g., Bill & Melinda Gates Foundation; the financial community; vaccine manufacturers; research and technical institutes; NGOs; and multilateral organizations such as WHO, UNICEF, and the World Bank.

The GAVI Alliance strategy (2011–2015) has four strategic goals:

1. Accelerate the uptake and use of underused and new vaccines
2. Contribute to strengthening the capacity of integrated health systems to deliver immunization
3. Increase the predictability of global financing and improve the sustainability of national financing for immunization
4. Shape vaccine markets

Eligible countries are those with gross national income (GNI) per capita <$1500. Eight countries account for two-thirds of the world's unimmunized children and are major GAVI recipients: India, Nigeria, Pakistan, Ethiopia, DR Congo, Sudan, and the Philippines.

Prompt 12: What Are the Strengths and Weaknesses of GAVI Alliance?

- GAVI Alliance has promoted the development of new vaccines, which has increased vaccine coverage. In its first decade, 280 million children have been immunized as a result, and WHO 2010 estimates more than 5 million child deaths have been prevented (Fig. 16.4). It has sped up the implementation of new vaccines and channeled private funding into vaccines.
- Despite its undoubted success, GAVI Alliance has received criticism from NGOs for its ties with pharmaceutical companies and for focusing on diseases individually, a so called "disease-siloed" approach. Recurrent costs (training, waste disposal, staff salaries, cold chains) receive little long-term funding and have to be repeated. Staff may be poached from national health services and employed on short-term basis undermining local services [22].
- GAVI Alliance only has remit for 5 years, which makes planning long-term funding of schemes difficult. New expensive vaccines are often prioritized over effective older cheaper ones, and the cost of new vaccines may be unsustainable leading to future funding crisis.
- GAVI Alliance reward systems for vaccine coverage often penalize countries with the most problems and may overlook essential elements such as cold chain and waste disposal. Broken cold chain linkages in rural areas are therefore not adequately monitored, and it probably encourages some countries to exaggerate coverage figures.

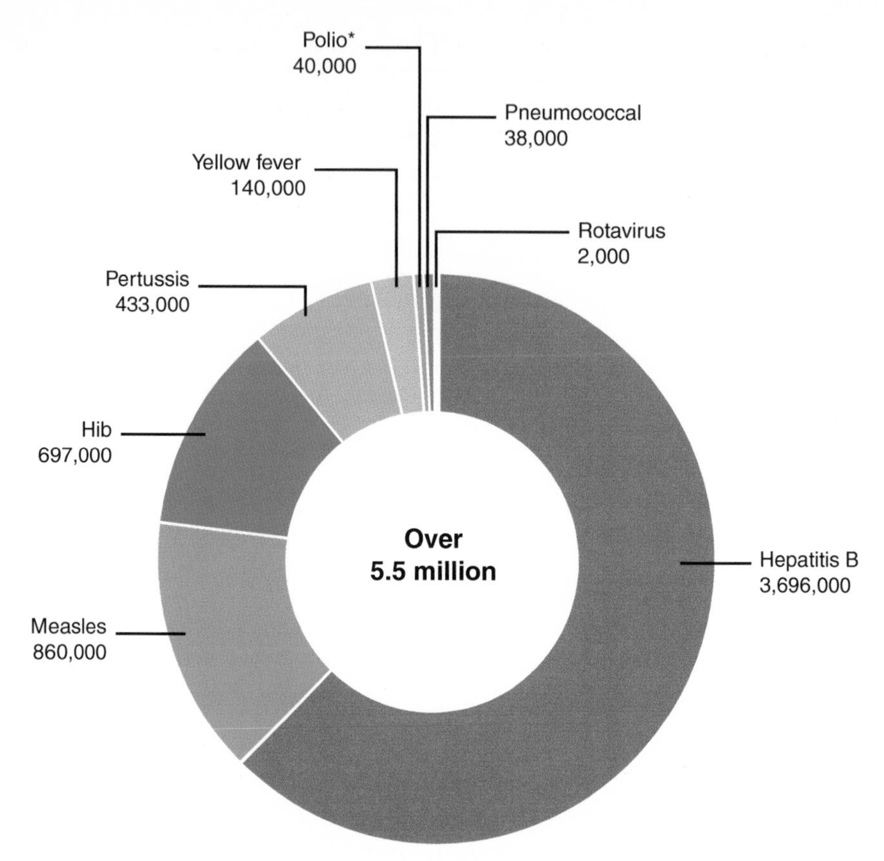

Fig. 16.4 Future deaths averted through GAVI support (2000–2010) [23] (*Source*: These estimates and projections are produced by the WHO Department of Immunization, Vaccines and Biologicals, based on the most up-to-date data and models available as of September 2011. Polio estimate includes deaths averted by vitamin A supplements supported by the GAVI Alliance)

- By far, the biggest problem with GAVI Alliance has been their failure to provide appropriate supportive research, especially for pneumococcal vaccine, which is beset by problems of serotype replacement.
- Global Health Partnerships have gone some way to respond to criticism and will continue to be part of the solution, although they will need to find ways

to be more efficient and sustainable in their use of resources in the next 10 years.

Prompt 13: What New Technology Is Available for Vaccination Program?

- New forms of vaccine storage boxes, autodisabled syringes, and incinerators will aid with programs. Vaccine vial monitors are also starting to be employed to ensure vaccine cold chains have not been disrupted.
- New heat-stable vaccines and multivalent vaccines may ease logistics by eliminating the need for cold chains and easing vaccine schedules [4]. Currently, new vaccines carry a price premium, which often outweigh savings that can be achieved, but if economies of scale can be properly harnessed, it could yield major breakthroughs.
- The lack of communication infrastructure is rapidly being overcome by global penetrance of mobile phone technology and the Internet. A new wave of software for logistics and epidemiology using mobile technology is also emerging which holds great promise, e.g., EpiSurveyor [24].

Prompt 14: What Are the Recommendations for Sustainable Development in Vaccines?

- Funding needs to be increased to meet the demands of an increased population and increased numbers of cost-effective vaccinations. The greatest costs of vaccination programs are the fixed cost of infrastructure and trained staff. Funding needs to be more reliable to allow staff and infrastructure to be retained and to improve negotiated contracts on vaccine supply [4].
- Ways of increasing efficiency of vaccination programs need to be developed. This can be through simple interventions such as revising the schedule of the EPI so that new vaccines can be added without additional visits. There also needs to be tailored vaccination schedules to address the different disease priorities in different countries [4].
- GAVI Alliance should cut costs by loosening ties with Western pharmaceutical companies and by investing in emerging nation producers that can produce vaccines at much lower prices. Development of meningitis A vaccine produced in India at $0.5 per dose provides a good model of how this can work.

Case Study: Angola

In August 2010, the Ministry of Health reported an outbreak of 19 cases of polio in six provinces. In addition to Angola's planned polio immunization campaign, UNICEF and WHO worked with the government to ensure that all 5.6 million children under five were vaccinated [25].

Polio cases originating in Angola spread across the border to the Democratic Republic of Congo and came close to wider international spread. Experts were worried that polio would become endemic in Angola and form a reservoir spreading polio to neighboring countries. Global experts also expressed concern about the risks of further spread and the high cost of conducting emergency response campaigns compared with routine vaccinations.

Angola's leaders took strong measures to respond to the epidemic, pooling financial support from multiple sources with a total of US $9.3 million committed to an emergency plan. This included support to routine immunization as well as additional nationwide campaigns to increase coverage to at least 90 %.

This case study shows the risks of incomplete coverage of childhood vaccination. Sadly, Angola together with Chad and the Democratic Republic of Congo currently have reestablished transmission.

At the same time, there is hope; with India for the first time no longer endemic with polio (no cases of polio in India in 2011). For polio eradication to make a long overdue breakthrough, increased political commitment is needed with secure funding, more resources, and increased technical ability [4].

If global efforts succeed in eradicating polio, this will be another massive victory for mankind, freeing up resources and inspiring efforts to eradicating other diseases such as pertussis, measles, and perhaps even malaria one day.

References

1. UNICEF: Millennium Development Goals 4. Reduce Child Mortality [Internet]. New York; Unicef [cited 2012 Apr 1]. Available from: http://www.unicef.org/mdg/childmortality.html.
2. UNICEF. Expanding immunization coverage [Internet]. New York; Unicef [cited 2012 Apr 1]. Available from: http://www.unicef.org/immunization/index_coverage.html.
3. Jamison DT, Breman JG, Measham AR, et al., editors. Disease control priorities in developing countries. 2nd ed. Washington, D.C.: World Bank; 2006.
4. GAVI Alliance. New and underused vaccine support [Internet] Geneva; GAVI Alliance [cited 2012 Apr 1]. Available from: http://www.gavialliance.org/support/nvs/.
5. World Health Organisation. Revolutionary new meningitis vaccine set to wipe out deadly epidemics in Africa. Press release OUAGADOUGOU; 2010, Dec 6 [cited 2012 May 12]. Available from: http://www.who.int/mediacentre/news/releases/2010/meningitis_20101206/.
6. Rotavirus Vaccine Program [Internet]. Seattle; Rotavirus Vaccine Program [cited 2012 Apr 1]. Available from: http://www.rotavirusvaccine.org/.

7. Nkowane BM, Wassilak SG, Orenstein WA, Bart KJ, Schonberger LB, Hinman AR, Kew OM. Vaccine-associated paralytic poliomyelitis. United States: 1973 through 1984. JAMA. 1987; 257(10):1335–40.
8. Profil L. Poliomyelitis world map – DALY – WHO2004 [Internet]. Using data from: Data from Death and DALY estimates for 2004 by cause for WHO Member States. Creative Commons. [cited 2012 Apr 1]. Available from: http://en.wikipedia.org/wiki/File:Poliomyelitis_world_map_-_DALY_-_WHO2002.svg.
9. Global Polio Eradication Initiative [Internet]. Geneva: World Health Organization. [updated 2012 Mar 27; cited 2012 Apr 1]. Available from: http://www.polioeradication.org/.
10. Donaldson L (Chair). Independent Monitoring Board of the Global Polio Eradication Initiative Report July 2011. [cited 2012 Apr 1]. Available from: http://reliefweb.int/node/427052.
11. Lipsitch M. Bacterial vaccines and serotype replacement: lessons from *Haemophilus influenzae* and prospects for Streptococcus pneumoniae. Emerg Infect Dis. 1999;5(3):336–45. PMID: 10341170.
12. Godlee F. The fraud behind the MMR scare. BMJ. 2011;342:d22.
13. Cohen J. Forensic epidemiology. Vaccine theory of AIDS origins disputed at Royal Society. Science. 2000;289(5486):1850–1.
14. WHO: Epidemiology [Internet]. Geneva; WHO [cited 2012 Apr 1]. Available from: http://www.who.int/topics/epidemiology/en/.
15. World Health Organization The world health report 2007: a safer future: global public health security in the 21st century. Geneva: The Organization; 2007.
16. Last J. Dictionary of epidemiology. Oxford: Oxford University Press; 1993.
17. Collier L, Oxford J. Human virology. 3rd ed. New York: Oxford University Press; 2006.
18. Global Immunization Vision and Strategy. Report by the Secretariat to the World Health Assembly 2011. Geneva: WHO; 2011 [cited 2012 Apr 1]. Available from: http://apps.who.int/gb/ebwha/pdf_files/WHA64/A64_14-en.pdf.
19. The Global Immunization Vision and Strategy (GIVS) [Internet]. New York; UNICEF: 2011 [cited 2012 Apr 1]. Available from: http://www.unicef.org/immunization/index_27089.html.
20. Wolfson LJ, Gasse F, Lee-Martin SP, Lydon P, Magan A, Tibouti A, Johns B, Hutubessy R, Salama P, Okwo-Bele JM. Estimating the costs of achieving the WHO-UNICEF Global Immunization Vision and Strategy, 2006–2015. Bull World Health Organ. 2008;86(1):27–39.
21. Mulholland EK, Griffiths UK, Biellik R. Measles in the 21st century. N Engl J Med. 2012;366(19):1755–7. PubMed PMID: 22571199.
22. Save the children UK. A Long Way to Go: a critique of GAVI's initial impact. London; Save the children UK: 2002. [cited 2012 Apr 1]. Available from: http://www.savethechildren.org.uk.
23. Gavi Alliance: Future deaths averted through GAVI support (2000–2010). [Internet] Geneva; GAVI Alliance [cited 2012 Apr 1]. Available from: http://www.gavialliance.org/about/mission/impact/.
24. Datadyne [Internet]. Washington, D.C; DataDyne Group LLC: 2012 [cited 2012 Apr 1]. Available from: http://www.datadyne.org/.
25. UNICEF. Angola, 4 August: Country launches nation-wide polio immunization campaign. New York; Unicef: 2010 [cited 2012 Apr 1]. Available from: http://www.unicef.org/esaro/5440_polio_immunization_campaign.html.

Chapter 17
Malaria in Children

James Houston

Learning Objectives

- Detail the history, examination, and assessment of a febrile child.
- Describe common differentials for febrile children in tropical world settings.
- Describe vector biology.
- Explain the investigation and management of malaria.
- Detail the treatment and complications of malaria.
- Describe how to prevent malaria.
- Describe public health initiatives that have been used to reduce the incidence of malaria (Fig. 17.1).

Initial Scenario

You have been based as a health worker in a rural sub-Saharan hospital for the last 6 months. It is a hot Monday morning and as you look out of the window at the queue of people waiting for the clinic, one of the nurses brings a child to your attention. Adie is a 2-year-old girl from one of the local villages. Her mother has walked for the last 4 h to take her to the clinic as she is worried about her child. Her mother mentions Adie has had a temperature for the last 2 days, which has not resolved with herbal remedies. While this is not completely out of the ordinary, you are concerned that Adie looks drowsy. You get one of the nurses to translate as you take a better history from the mother.

J. Houston, MBBS, MEng
FY2 Doctor, Department of Surgery,
Chelsea and Westminster Hospital,
London, UK
e-mail: jameshouston@doctors.org.uk

D. MacGarty, D. Nott (eds.), *Disaster Medicine*,
DOI 10.1007/978-1-4471-4423-6_17,

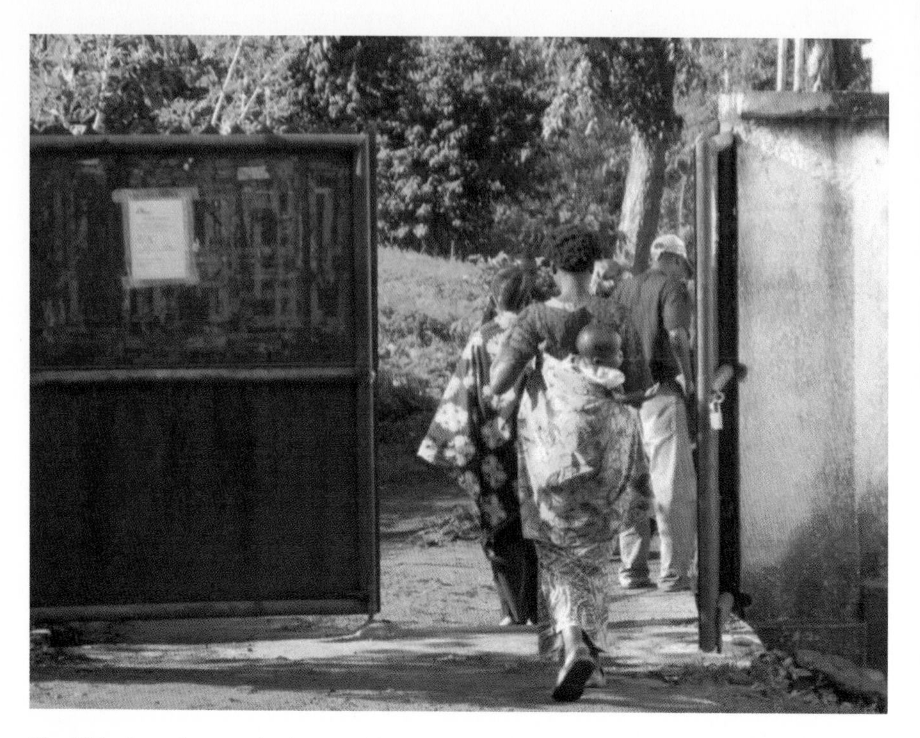

Fig. 17.1 A mother carrying her child from a hospital in the Congo (Picture by David Nott)

Prompt 1: Describe How to Take a History of a Febrile Child in Sub-Saharan Africa

Fever is a nonspecific symptom that can be caused by a large variety of conditions. It is a common presentation in tropical areas, especially in children. In the developing world, many standard investigations may not be available. Thus, a thorough history and examination are crucial to providing a differential diagnosis.

History [1]

The history can be split up into separate parts: assessing the presenting complaint and then broadening out to cover a standard medical history.

Fever

Questions about the fever itself should include its duration and severity, as well as its character (continuous or remitting), and its progression (worsening or improving).

Associated Symptoms

Such symptoms can be split up according to different body systems. These include neurological symptoms such as a headache, photophobia or fitting, respiratory symptoms such as a cough (include whether it is productive), and GI symptoms such as diarrhea (ask about blood in the stools) and loss of weight or appetite. Never forget to ask if the mother has noticed a rash. You should also ask about more general symptoms such as rigors, night sweats, irritability, and lethargy and those of coryza. Find out whether the child has been feeding/drinking and passing urine.

Past Medical and Family History

Further general questions should include that of the child's development and whether they have had any immunizations. Ask about any past medical issues that the child may have that include HIV, malaria, and chronic disease. Questions about these diseases should also extend to the mother and close family, as well as asking about any acute family illnesses.

Social History

The history should be taken relative to the environment; has the child been drinking clean water, are there malaria nets at home that are being used properly, and has the child been bathed in or drank freshwater that might harbor disease. Practical use of epidemiology is very important in the absence of sophisticated tests; find out the endemic conditions and timings for seasonal outbreaks.

Prompt 2: Describe the Examination and Assessment of a Sick Febrile Child in a Resource-Poor Setting

A comprehensive pediatric exam may help pinpoint the source of infection. Assessment of any sick child should first follow an ABC approach. Common equipment such as blood pressure cuffs and pulse oximetry may not be available, which makes the examination all the more important.

- Airway. Is the child crying (generally sign of a patent airway) or comatose? Is the child making an obstructive sounding noise as she tries to breathe? The child may lose an airway from obtundation due to severe illness or neurological infection. Another common cause is upper respiratory tract infection (e.g., croup, epiglottitis).

- Breathing (with respiratory examination). Does the child bear signs of respiratory distress such as grunting, head bobbing, sternal indrawing, or making use of accessory muscles of respiration? What is the respiratory rate relative to the child's age? Respiratory distress is a sensitive marker of an unwell child. It is not, however, specific to respiratory pathology.
- Circulation (with cardiovascular examination). Does the child have a delayed peripheral or central capillary refill time? Sunken eyes or fontanelle may also indicate profound dehydration.
- Disability (with neurological examination). An AVPU scale (alert, voice, pain & unresponsive) is a simple way of assessing disability in a child where formal GCS may be difficult.

A further comprehensive exam could then be attempted in conjunction with measuring blood glucose. The exam should be similar to the standard exam for an adult but also take into account some of the following points bearing in mind the age of the patient and particular signs that may be seen in the developing world:

- Ears. Examining with an otoscope, one may find inflammation and point to the origin of an infection.
- Mouth. May reveal dehydration or candidiasis secondary to other pathology (e.g., HIV).
- Lymph Nodes. Widespread lymphadenopathy may point toward HIV, lymphoma, or EBV, while localized nodal involvement may suggest viral infection.
- Skin. Darker skin may be more difficult when differentiating changes; the child should be undressed completely to examine for meningococcal rashes (non-blanching). Changes in skin temperature may point toward cellulitis if local or septic shock if generalized.
- Abdominal Examination. A locally tender abdomen may point to focal sources such as appendicitis or liver abscess. Generalized tenderness or peritonism may present from worsening symptoms of the above or from perforation (e.g., in typhoid). Organomegaly results from many developing world conditions; hepatomegaly may be seen in malaria, schistosomiasis, and hepatitis, while splenomegaly may also present in malaria but also lymphoma, leishmaniasis, and HIV. You should examine for ascites and presence of bowel sounds.
- Weight and mid-upper arm circumference (MUAC). Malnutrition is very common, a risk factor for mortality and easily assessed. (See chapter on Malnutrition.)

During the examination, routine observations can be made of the child, which should complement other signs elicited. These include heart and respiratory rate, which should be measured against standard values for their age. A thermometer should hopefully be available to measure for fever. Blood glucose is essential. While campaigns have been made to supply developing hospitals with simple equipment such as pulse oximeters and blood sugar monitors, clinical examination will often provide the primary observations in resource-poor settings.

Prompt 3: Describe Diseases Commonly Found in a Tropical, Developing World Setting Causing Fever

- While some tropical and developing world pathology may be very different from developed countries, much of it is also very similar. Thus, high up on the list should be viral upper respiratory tract infections, middle ear infections, and urinary tract infections. Meningitis and resulting meningococcal septicemia is rarer but more dangerous.
- Diseases more specific to the tropics include malaria and arbovirus infections like dengue fever and chikungunya. Dengue fever is caused by a virus transmitted by mosquitoes and is generally treated by using supportive measures such as rehydration. All three diseases can largely be prevented by adequate use of mosquito nets.
- Diseases preventable by effective immunization programs include measles and typhoid. Mass immunization regimes have previously helped almost eradicate typhoid, a feco-orally spread disease that can cause intestinal perforation and resulting septicemia. Common problems seen in the developing world such as poor nutrition and poor sanitation are risk factors for measles and typhoid, respectively.
- HIV seroconversion can produce fever independently, as well as coexisting HIV making the patient more vulnerable to all the above diseases. HIV-positive individuals may be less symptomatic than expected from infections due to immune "anergy" – a weakened immune system producing a dampened response to infection.
- Rarer diseases include brucellosis, viral leishmaniasis, amoebiasis, trypanosomiasis, and acute schistosomiasis, whose scope is sadly outside the remit of this introductory book.

Prompt 4: What Investigations Are Generally Available for Evaluating a Febrile Child in Developing Countries?

Some of the earlier differentials such as URTI and otitis media can be picked up without the need for investigation. In malaria, growing resistance and the need to monitor outbreaks, has made prior investigation and definitive diagnosis generally preferable to empirical treatment.

Rapid Diagnostic Tests (RDTs)

- Used for malaria and HIV. These are increasingly being used as they require very little training or equipment and are useful in austere settings. Commonly used RDTs for malaria can give results in under an hour [2], and some have been found in trials to have a sensitivity of 100 % for *P. falciparum* and 90.7 % for other plasmodium species [3]. Some RDTs can differentiate falciparum infection from non-falciparum malaria species according to which malarial enzymes or

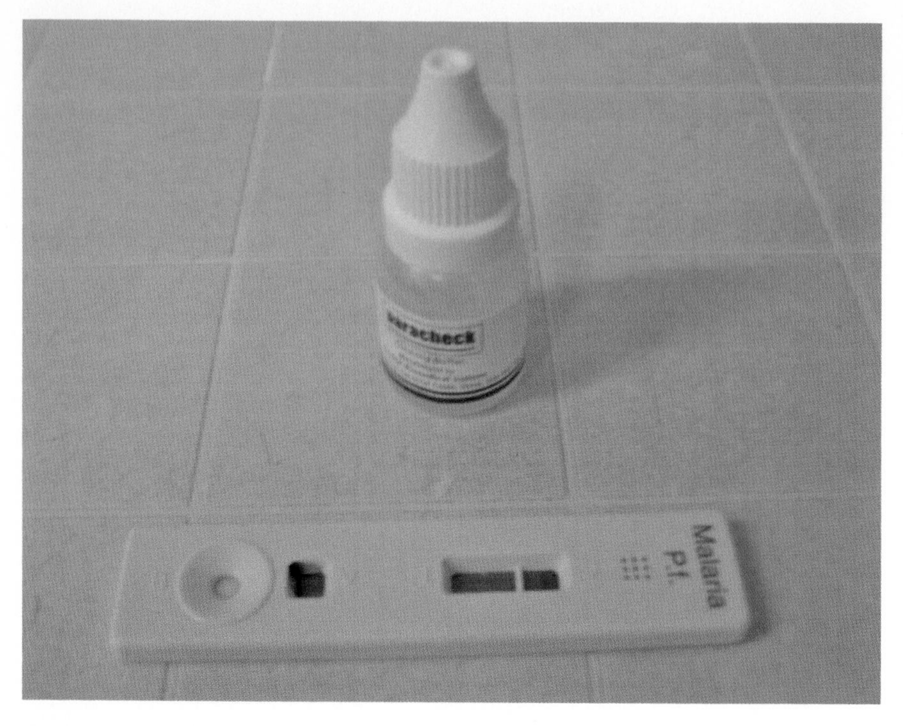

Fig. 17.2 A rapid diagnostic testing set for malaria (Picture by David Nott)

proteins are present. Some RDTs are able to differentiate between the non-falciparum species. A set is shown in Fig. 17.2 below.

Malaria Blood Films

- *Thick blood films* are the most sensitive test for malaria parasites.
- *Thin blood films* are used to identify the species of parasite, but may miss a diagnosis if the parasite density is low.
- Examination of blood films requires training and equipment, and the reliability of these tests is very dependent on the staff performing them.
- Ideally, three blood films should be taken for increased sensitivity,
- Negative blood films do not rule out malaria.
- Microscopy remains the gold standard if done by an expert.

Further tests may or may not be available. If possible, these could include:

- Full Blood Count. Anemia and thrombocytopenia are common in malaria. Raised leukocytes may be seen in infection or leukopenia in immunosuppression. If no full blood count is available, a hematocrit can give an estimate of hemoglobin.
- Urea and Electrolytes. Dehydration may cause acute kidney injury.
- Liver Function Tests. These could be deranged in hepatitis, EBV, or as the result of treatment for disease (e.g., hepatotoxicity from anti-TB medication).
- Stool microscopy

In a better resourced setting you may request more tests as part of a septic screen. While they should only be used if indicated, they may include:

- Blood cultures
- Urine cultures or dipstick
- Chest x-ray
- Sputum samples (if productive cough)
- Lumbar puncture – if there is suspicion of meningitis
- Ultrasound scans – may be useful to examine enlarged livers or spleens

Further Information 1

The history regarding Adie is nonspecific. She had a fever about 2 days ago although this now seems to have passed. At the time of this, Adie seemed to shake and then sweat profusely. She has not been feeding properly for the last couple of days. Previously, she has been otherwise well and lives at home with her 4 brothers. There has been no weight loss, and there is no history of other serious diseases in the family. Her siblings have had fevers like Adie's before, but they never seemed to be so severe.

Adie opens her eyes to your voice. She cries and is irritable when you examine her. She has a respiratory rate of 30 although her lungs are clear. You think you can feel a slightly enlarged spleen on an otherwise normal abdomen. She has some pallor of the conjunctiva and has dry mucous membranes. There is no sign of otitis media, lymphadenopathy, or rash. She weighs 10 kg, and her temperature is 38.5 °C. Her blood glucose is 5 mmol/L.

Malaria is endemic in your area and is your main differential. You send off for an RDT. The FBC result will take 2 days to come back. No other tests are available. While you wait for the results, you insert a cannula and administer some fluids.

Prompt 5: What Are Vectors and Zoonotic Diseases, and How Is This Relevant to Malaria?

A vector is an organism that carries a pathogen between hosts.

Examples of vectors include many arthropods such as mosquitoes, ticks, and flies that transmit malaria, Lyme disease, and leishmaniasis, respectively. A hematophagous vector is one that feeds on blood. Such vectors can transmit the pathogen during this process.

A zoonotic disease is one that can be transmitted between animals and humans. Transmission may be via direct contact with the animal, via contamination of infected produce, or via a vector between the two species. Examples of zoonotic disease are rabies via being bitten by an infected dog and E. coli via eating poorly cooked poultry.

Malaria is an acute febrile illness caused by the parasites from the genus Plasmodium. Female anopheles mosquitoes transmit the parasite to humans at the time of biting. Mosquitoes are known as vectors since they carry the disease between infected parties. Thus, reducing the numbers and disease transmissibility of mosquitoes, known as vector control, is one of the main tenets of reducing mortality and morbidity in malaria [4].

Five species of plasmodia cause human disease. There are four species (*P. falciparum*, *P. ovale*, *P. vivax*, and *P. malariae*) that infect only humans and a fifth (*P. knowlesi*) that is normally a disease of macaque monkeys but which can be transmitted to man. Since *P. knowlesi* can be transmitted between different species, it is known as a zoonosis, whereas the other species of plasmodia are not.

While *P. vivax* is responsible for the largest number of malaria infections worldwide, *P. falciparum* is more lethal and accounts for about 90 % of malarial deaths.

Malaria was once thought to arise from "bad air" and so its name is derived from Italian (*mal aria*). Today, half the world's population (3.3 billion people) live in endemic malarial areas. Malaria is one of the world's most devastating diseases with around 216 million infections every year [5]. An estimated 655,000 [5] million people died from malaria in 2010, where most were young children in Africa. Those at greatest risk of dying are children in sub-Saharan Africa.

Prompt 6: What Are the Presenting Features and Pathophysiology of Malaria?

There is no definitive way of diagnosing malaria through symptoms alone. Malaria classically presents in febrile paroxysms, known as such due to their sudden onset.

These occur in three stages:

- Initial cold stage with shivering, shaking, or rigors
- Secondary hot stage with high fever
- Final sweating stage with return to original temperature and lethargy

The time to progress through all three stages takes between 4 to 6 h. There may often be a prodrome of muscle ache/pain. The fevers in malaria can occur in repetitive cycles. Classically, *P. vivax* will repeat every three days with *P. falciparum* varying from a 2-day cycle to continuous fever. It is important to note that a patient with malaria may well not be febrile on presentation. It is an account of previous febrile illness that is important to note in the history.

Pathophysiology

The parasite known as a sporozoite moves from the puncture site through the bloodstream from to the liver where it multiplies asexually. No symptoms occur during this hepatic stage. Sporozoites form schizonts which rupture to release merozoites in the bloodstream. Fevers occur as host cytokines such as IL6 are secreted as inflammatory response, which slow the growth of mature parasites. Merozoites go on to infect red blood cells, feed on hemoglobin, and cause cell rupture and hemolysis with resulting anemia and jaundice. They also reproduce asexually again and go on to infect other blood cells. Further signs such as splenomegaly are caused when red cells infected with falciparum malaria bind to endothelial cells in deep tissues leading to the *sequestration* of large numbers of mature parasites.

Prompt 7: Apart from Children, What Other High-Risk Groups Are Vulnerable to Malaria?

Malaria in Pregnancy

Women are particularly at risk in their first pregnancy. Malaria increases the risk of stillbirth, spontaneous abortion, low birth weight, and neonatal death. Maternal anemia can make the perils of postpartum hemorrhage in the developing world even more dangerous. WHO estimates suggest that malaria in pregnancy causes 10,000 maternal and 200,000 infant deaths annually. WHO guidelines suggest that pregnant women living in areas of high malaria transmission should receive two doses during pregnancy after the second trimester of intermittent preventative treatment such as sulfadoxine-pyrimethamine as well as receiving insecticide-treated nets [6].

Malaria in HIV/AIDS

HIV and malaria are frequently concentrated in the same geographical areas with the overlap particularly affecting female adolescents [7]. Those infected with HIV are particularly vulnerable from malaria and should be provided with insecticide-treated nets. Likewise, in areas of high HIV prevalence, people who present with recurrent fevers should also be offered HIV testing as opposed to blindly treating for malaria. New antimalarials should also be trialled for their effect on HIV immunosuppressed patients prior to release. The WHO advocates more integration of HIV and malaria prevention and control strategies [8].

Further Information 2

The RDT comes back positive for Plasmodium falciparum parasites in Adie's blood sample. You plan to begin antimalarial therapy. As you review her again, she still looks particularly drowsy and now cannot seem to sit up. You are concerned as the disease appears severe and she may be showing cerebral complications.

Prompt 8: How Can Malaria Be Treated?

The mainstay of treatment for malaria should include:

- Antimalarial chemotherapy
- Analgesia and antipyretics

There are many different antimalarial chemotherapy drugs available which have a variety of side effects and degrees of effectiveness. The mainstay of treatment for falciparum malaria is through artemisinin derivatives.

- *Artemisinin Derivatives*
- Sourced from the plant Artemisia annua, these drugs include artesunate and artemether.
- Artesunate has the added advantage over artemether that it can be used intravenously.
- These medications have been shown in recent years to be superior to quinine for treatment of severe falciparum malaria in both adults [9] and children [10].
- The WHO recommends the use of artemisinin combination therapies to treat uncomplicated malaria.

Treatment of Falciparum Versus Non-falciparum Malaria

Disclaimer: Medication regimes are liable to change. Please consult your own, or the WHO's, current guidelines before prescribing any medications.

Severe Falciparum Malaria [11]
- Parenteral (IV/IM) medication is required for at least the first 24 h.
- Artesunate is considered the first choice in treatment.
  - 2.4 mg/kg IV or IM on admission and then at 12 h and at 24 h.
  - Following this, it can be given every 24 h.
- Quinine or artemether should be considered if parenteral artesunate is not available.
  - Quinine
    - 20 mg salt/kg loading dose as an infusion then 10 mg/kg every 8 h.
    - Infusion rates should not exceed 5 mg salt/kg/h.

- Artemether
    - 3.2 mg/kg IM on admission then 1.6 mg/kg/day

Uncomplicated Malaria
Artemisinin combination therapies (ACTs) are recommended as first-line treatment for uncomplicated malaria by the WHO to delay the development of resistance.

- The second drugs that are added have a longer half-life and make sure that the remaining parasites are destroyed. Examples include:
    - ASMQ (artesunate given with mefloquine).
    - ASAQ (artesunate given with amodiaquine).
    - Coartem (artemether given with lumefantrine).
    - These ACTs can now be given as single tablets which will improve compliance and help reduce resistance.

Oral quinine is an alternate treatment for uncomplicated malaria but must be taken for 7 days. Fortunately, quinine resistance is rare, but the medicine itself is poorly tolerated. It should be given with clindamycin or doxycycline.

Non-falciparum Malaria

- A 3-day course of oral chloroquine is the treatment of choice [12].
- Hypnozoites can reside in the liver and should be treated with primaquine. This treatment however must be avoided in people with G6PD deficiency due to the risk of hemolysis or those that are pregnant due to risks to the fetus.

Side Effects Associated with Antimalarials

As with most drugs, the most common side effects are nausea, diarrhea, and vomiting. Quinine is poorly tolerated due to its taste and is associated with hearing problems and cinchonism, which includes hot flushes, vertigo, and tinnitus. Chloroquine is associated with itching. Few serious side effects are associated with artemisinin relative to the other drugs. Side effects are generally mitigated by stopping and changing the drug.

Antipyretic and Analgesic Therapy

The mainstay of antipyretic therapy is paracetamol. This also acts as an analgesic. Aspirin is generally discouraged in young children due to its association with Reye's syndrome. Antipyretics only serve as symptom control and do very little to clear the underlying pathology.

Prompt 9: What Constitutes Severe Malaria and What Complications Are Seen?

The WHO classifies the severity of malaria in children according to symptoms [13]. The most severe forms include children that are prostated (where a child is unable to sit up if normally able to do so, or if the child is unable to drink if too young to sit) or those that show signs of respiratory distress, such as marked indrawing or sustained nasal flaring. These children are at risk of dying and require immediate parenteral antimalarial drugs and supportive therapy. Other clinical indicators of severe malaria include impaired consciousness, failure to feed, multiple convulsions, anemia and hypoglycaemia.

The most serious complication of the disease is cerebral malaria and is associated with Plasmodium falciparum infection. Other complications that might be observed and treated in austere environments are also listed below.

Cerebral Malaria

Noted by reduced levels of consciousness or posturing, this is the most serious of complications of malaria and has up to a 20 % mortality rate. Its pathophysiology is still not completely understood. Prompt treatment with antimalarials is essential. Associated convulsions may be treated with benzodiazepines such as diazepam. Treatment should be complemented with supportive management for coma (such as maintaining airway) as available.

Anemia

Due to hemolysis and bone marrow suppression. The anemia is normocytic. There is some controversy in giving blood transfusions for anemia in malaria in the developing world particularly when also considering the risk of transmission of blood-borne viruses. A Cochrane review found, unless there was respiratory distress, the clinical evidence in transfusing anemic children with malaria to be insufficient [14].

Hypoglycemia

Measured by routine blood glucose. Reduced liver function leads to impaired gluconeogenesis (formation of glucose) and therefore hypoglycemia. Low blood glucose can also be caused by quinine-induced insulin secretion [15]. Treatment is usually via the use of dextrose in fluids, where if glucose is less than <2.2 mmol/l, then it should be treated with 0.3 g–0.5 g/kg of glucose [11].

Other acute complications include renal failure, which is more commonly seen in adults, and metabolic acidosis, which often manifests itself through tachypnea.

Longer-term complications include hepatosplenomegaly, parasitic persistence (recrudescence) that can cause severe anemia, and increased severity of coexisting infections (e.g., HIV, pneumonia)

Further Information 3

You place Adie in the recovery position. Fortunately, the hospital is well stocked, and Adie is started immediately on 25 mg IV artesunate. She improves over the next 48 h and becomes well enough to tolerate ACT tablets. Her Hb returns as 6 g/dL. Within a week, she has recovered without any lasting impediment. You note that many children are not as lucky as Adie and wonder whether this event could have been prevented.

Adie's mother has her net packed away at home and normally uses herbal remedies to ward away fevers. On discharge, you ask a trained nurse to explain to Adie's mother about the role of mosquitoes in malaria and to give advice on how to reduce bites. Time is also taken to warn about the symptoms of malaria for future recognition and the importance of taking extra care should she become pregnant. Leaflets are given to pass on to other people in their village.

Prompt 9: Discuss the Importance of Vector Control in Managing Malaria Outbreaks?

Vector control in malaria aims to reduce transmission levels in malaria by removing or killing the mosquitoes and their larvae. It is regarded as one of the most effective means of reducing the levels of transmission [16] and is a crucial component in the fight against reducing morbidity and mortality.

Forms of Vector Control

- Insecticide-Treated Nets (ITNs). Perhaps the simplest and most cost effective way of reducing mortality and morbidity associated with malaria. The nets generally last for 6 months as standard and when used properly can reduce malaria cases by up to 50 % and child mortality by 18 % [17]. Growing insecticide resistance to pyrethroids, the most commonly used chemical in ITNs, will make future research into new classes of insecticides a priority [18]. Now, an estimated 50 % of all households in sub-Saharan Africa have at least one bed net with 145 million nets being handed out in 2010 [19]. Examples of nets are seen in Figs. 17.3 and 17.4.

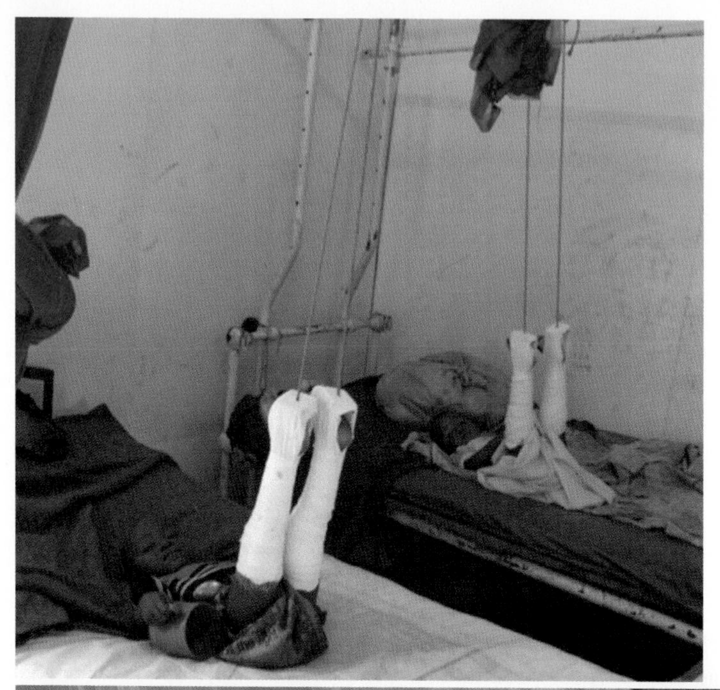

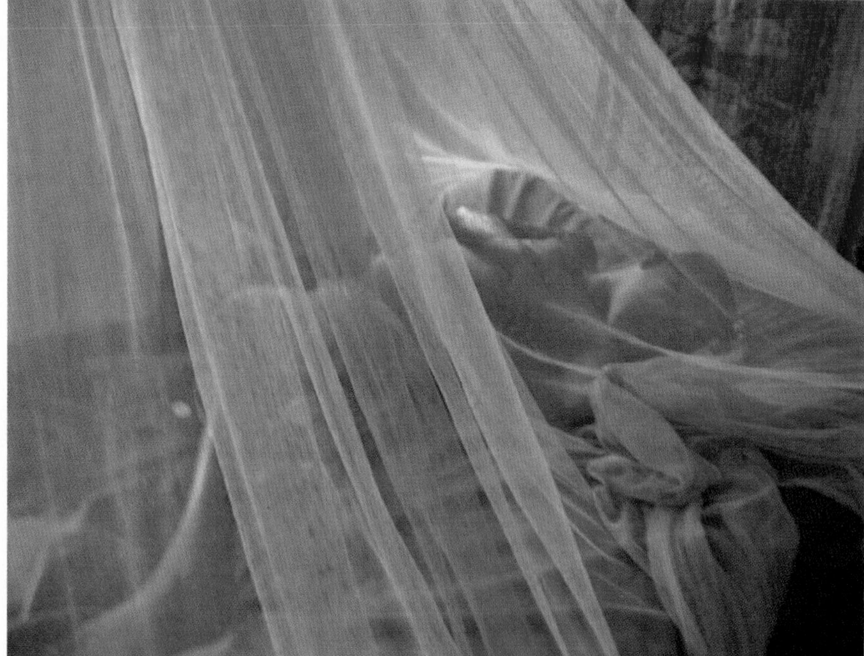

Figs. 17.3 and 17.4 Rudimentary nets used to protect children in hospital from disease vectors (Picture by David Nott)

- Indoor Residual Spraying (IRS). This uses insecticides on indoor walls to kill insects that might reside on them. Long-acting insecticides lower transmission by reducing the lifespan and density of vector mosquitoes [20]. Some controversy exists with the use of DDT for spraying, but its use within established guidelines for malaria eradication is supported by the WHO and is allowed under the Stockholm Convention (2004) [20]. An estimated 6 % of the global population and 11 % of the sub-Saharan African population are protected through IRS [19].
- Removal of Breeding Grounds. This can be achieved by eradication of swamps that house the larvae, covering the water, or use of fish in the water to eat them. Occasionally, larvicidal treatment can be used, but this may have other environmental costs.

Prompt 10: What Other Methods and Strategies Could Be Used to Reduce the Burden of Malaria?

Education

As with many other diseases, it is imperative that those at risk are aware of the causes. Those at risk should be encouraged to avoid being bitten such as using ITNs or IRS, as well as covering up exposed skin where possible. This is especially important during dusk and dawn when the mosquitoes feed. Likewise, mothers can be advised of the symptoms of malaria to encourage prompter referral to medical help.

Medication

While medication is used for the treatment of malaria, it is not feasible to use across Africa as a means of prophylaxis. Much simpler and cheaper methods can be used to reduce the transmission of malaria.

Malaria Vaccines

While there are no current licensed vaccines for malaria, indeed none exists for any parasites in humans; a number are currently in clinical trials. The most promising is the RTS,S vaccine which aims to provide cover against *P. falciparum* although offers no protection against *P. vivax*. Some preliminary results were released in late 2011, showing a 55 % reduction in the frequency of malaria episodes in children aged between 5 and 17 months [21]. Much more data will follow in the coming years, in particular the length of protection inferred by the vaccine and its protection for younger children. While future results need to be thoroughly analyzed before new policy is made, the first results are certainly encouraging and may pave the way for a new approach against such a devastating disease.

Global Strategies

While some progress has been made on preventative techniques in malaria as well as improving medical treatment, real progress can only be made toward eradicating the disease through coherent regional, national, and international strategies. These are frequently coordinated by UNICEF, the WHO, and, more recently, "The Global Fund to Fight AIDS, Tuberculosis and Malaria." UNICEF identifies key actions such as clear and timely policy guidance, integration of malaria control into existing maternal and child health programs, and improvement in forecasting as key to achieving global malaria goals [22]. The WHO's recently released initiative *T3: Test. Treat. Track* refers to a three-pronged approach to tackling malaria, aiming to provide universal access to both testing and treatment, as well as providing stronger malaria surveillance systems [19]. Even with an estimated 88 million RDTs delivered in 2010, the number of diagnostic tests was still less than half the number of ACTs procured. Treatment must only be used where necessary and combination therapies should be used where possible in order to combat resistance. Funding from initiatives similar to the above has meant that 60 countries provided ACTs free of charge to all age groups in 2010. With coordinated strategies such as those above, progress can be made; since 2000, the estimated global incidence of malaria has been reduced by 17 %, and malaria-specific mortality rates have fallen by 26 % [19].

Case Study: Zambia

Zambia has made significant leaps forward to reducing the impact of malaria in the last 10 years. The sub-Saharan country is one of the poorest in the world with endemic malaria accounting for around 36 % of hospital admissions [23]. The National Malaria Control Program has aimed to reduce disease rates through simple control measures such as insecticide-treated nets, adequate medicines provision, and preventative treatment in those in high-risk groups. Overall malaria deaths decreased by 37 % between 2001 and 2006, and it is estimated that 75,000 child deaths have been avoided [24]. A new plan between 2006–2010 was implemented which handed out more than six million nets, and parasitemia prevalence in children under five further reduced from 22 to 16 %. However, a decrease in funding also showed some effects between 2008 and 2010 with rebounds in parasitemia [25]. Thus, while funding can make significant progress, support must remain to ensure a permanent impact is made on such a devastating illness.

References

1. Eddleston M. Oxford handbook of tropical medicine. Oxford: Oxford UP; 2008. Print.
2. Murray CK, Gasser Jr RA, Magill AJ, Miller RS. Update on rapid diagnostic testing for malaria. Clin Microbiol Rev. 2008;21(1):97–110. Review.
3. Gatti S, et al. Gispi Study Group. A comparison of three diagnostic techniques for malaria: a rapid diagnostic test (NOW Malaria), PCR and microscopy. Ann Trop Med Parasitol. 2007;101(3):195–204.
4. WHO. Vector control of malaria. http://www.who.int/malaria/vector_control/en/. Accessed 18 May 2012.
5. WHO. World malaria report: 2011. Geneva: WHO Press; 2011.
6. WHO. Malaria in pregnancy, guidelines for measuring key monitoring and evaluation indicators. Geneva: WHO Press; 2007.
7. Brabin L, Brabin BJ. HIV, malaria and beyond: reducing the disease burden of female adolescents. Malar J. 2005;4:2.
8. WHO. Malaria and HIV/AIDS interactions and their implications for public health policy, report of a Technical Consultation, 23–24 June 2004. Geneva; 2005.
9. Dondorp A, Nosten F, Stepniewska K, Day N, White N. Artesunate versus quinine for treatment of severe falciparum malaria: a randomised trial. Lancet. 2005;366(9487):717–25.
10. Dondorp AM, Fanello CI, Hendriksen IC, et al. Artesunate versus quinine in the treatment of severe falciparum malaria in African children (AQUAMAT): an open-label, randomised trial. Lancet. 2010;376(9753):1647–57.
11. World Health Organization. Guidelines for the treatment of malaria. Geneva: World Health Organization; 2010. Print.
12. Lalloo DG, Shingadia D, Pasvol G, Chiodini PL, Whitty CJ, Beeching NJ, Hill DR, Warrell DA, Bannister BA. UK malaria treatment guidelines. Journal of Infection. 2007;54(2):111–21. Print.
13. World Health Organization. Communicable Diseases Cluster, Severe falciparum malaria. Trans R Soc Trop Med Hyg. 2000;94 Suppl 1:S1–90. Review.
14. Meremikwu M, Smith HJ. Blood transfusion for treating malarial anaemia. Cochrane Database Syst Rev. 2000;(2):CD001475. Review.
15. White NJ, Warrell DA, Chanthavanich P, Looareesuwan S, Warrell MJ, Krishna S, Williamson DH, Turner RC. Severe hypoglycemia and hyperinsulinemia in falciparum malaria. N Engl J Med. 1983;309(2):61–6.
16. WHO. Vector control. http://www.who.int/malaria/vector_control/en/. Accessed 18 May 2012.
17. Lengeler C. Insecticide-treated bed nets and curtains for preventing malaria. Cochrane Database Syst Rev. 2004;(2):CD000363.
18. Moszynski P. Insecticide resistance threatens malaria control programmes, WHO says. BMJ. 2012;344:e3416.
19. WHO. T3: Test Treat Track. Scaling up diagnostic testing treatment and surveillance for malaria. 2012., http://www.who.int/malaria/publications/atoz/test_treat_track_brochure.pdf. Accessed 19 May 2012.
20. WHO. Indoor residual spraying, use of indoor spraying for scaling up global malaria control and elimination. Geneva: WHO; 2006.
21. RTS,S Clinical Trials Partnership. First results of phase 3 trial of RTS,S/AS01 malaria vaccine in African children. N Engl J Med. 2011;365(20):1863–75.
22. UNICEF. Malaria and children, progress in intervention coverage. New York; 2007.
23. National Malaria Control Centre. Zambia: http://www.nmcc.org.zm/malaria_control.htm. Accessed 17 May 2012.
24. The Gates Foundation: Progress against malaria. 2009. http://www.gatesfoundation.org/livingproofproject/Documents/progress-against-malaria.pdf. Accessed 17 May 2012.
25. WHO. Rollback Malaria 2011. http://www.rollbackmalaria.org/ProgressImpactSeries/docs/report7-en.pdf. Accessed 18 May 2012.

Chapter 18
Cholera: An Infectious Waterborne Disease

David MacGarty

Reviewed by Daniele Lantagne

Learning Objectives

- Discuss the infection risk associated with poor sanitation.
- Outline the common diseases transmitted through the fecal-oral route.
- Describe the clinical presentation of a cholera patient.
- Outline the pathophysiology and clinical course of cholera infection.
- Explain the treatment of severe dehydration.
- Identify the initial management of a cholera outbreak.
- Outline a policy for planning for a cholera epidemic.

Initial Scenario

With sweaty palms and a thousand butterflies dancing in your stomach you wait outside the interview room. Having completed your GP training, you decided to work abroad for a year and following reports of an earthquake you knew you had to apply. Hundreds of thousands of survivors are displaced and living in overcrowded camps. Waterborne diseases are rife due to damaged sanitation and drinking water supplies. You knock and enter the room.

The interviewers describe the situation on the ground. They tell you many responders who deploy are a resource burden who consume more than they contribute. "How will you be different?"

D. MacGarty, MBBS, BSc
FY2 Doctor, Department of Obstetrics and Gynaecology,
St Peter's Hospital, Chertsey, Surrey, UK
e-mail: dmacgarty@hotmail.com

D. MacGarty, D. Nott (eds.), *Disaster Medicine*,
DOI 10.1007/978-1-4471-4423-6_18, © Springer-Verlag London 2013

While acknowledging your inexperience, you describe how you would use your medical and technical skills and knowledge in a practical way. The interviewees seem ambivalent.

Later that day, you receive the call you hoped for. You will be working in an improvised health center in a damaged town near the capital. It is time to buy your ticket.

Prompt 1: Why Does Poor Sanitation Pose an Infection Risk?

- Poor sanitation is common in overcrowded camps following disasters and conflict where the swell of survivors overwhelms existing sanitation facilities. Efforts to maintain Sphere Standards for the provision of water and sanitation frequently fail [1, 2].
- Poor sanitation results in the improper disposal of feces and the subsequent contamination of water used for drinking, cooking, and cleaning.
- Through eating or drinking, fecal matter and the associated waterborne pathogens are consumed resulting in infection. The infected individual then spreads the infection through their own feces. This is the fecal-oral route of disease transmission.

Prompt 2: List and Summarize the Most Important Waterborne, Fecal-Oral Diseases

Typhoid

- An acute infectious enteric fever caused by the gram-negative, motile bacillus *Salmonella typhi*. The disease has an insidious onset with malaise, headache, lack of appetite, and nausea followed by fever. Fever increases slowly and gradually reaches a peak in the second week. The fever may continue for a third week, with the patient recovering in week 4. Severe disease may result in bowel perforation which is a common complication in sub-Saharan Africa.

Giardia

- *Giardia* is a protozoan parasite that colonizes the upper portions of the small intestine. The disease is characterized by the sudden onset of explosive, watery, foul-smelling diarrhea. Stools associated with *Giardia* infection are loose, bulky, and frothy with the absence of blood or mucus. Patients suffer from flatulence, bloating, anorexia, cramps, and foul belching.

Dysentery

- Dysentery is an enteric illness caused by pathogenic bacteria or parasitic protozoa which is characterized by bloody diarrhea. Bacterial dysentery is caused by a gram-negative, rod-shaped bacterium called *Shigella*, whereas parasitic dysentery is caused by the amoeba *Entamoeba histolytica.* Pathogens invade the epithelial cells of gut mucosa causing tissue damage resulting in inflammation and bleeding with fever and severe abdominal pain. The diarrhea is mixed with mucus and blood, and defecation is painful.

Cholera

- Cholera is an acute diarrheal disease caused by infection with the *Vibrio cholerae* bacterium. After entry into the gut, the bacteria attaches to the small intestine, multiplies rapidly, and in the process produces cholera toxin. The toxin results in profuse watery stool and rapid and severe dehydration of the body due to loss of large quantities of fluid and electrolytes with the stool.

Hepatitis

- Hepatitis A is an acute infectious disease of the liver caused by the hepatitis A virus. Early symptoms can be mistaken for influenza and include fatigue, fever, abdominal pain, nausea, jaundice, and clay-colored feces. Some sufferers, especially children, exhibit no symptoms at all.

Polio

- The poliovirus invades and then resides in the intestinal tract and the mucus of the nose and throat. Up to 95 % of people infected with poliovirus will have no symptoms, but approximately 1 % of those infected get paralytic poliomyelitis and 1–2 % will get aseptic meningitis [3].

Further Information 1

You are welcomed by representatives of the NGO and are brought to a tented treatment center on the edge of town. There are hundreds of people awaiting treatment – you will start immediately.

During the morning, a lady presents you with a child suffering with sudden onset diarrhea which began that morning. Her family lives in a camp for displaced people 10 miles away. Nobody else in the family has had diarrhea. The mother says the family uses a collection tank in the camp for drinking water. She does not let her daughter use the latrines because they are too dangerous.

Prompt 3: What Information Do You Want to Elicit in the History?

General Information

- How has the child been? A drowsy, lethargic, and/or irritable child may be dehydrated and will require prompt treatment.

Time Course of the Diarrhea

- Is the disease acute or chronic? Acute diarrhea is defined as a greater number of stools of decreased form than normal lasting for less than 14 days.

Specific Diarrhea Symptoms such as Stool Consistency, Frequency, Volume, and Blood

- What is the volume produced? Large volumes of watery diarrhea suggest small bowel or proximal colonic disease.
- What is the frequency? Small frequent stools with urgency are associated with left colon or rectal disease.
- Is it dysentery? The presence of blood is suggestive of infection by invasive organisms and inflammation.
- What is the color? Pale stools suggest biliary and/or hepatic disease.

Associated Symptoms such as Nausea and Vomiting, Pain, or Fever

- Diarrhea with severe nausea and vomiting may suggest toxigenic infection or the ingestion of external toxins.
- Diarrhea with severe abdominal pain and high fever may suggest infection with invasive bacteria or organisms that produce cytotoxins.

Drug History and Diet

- Many drugs (e.g., antibiotics), foods (e.g., milk products and shellfish), and nutritional supplements can cause acute diarrhea.
- Ask about food hygiene.

Family and Social History

- Are other family members affected? Infectious acute diarrhea is contracted through ingestion of contaminated food and water which are generally shared by the family.
- The place of residence gives an indication of available drinking water and demands on sanitary facilities (see Fig. 18.1).

Past Medical History

- Has the child had diarrhea before? The diarrhea may be due to an underlying condition such as inflammatory bowel disease or celiac disease [4].

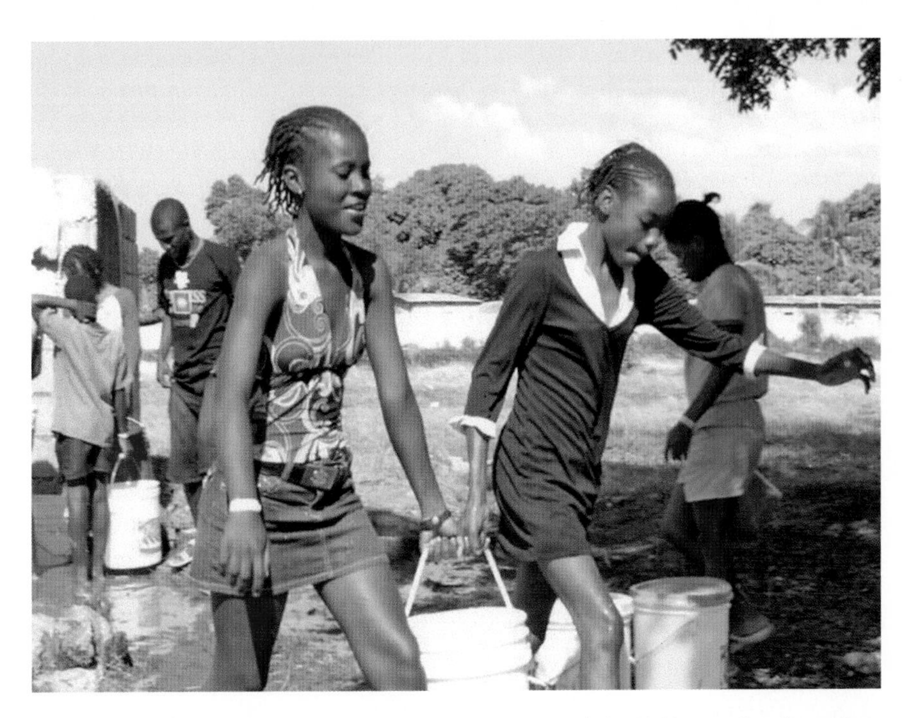

Fig. 18.1 Collecting safe drinking water. In the aftermath of the Haitian earthquake, tankers brought drinking water into displacement camps for distribution (Reproduced with permission from SOS children's villages worldwide)

Further Information 2

The child's name is Eva, and she is 7 years old weighing 19 kg. She has been voiding large quantities of watery diarrhea since this morning (6 hours ago) and had several bouts of vomiting. There is no blood in the diarrhea.

On examination, she looks drowsy and lethargic. She is very dry with sunken eyes and reduced skin turgor. Her heart rate is high, and her blood pressure low. You cannot feel her radial pulse.

You look for a WHO leaflet regarding treatment of dehydration. You read:

Cholera should be suspected when:

- *A patient older than 5 years develops severe dehydration from acute watery diarrhea (usually with vomiting) or*
- *Any patient above the age of 2 years has acute watery diarrhea in an area where there is an outbreak of cholera*

You explain you must keep the child in hospital overnight as she may need urgent IV fluids to restore her fluid balance. You start her on oral rehydration solution (ORS). Strongly suspecting cholera, you take a stool sample and send it to the lab for analysis. You call the Ministry of Health and the regional PAHO (WHO) office to let them know. Before dusk, there is an influx of 50 patients, all complaining of watery, voluminous, acute diarrhea.

Prompt 4: How Is Information Managed in a Suspected Cholera Outbreak?

- Under the terms of the International Health Regulations (1969), it is mandatory for health authorities to notify the WHO of a cholera outbreak. Often, countries fail to do this because they fear it will damage tourism and interfere with exports [5]. Laboratory confirmation should be sought as soon as possible.
- If a cholera outbreak is confirmed, the health authorities must make weekly reports to the WHO. Reports must confirm the number of new cases and deaths since the last report, and the cumulative death totals for the year [5].

Prompt 5: What Is the Clinical Course of Cholera Infection?

- Most people infected with *V. cholerae* do not become ill, but everyone infected can spread the disease. The reason for individual resistance to the disease is not known though individuals may differ in the availability of intestinal receptors for binding the bacterium and its toxin. Previously infected individuals have a lower risk of illness following reinfection.
- Of those who become ill, fewer than 20 % develop signs of moderate or severe dehydration. The rest have symptoms indistinguishable from gastroenteritis.
- For those who become ill, symptoms begin following a 24–48-h incubation period.
- Fluid volume depletion can lead to hypovolemic shock and death without adequate replacement of fluids and electrolytes.
- The bacterium remains present in feces for 7–14 days.
- Strains of *V. cholerae* vary in virulence. Some strains can cause death within 4–6 h of the onset of symptoms.
- In a well-managed outbreak, <1 % case fatality rate (CFR, total number of registered deaths/total number of registered cases) is considered good treatment [6, 7].

Prompt 6: Outline the Pathophysiology of Cholera Infection

1. Following ingestion, the bacterium colonizes the mucosa of the small bowel (duodenum and upper jejunum).
2. The bacterium produces enzymes which allow its enterotoxin to bind with receptors on the surface of intestinal mucosa cells.

3. The toxin enters the cell, and once inside, it immediately increases the rate at which cAMP is produced.
4. cAMP stimulates mucosal cells to pump large amounts of Cl^- into the intestinal lumen.
5. Water, Na^+, and other electrolytes follow the Cl^- due to the osmotic and electrical gradient.
6. The lost water and electrolytes in the mucosal cells are replaced from blood plasma.
7. The process continues with mucosal cells continually pumping water and electrolytes into the intestinal lumen.
8. The colon remains in a state of absorption but is overwhelmed by the large fluid volumes resulting in copious watery diarrhea isotonic with blood plasma.
9. Water and electrolyte loss from plasma causes dehydration and volume depletion [8].

Prompt 7: How Should a Severely Dehydrated Child with Cholera Be Treated?

The following guidelines for the treatment of cholera have been reproduced with permission from the WHO [9]:

Step 1: Assess the level of dehydration using Table 18.1.
Step 2: Rehydrate the patient, and monitor frequently. Then reassess hydration status.
Step 3: Maintain hydration: replace continuing fluid losses until diarrhea stops.
Step 4: Give an oral antibiotic (doxycycline) to patients with severe dehydration (co-trimoxazole in children).
Step 5: Feed the patient.

Table 18.1 WHO guidelines for assessment of dehydration in a diarrheal patient

	Level of dehydration		
	No sign	Some	Severe
Condition	Well, alert	**Restless, irritable**	**Lethargic or unconscious, floppy**
Eyes	Normal	Sunken	Very sunken and dry
Tears	Present	Absent	Absent
Mouth and tongue	Moist	Dry	Very dry
Thirst	Drinks normally, not thirsty	**Thirsty, drinks eagerly**	**Drinks poorly or not able to drink**
Skin pinch	Goes back quickly	**Goes back slowly**	**Goes back very slowly**
Decide	The patient has no signs of dehydration	If the patient has 2 or more signs, including at least one major sign (**bold**), there is some dehydration	If the patient has two or more signs, including at least one major sign (**bold**), there is severe dehydration

In adults and children older than 5 years, other major signs for severe dehydration are **absent radial pulse** and **low blood pressure**. The skin pinch may be less useful in patients with malnutrition, or obese patients. Tears (or lack of) are a useful sign for infants and young children only

The information in the table suggests Eva has severe dehydration. Patients with "severe" dehydration should be given IV fluid immediately to replace their fluid deficit. Ringer's lactate is recommended (higher sodium concentration), but normal saline is acceptable. The WHO guidelines state patients aged 1 year and older should be given:

- 30 ml/kg as rapidly as possible (within 30 min) (for Eva, 30 × 19 = 570 ml)
- 70 ml/kg in the next 2.5 h (for Eva, 70 × 19 = 1,330 ml)

Eva is able to drink and so she should be given oral rehydration (ORS) solution (5 ml/kg/h = 5 × 19 = 95 ml/h) and must be monitored frequently. She should be reassessed after 3 h using Table 18.1 and retreated as necessary. Antibiotics should be started once she is adequately hydrated (4–6 h).

Patients with "some" dehydration should be given ORS solution in an amount suitable for patient age and weight and must be monitored frequently. They should be reassessed after 4 h using Table 18.1 and retreated as necessary.

Patients with no obvious signs of dehydration can be treated at home. They should be given enough ORS packets for 2 days and instructed to return if they develop further symptoms of cholera or dysentery.

Further Information 3

In the next 48 hours, the treatment center receives 1,500 further patients complaining of acute diarrhea. The center is completely overwhelmed, lacking the staff, resources, and materials to cope. You work around the clock to deal with the patient load, but many patients die before you can see them. The stool sample comes back from the lab positive for Vibrio cholerae.

You contact the directors of the nearest hospital to find out what protocols are in place to deal with the outbreak. They explain that the region has not experienced a cholera epidemic for over 100 years. This epidemic was completely unexpected, and there are no plans in place for dealing with it.

Meanwhile, since her rehydration therapy, Eva has developed tachypnea and tachycardia and is coughing up frothy pink secretions. You sit her up and give oxygen, and she gradually improves. She makes a full recovery.

Box 18.1: Minimum Supplies Needed to Treat 100 Patients During a Cholera Outbreak [8]

Rehydration supplies:

- 650 packets oral rehydration salts (for 1 l each)
- 120 bags Ringer's lactate solution, 1 l, with giving sets
- 10 scalp vein sets
- 3 nasogastric tubes, 5.3 mm OD, 3.5 mm ID (16 French), 50 cm long for adults
- 3 nasogastric tubes, 2.7 mm OD, 1.5 mm ID (8 French), 38 cm long for children

Antibiotics:

Adults

- 60 capsules doxycycline, 100 mg (3 capsules per severely dehydrated patient)

Children

- 300 tablets co-trimoxazole, each tablet trimethoprim 20 mg + sulfamethoxazole 100 mg (15 tablets per severely dehydrated patient)

Other treatment supplies:

- 2 large water dispensers with tap (marked at 5- and 10-l levels) for making ORS solution in bulk
- 20 bottles (1 l) for oral rehydration solution (e.g., empty IV bottles)
- 20 bottles (0.5 l) for oral rehydration solution
- 40 tumblers, 200 ml
- 20 teaspoons
- 5 kg cotton wool
- 3 reels adhesive tape

The supplies listed are sufficient for IV fluid followed by oral rehydration salts for 20 severely dehydrated patients and for oral rehydration salts alone for the other 80 patients.

If Ringer's lactate solution is unavailable, normal saline may be substituted.

Prompt 8: What Are the Complications of Rapid Rehydration Therapy?

- Pulmonary edema is caused by giving too much IV fluid too quickly. Rapid fluid replacement overwhelms the heart's ability to pump the fluid and leads to buildup in the pulmonary circuit causing respiratory distress and pink frothy sputum. Cerebral edema (brain swelling) may also result from the rapid fluid shifts in electrolyte imbalances during rehydration therapy.
- Metabolic acidosis is another complication of rapid administration of normal saline. This is a hyperchloremic acidosis which occurs when the kidneys are unable to generate enough HCO_3^- to compensate for the increase in chloride.
- Acute kidney injury occurs when too little fluid is given and shock is not rapidly corrected or is allowed to recur. Renal failure is rare when severe dehydration is rapidly corrected and normal hydration is maintained according to guidelines.
- Generally, the more acute the fluid loss, the more acutely it can be replaced. When the guidelines for IV rehydration are followed, pulmonary edema should not occur. Oral rehydration solution (ORS) never causes pulmonary edema [9].

Prompt 9: What Are the Local Priorities in Managing a Cholera Epidemic?

Early detection, treatment, and health education are the best control measures in a cholera outbreak. In countries with inadequate rural health services and no experience in controlling cholera, there is a delay in initiating these processes. The WHO recommends the formation of local mobile teams of skilled health workers, epidemiologists, engineers, and educators to work in collaboration with existing or newly arrived NGOs [9].

Early Detection

- As soon as a cholera outbreak is suspected, local authorities should be notified so that plans can be initiated.

Treatment

- Engineers should supervise the construction of emergency treatment centers and rehydration posts and ensure the provision of appropriate environmental sanitary measures and disinfection. These centers provide rapid and efficient treatment for a large number of patients in areas inaccessible to existing health facilities. Cholera beds should be constructed. These beds have a hole with a bucket underneath to collect diarrhea during treatment. (See Fig. 18.2)
- It is not necessary to impose quarantine or strict isolation measures although it is best to restrict contact between patients and community to a minimum. There

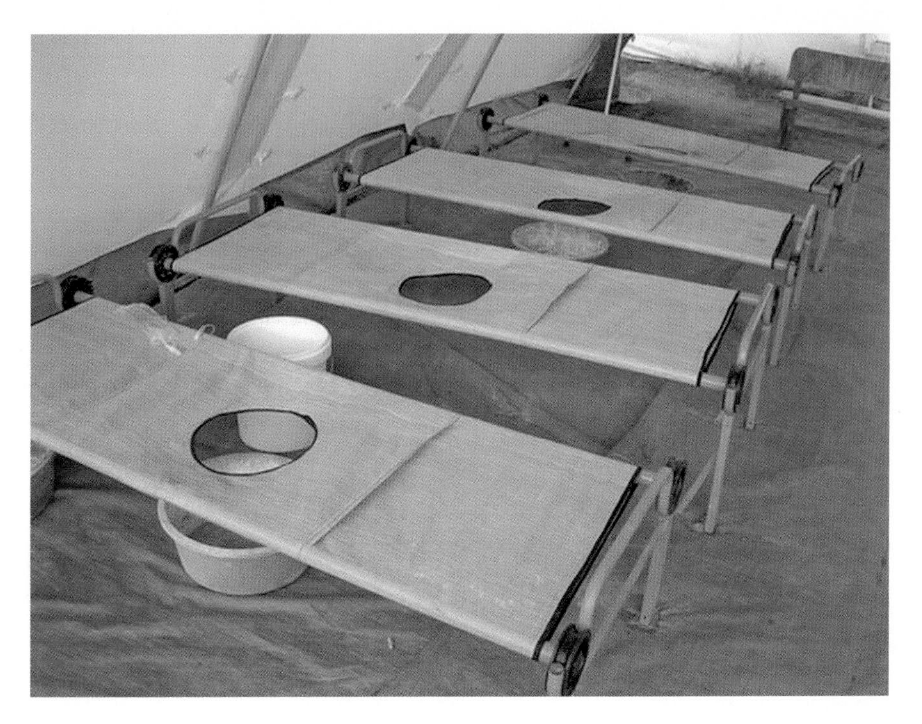

Fig. 18.2 Cholera beds (Photo taken by Taseum)

must be convenient hand-washing facilities for people working with cholera patients, and the safe disposal of excreta and vomit is essential.

Education

- Health workers should provide on-the-spot training in case management for local health staff. Educators should carry out health education activities and disseminate information to the public to prevent panic. Safe hand washing, drinking water safety/treatment, and food preparation practices must be taught.

Investigation of Outbreak

- Epidemiologists should establish the mode of disease transmission through investigation of outbreaks and assessment of local infrastructure. In reality, stool samples and environmental specimens rarely help with identifying the route of transmission as the data is too variable. Case-control studies are more effective in identifying cholera transmission routes.
- Recording the time and place of suspected and confirmed cases, preferably on a spot map, can help identify sources and routes of infection and spread.
- Adults are more frequently affected in cholera outbreaks due to their greater exposure to sources of contamination, such as food or drinks taken outside the home. A prevalence of cases in children suggests that the disease is endemic in the area [8].

Further Information 4

One month after the first case of cholera, over 1,000 people have died, and 100,000 have been affected by the disease. You feel aggrieved that resources and reinforcements took so long to reach the communities around the health center. The government has been much maligned for its poor preparatory measures, and there is strong feeling that many deaths could have been prevented. This has prompted the Ministry of Health to begin planning for future epidemics.

Prompt 10: How Should Nations Plan for Future Cholera Epidemics?

Once cholera is established, it can lay dormant for years before reemerging. Emergency measures are needed to minimize the risk of recurring outbreaks developing into epidemics. Improvements in both the water supply and sanitation are the best means of preventing cholera, but in resource-poor countries, this cannot be achieved. Affordable short- and medium-term preparations are the priority. The WHO has suggested a program for the Control of Diarrheal Diseases (CDD) involving education, resource, and surveillance measures [9].

Training and Education

- Medical personnel must be familiar with the most effective techniques for managing patients with acute diarrhea, including cholera. Public health education programs must continually stress the principles of good personal hygiene and safe food preparation while stressing the importance of using safe water sources and the safe disposal of excreta.

Resources

- Stocks of rehydration salts, IV fluids, and antibiotics must be maintained at appropriate points in the drug delivery system. Stocks should be kept in local health facilities in addition to district levels with an adequate emergency stock at a central distribution point (see Box 18.1).

Surveillance

- Daily records should be maintained of diarrheal cases seen in health facilities and by health workers in the community. When changes in the pattern of diarrheal disease occur, the nearest referral facility should be notified. Epidemiological investigation, such as case-control studies, should be promptly arranged to determine the cause of the outbreak, and the manager of the national CDD program should be informed [6, 9].

Case Study: The Haiti Cholera Epidemic 2010

Nine months after the Haitian earthquake (2010), a cholera outbreak emerged in the Centre Department (region) of central Haiti. The epidemic was precipitated by an influx of earthquake survivors fleeing the capital Port-au-Prince into the Centre and Artibonite departments. Sanitation and drinking water provision were poor in these departments prior to the earthquake, and the influx increased the exposure of populations to fecal-oral disease transmission. Within 48 h of the cholera outbreak, 1,500 cases were recorded [1].

Epidemiological studies mapped the outbreak along the course of a large river in the Centre and Artibonite Departments. The outbreak was blamed on UN workers from Nepal whose compound backed onto the river. Although not scientifically proven, it was suspected that Nepali workers inadvertently introduced endemic Asian cholera into the river.

Given the availability of safe drinking water (transported by tanker trucks) in the displacement camps, the camps were somewhat protected from severe cholera outbreaks. The major outbreaks were found in existing communities in the Artibonite delta and mountainous areas and in the non-displacement camp slums in Port-au-Prince (Daniele Lantagne, 2012).

Between October 20th and November 9th, the NGO "Partners in Health" recorded 7,159 cases of cholera, of which 161 died in 7 hospitals in the Centre and Artibonite departments (a case fatality rate (CFR) of 2.2 %) [1].

Forty-eight hours after Hurricane Tomas hit (November 6th), Partners in Health reported seven clinical cases of cholera in a large displacement camp, and MSF reported seeing 200 patients with cholera in the nearby Cite Soleil slum where tanker truck water was unavailable. By November 9th, the Ministry of Health reported 11,125 hospitalized patients and 724 confirmed deaths [1].

Relief efforts were hampered by the speed with which the epidemic spread and by Haiti's inexperience in dealing with cholera. Haiti had very little institutional knowledge about cholera, and it took time to train health workers (who had no prior experience of the disease) to put in place suitable containment and disease treatment measures. The CFR was 10 % in the first 48 h of the outbreak which reflects the delay in appropriate management. Hospitals were completely overwhelmed, and many patients died before treatment [1].

Between the 20th and 26th February 2011, 7,664 new cases and 52 new deaths were registered, and the overall case fatality rate was 1.9 %. Case fatality rates varied widely between regions (Port-au-Prince having 0.9 % and the Sud-Est Department having 8.5 %) which is most likely due to both the variation in logistical reality of accessing healthcare and the variation in the human capacity to deliver training and healthcare in different regions [10].

References

1. Walton DA, Ivers LC. Responding to cholera in post-earthquake Haiti. New England Journal of Medicine. 2011;364:3–5.
2. "We've been forgotten": Conditions in Haiti's displacement camps eight months after the earthquake, 2010, Joint report from University of San Francisco, Institute for Justice and Democracy in Haiti and The LAMP for Haiti Foundation. (http://ijdh.org/wordpress/wp-content/uploads/2010/09/IDP-Report-09.23.10-compressed.pdf).
3. Ananda Pokhrel. 2003. How to promote measures to prevent water-borne diseases, Nepal Water for Health in: IRC International Water and Sanitation Centre library (Assessed in 2011 at: http://www.irc.nl/page/8904).
4. Lever D, Soffer E. 2010. Acute Diarrhea, Cleveland Clinic: Center for Continuing Education (Assessed in 2011 at: http://www.clevelandclinicmeded.com/medicalpubs/diseasemanagement/gastroenterology/acute-diarrhea/).
5. WHO. International Health Regulations, 1969, Third annotated edition; 1983 (http://whqlibdoc.who.int/publications/1983/9241580070.pdf).
6. Global Task Force on Cholera Control. Cholera outbreak: assessing the outbreak response and improving preparedness, WHO publications; 2010. (WHO reference number: WHO/CDS/CPE/ZFK/2004.4).
7. WHO heath topics: Cholera (www.who.int/topis/cholera/about/en/index.html).
8. Wachsmuth K, Blake PA, Olsvik O. Vibrio cholerae and cholera: molecular to global perspectives. Washington D.C.: ASM Press; 1994.
9. Guidelines for Cholera Control. Geneva: World Health Organization; 1993.
10. PAHO. Epidemiological alert: weekly update on the cholera situation. Epidemiological Week 8 (Feb 20-26 2011) published 17 Mar 2011.

Chapter 19
HIV/AIDS

Shao Foong Chong and Michael Brown

Learning Objectives

- Recognize common presentations of HIV
- Outline the clinical complications associated with HIV
- Describe the clinical and immunological stages of HIV infection
- Discuss what investigations and treatment can be offered for people with HIV in developing countries
- Outline WHO's new antiretroviral therapy guidelines
- Discuss issues that arise from HIV/TB coinfection
- Recognize the problem with MDR- and XDR-TB
- Describe the epidemiology of the HIV/AIDS epidemic
- Outline global initiatives to fight HIV/AIDS

Initial Scenario

Mr. B, a 26-year-old long-distance lorry driver living in a township, is admitted to a local hospital severely ill and bed bound for the last 10 days, complaining of coughing up blood-stained sputum, headache, and a low-grade fever. Given that he lives in a township where the population prevalence of HIV is over 50 % and he is in a specific at-risk group, you suspect that his illness may be related to HIV. You are the attending doctor.

S.F. Chong, MBBS, MA (Oxon) (✉)
FY2 Doctor, Department of Emergency Medicine,
St George's Hospital, Tooting, London, UK
e-mail: shaofoong@hotmail.com

Michael Brown, BA (Oxon), BM BCh, MRCP, PhD, DTM&H
Consultant Physician, Hospital for Tropical Diseases, London, UK

D. MacGarty, D. Nott (eds.), *Disaster Medicine*,
DOI 10.1007/978-1-4471-4423-6_19,

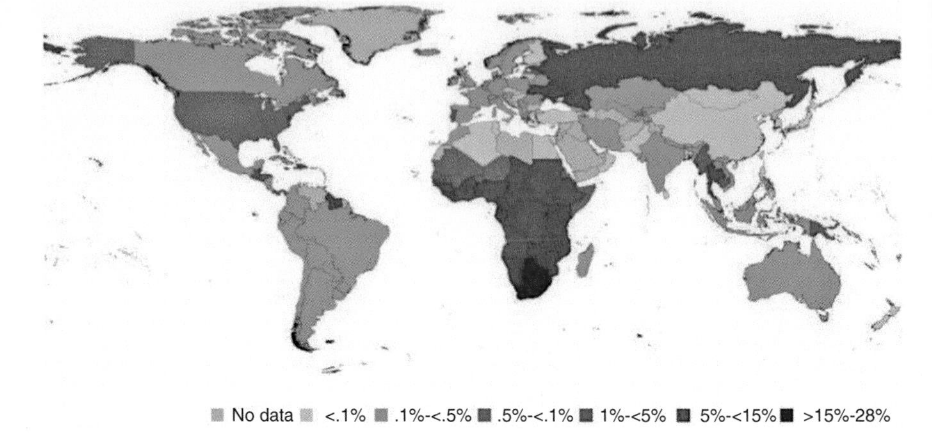

Fig. 19.1 Global prevalence of HIV, 2009 (Source: UNAIDS [1])

Prompt 1: What Information Would You Like to Elicit in the History?

How Long Has the Cough and with Red Sputum Been Present? Any Chest Pain? Smoking History?

- Sudden onset of hemoptysis under 2 weeks may occur with acute respiratory tract infections and pulmonary embolism, while a chronic recurrent course may occur with other conditions like lung neoplasm or tuberculosis (TB). Chronic dry cough and breathlessness are found in *Pneumocystis jirovecii*, although this is uncommon in adults in Africa [2]. Pleuritic chest pain is not uncommon in pneumonia or TB. Smoking history predisposes him to chest infections, to TB, and, if he were older, to lung cancer.

Other Sites of Bleeding: Hematuria, Dysentery, or Epistaxis?

- Hematuria is associated with Goodpasture's syndrome, dysentery may occur with parasitic disease such as amoebiasis or bacterial infections, and epistaxis with Wegener's granulomatosis and hereditary hemorrhagic telangiectasia.

Characteristics of the Headache?

- Worsening headache associated with photophobia, neck stiffness, vomiting, and non-blanching rash are sinister signs for meningoencephalitis. Early morning headaches may be caused by an intracerebral space-occupying lesion or hydrocephalus.

Previous History of Opportunistic Infections?

- Often, there is a history of shingles, pneumonia, or, if someone has advanced HIV disease, concurrent oral lesions, unexplained persistent diarrhea, fever, and severe weight loss.

Prompt 2: What Aspects on Examination Should You Look for to Confirm HIV/AIDS?

General Examination

- Fevers, wasting, and anemia – Signs of disseminated infection. "Slim disease" is sometimes equated with African AIDS [2].
- Generalized lymphadenopathy – May be found in a number of conditions such as HIV, TB, or lymphoma.

Respiratory

- Lobar consolidation with bronchial breathing may be heard with pneumonia, most likely pneumococcal.
- Inspiratory crepitations audible bilaterally over the upper lungs is suggestive of TB.

Abdominal

- Oral or esophageal thrush due to *Candida albicans*. Oral hairy leukoplakia is a white patch usually occurring along the sides of the tongue with a corrugated or hairy appearance, associated with Epstein-Barr virus.
- Abdominal pain and chronic diarrhea are present in colitis due to underlying HIV infection, widespread metastatic disease, or disseminated TB infection or cytomegalovirus.

Neurological

- Headache, neck stiffness, and confusion may be caused by cerebral toxoplasmosis, cryptococcal meningitis, CNS lymphoma, cytomegalovirus encephalitis, progressive multifocal leukoencephalopathy, and cerebral abscesses.
- Rapid painless visual field loss can occur in late stage of HIV infection due to cytomegalovirus retinitis, where fundoscopy would be useful.

Skin

- Examine for burrows in the hand and groin for scabies.
- Blistering rash in a dermatome distribution from an eruption of *Herpes zoster*.
- Painless purple/violet raised plaques typically found in the palate from Kaposi's sarcoma.

- Chronic itchy maculopapular rash that may be hyperpigmented or nodular in dark skin for HIV dermatitis.
- Genital ulcers, warts, etc.

Further Information 1

You find out that Mr. B has had a cough, hemoptysis, night sweats, fatigue, and weight loss of almost 10 kg for 1 month, with a 10-pack-year smoking history. He lives alone in the township and does a lot of long-distance driving for his work.

On examination, you notice he appears lean and pale with oral candidiasis, supraclavicular lymphadenopathy, and inspiratory crepitations bilaterally over the upper zones.

Your impression is that his HIV infection has caused significant immune deficiency, which has laid him vulnerable to bacterial pneumonia, oral thrush, and opportunistic infections, in particular TB.

Prompt 3: Define HIV and AIDS

- *Human immunodeficiency virus* (*HIV*) – An RNA retrovirus that causes the loss of function and depletion of CD4 T-helper lymphocytes, which disrupt both cell-mediated and humoral immunity. As HIV progresses and CD4 count falls, opportunistic infections happen. Without treatment, the average survival time after HIV infection is estimated to be 10 years.
- *Acquired immune deficiency syndrome* (*AIDS*) – End stage of HIV disease due to advanced immunosuppression associated with certain severe life-threatening opportunistic infections or cancers. The progression to AIDS is diagnosed when any condition listed in clinical stage 4 is diagnosed and/or the CD4 count is less than 200×10^6 cells/L or a CD4 percentage less than 15. Prognosis is no more than 2 years without medication.

Prompt 4: Outline the Difference in Presentation of Opportunistic Infections Commonly Associated with HIV/AIDS Between Developing and Developed Countries

- Opportunistic infections are defined by pathogens of relatively low virulence that take the opportunity to cause disease when their host has a compromised immune system.
- In the developing world, patients may initially present with opportunistic disease associated with later stages of HIV disease as time has allowed more severe immunosuppression to develop. Opportunistic infections such as tuberculosis, cerebral toxoplasmosis, or cryptococcal meningitis may be present.

- In the developed world, patients will generally seek medical advice earlier with symptoms. Therefore, conventional pathogens such as Mycobacterium tuberculosis, *Pneumocystis jirovecii* pneumonia, esophageal *Candida albicans*, and Kaposi's sarcoma-associated human herpes virus 8 may be the initial presentation.

Prompt 5: Describe the Natural Course of HIV Infection

Group 1 – Primary HIV Infection

- During primary HIV infection, also known as acute seroconversion illness, there is wide dissemination of virus, seeding of lymphoid organs, and a marked fall in CD4 count, and very high viral load making patients very infectious. This occurs 2–6 weeks after exposure, while some people remain asymptomatic; between 25 and 65 % of people have a transient flulike illness complaining of fever, headache, tiredness, and enlarged neck lymph nodes similar to glandular fever [3].

Group II – Asymptomatic Infection

- After seroconversion, the CD4 count returns to near normal levels or above 350×10^6, and the individual is asymptomatic. There is slow but silent virus replication in lymph nodes during this phase, and viral load assays can be used to quantify this. This phase of the illness varies widely among individuals from a few months to over 10 years before immune system dysfunction produces symptoms.

Group III – Persistent Generalized Lymphadenopathy

- HIV-related lymphadenopathy, which is defined as enlarged lymph nodes in at least two extra-inguinal sites that persist for at least 3 months, may present with people with HIV infection who are otherwise well.

Group IV – Symptomatic infection/AIDS

- Progressive depletion of CD4 cells is associated with progression of HIV disease and increased replication from latent sites (Fig. 19.2). This results in a weakened immune system that is susceptible to AIDS-defining opportunistic infections or unusual HIV-related tumors (Table 19.1). In tropical regions, people with HIV disease living in poor overcrowded communities are particularly vulnerable to respiratory and diarrheal opportunistic infections.

Prompt 6: Outline the Clinical Stages of HIV Infection win the Africa Region

In resource-limited settings, CD4 and viral load tests are not readily available to determine the right time to begin antiretroviral treatment. Thus, the World Health Organization (WHO) has developed a staging system for HIV disease based on

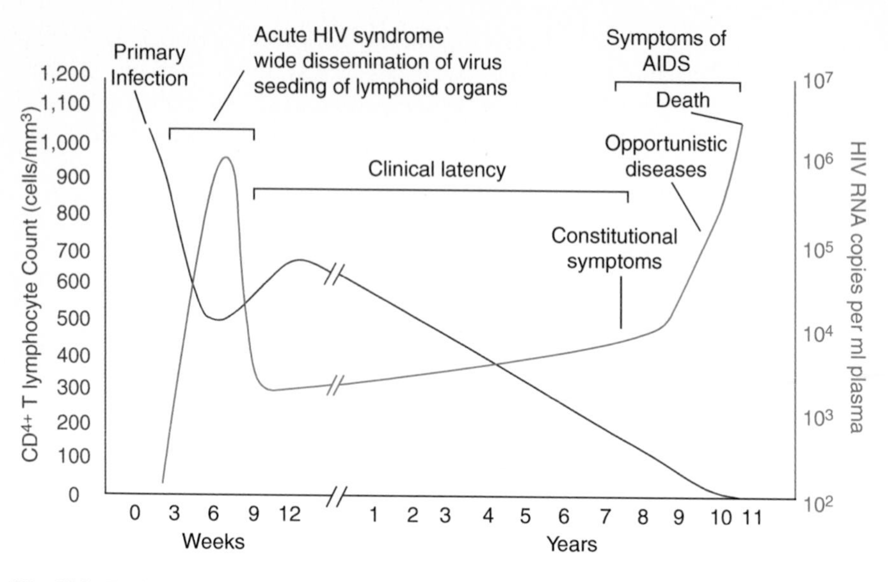

Fig. 19.2 Typical course of HIV infection (Adapted from Panaleo et al. [3])

Table 19.1 WHO clinical staging of established HIV [4]

WHO clinical stage	HIV-related conditions
1. Asymptomatic	Asymptomatic
	Persistent generalized lymphadenopathy
2. Mild symptoms	Moderate unexplained weight loss (<10 % of presumed or measured body weight)
	Recurrent respiratory tract infections
	Herpes zoster
	Papular pruritic eruptions
3. Advanced symptoms	Unexplained severe weight loss, chronic diarrhea, or persistent fever for longer than 1 month
	Persistent oral candidiasis
	Pulmonary tuberculosis (current)
	Severe presumed bacterial infections (e.g., pneumonia, empyema, pyomyositis, bone or joint infection, meningitis, bacteremia)
	Unexplained anemia (<8 g/dL) and/or neutropenia (<500/mm^3) or chronic thrombocytopenia (<50,000/mm^3)
4. Severe symptoms	HIV wasting syndrome
	Pneumocystis pneumonia or extrapulmonary TB
	HIV encephalopathy, central nervous system toxoplasmosis, extrapulmonary cryptococcosis including meningitis
	Chronic cryptosporidiosis or isosporiasis
	Cytomegalovirus infection (retinitis or of other organs)
	Kaposi's sarcoma
	Recurrent non-typhoidal salmonella septicemia
	Lymphoma (cerebral or B cell non-Hodgkin)
	Invasive cervical carcinoma

Table 19.2 Immunological staging of HIV infection

Stage of immunosuppression	CD4 count × 10^9 per liter
None or not significant	>500
Mild	350–499
Advanced	200–349
Severe	<200 or <15 %

clinical symptoms to guide management, monitoring, and surveillance. N.B. Table 19.1 includes a selected number of clinical conditions.

Prompt 7: Describe the Immunological Stage of HIV Infection

- Long-term prognosis has been shown to be related to the CD4 count (Table 19.2); opportunistic infections and other HIV-related conditions are increasingly likely with CD4 counts below 200.
- Where facilities are available, CD4 testing is useful for determining the degree of immunocompromise and support clinical decision making. CD4 levels are not necessary for start treatment but can be used in conjunction with clinical stages to provide a better idea of the severity of HIV infection.

Further Information 2

You inform Mr. B that you would like to do some tests on him. You counsel him that you believe he has HIV and a number of associated diseases. You would like his consent to having an HIV test. At first he is resistant, but you explain the results will be kept confidential and, if diagnosed, HIV can be treated preventing progression to AIDS. You explain there is funding for treatment, and so later he agrees. You assess his HIV infection as stage 3 with advanced symptoms and would like to immediately start him on antiretroviral treatment.

Prompt 8: Outline How to Test for HIV in the Developing World

- Voluntary counseling and testing (VCT) facilities should be accessible to the general population where information about the purpose of the test and implications of a positive or negative result are provided in confidence. But particular focus should be targeted toward specific at-risk groups, such as commercial sex workers, long-distance lorry drivers, and intravenous drug users.

- Provider-initiated HIV testing and counseling (PITC) occurs in health facilities to support increased uptake and improve access to HIV prevention and treatment. In high HIV-prevalence settings, all patients who present to hospitals with opportunistic infections should be tested for HIV.
- HIV infection is diagnosed with a positive HIV antibody test, which uses blood, saliva, or urine to provide an antibody/antigen measurement. There are a variety of methods that can identify anti-HIV antibodies, but local policies on HIV testing ought to reflect local resources, which may exclude expensive techniques such as Western blotting. WHO recommends a combination of rapid point of care tests (POCTs) using rapid test devices, which can provide results within about 20 minutes of a specimen being taken, so results are available within a single clinic session, as well as enzyme-linked immunosorbent assay (ELISA) methods in the laboratory [2].
- Sensitivity of these HIV tests is high, and while ELISA specificity is good, POCT specificity testing is lower. Therefore, WHO recommends a second HIV antibody test relying on different antigens or of different operating characteristics to confirm HIV [4].
- Tests for CD4 count should be performed where possible to decide when to initiate antiretroviral therapy although therapy can be started on clinical suspicion alone. Viral load estimation is helpful in monitoring response to treatment but is expensive and may not be available in developing countries.

Prompt 9: What Investigations Should Be Performed for Opportunistic Infections and Diseases Commonly Associated with HIV/AIDS?

- *Sputum sample* – Gram staining of sputum is useful in confirming types of bacterial pneumonia. A sample should be tested for Ziehl-Neelsen stain which is a rapid and sensitive microscopical test looking for acid-fast bacilli (this does require trained personnel). TB culture on Lowenstein-Jensen medium adds very little for initial management as it typically takes 4–6 weeks to identify *M. tuberculosis* but should be performed for patients at high risk of drug-resistant TB. Increasingly, liquid culture methods (DOTS and MGIT) and molecular methods (Xpert MTB/rif) are available.
- *Chest X-ray* – Consolidation is likely due to bacterial infection or empyema. Tuberculosis (TB) infection is classically seen as upper-lobe cavitations. In HIV, the X-ray may be normal or otherwise atypical for TB. *Pneumocystis jirovecii* demonstrates widespread pulmonary infiltrates.
- *CT head* – Unlikely in a rural setting.
- *Lumbar puncture – Examination of* cerebrospinal fluid may provide useful information with white blood cell count and total protein. Microscopy with India ink may diagnose cryptococcal meningitis.

Prompt 10: What Are the Guidelines for Antiretroviral Treatment (ART)?

When to Start Therapy

- The decision to start ART may be based on WHO staging of clinical symptoms +/– CD4 count. The objective is to reduce and sustain low plasma viral load concentrations, keep the CD4 cell count high, and reduce the rate at which resistance develops.
- There is strong evidence of the clinical benefit of ART in HIV-positive adults with advanced and severe symptoms [2]. Thus, in resource-limited settings where CD4 counts are not available, all patients with WHO clinical stages 3 and 4 disease should start ART irrespective of their CD4 cell count.
- In 2010, WHO revised ART guidelines in response to research which showed ART with advanced immunodeficiency had better virological outcomes than those with more severe immunodeficiency. Thus, where CD4 counts are available, any patients with HIV infection with a CD4 count $<350 \times 10^9$ should start on therapy, regardless of the presence or absence of clinical symptoms [5].
- There is an impetus to improve management of coinfections between HIV and TB or hepatitis B. Thus, all people living with HIV who have active TB and chronic active hepatitis B disease should be started on ART as soon as possible, irrespective of CD4 cell counts.

Recommended Regimens

- A public health approach has been advocated in developing settings where individually tailored ART delivery is not feasible. Where HIV clinics are run by various health-care professionals ranging from doctors to social workers, simple protocols allow ART be prescribed to a large number of clients safely. It is hoped that the use of less toxic drugs and fixed-dose combinations will reduce the risk of adverse events and improved adherence.
- There are three classes of drugs: nucleoside reverse transcriptase inhibitors (NRTI), non-nucleoside reverse transcriptase inhibitors (NNRTI), and protease inhibitors (PI). First-line therapy should consist of an NNRTI and 2 NRTIs, one of which should be zidovudine or tenofovir. An example of a fixed-dose combination may be zidovudine (NRTI) and lamivudine (NRTI) plus efavirenz (NNRTI). Stavudine, an NRTI, should be avoided in first-line regimens because of its well-recognized toxicities. Second-line therapy should consist of a ritonavir-boosted PI plus 2 NRTIs [5].

Prompt 11: How Do You Treat This Opportunistic Infection?

- Treatment of pneumonia is with a 5–7-day course of benzylpenicillin. If the patient does not respond and you suspect that he has pulmonary TB, attempt to obtain a sputum sample for microscopy, and if confirmed, start him on the WHO

DOTS (Directly Observed Therapy, Short-course) 6-month course of antituberculosis chemotherapy. A decision will have to be made as to whether to start treatment if there is no facility for microscopy or if the microscopy is negative.
- Oral candida can be treated with antifungal agents such as nystatin drops, miconazole gel, or fluconazole tablets.
- Cryptococcal disease can be treated with intravenous amphotericin B or high-dose fluconazole, if this is unavailable, and cerebral toxoplasmosis with oral cotrimoxazole.
- Cotrimoxazole prophylaxis is generally given to all patients living with HIV in Africa with CD4 counts $< 500 \times 10^6$/L or with WHO clinical stage 2, 3, or 4 [2]. Studies suggest it has a protective effect against *Isospora belli*, *Pneumocycistic jirovecii*, and *Toxoplasma gondii* but also against common bacterial infections and malaria.

Further Information 3

Sputum samples taken on three consecutive mornings are put under a light microscope and are not smear positive for acid-fast bacilli (AFB). You make a presumptive diagnosis of smear-negative pulmonary TB (and 3 weeks later, the cultures come up positive for M. tuberculosis. You explain that he is coinfected with TB and HIV.

Prompt 12: What Is the Relationship Between TB and HIV?

- Mortality in coinfected patients is much higher than in patients only suffering TB. Sometimes, TB infections remain latent, but it may later become active where the bacteria multiple and spread within the body to other people by airborne transmission. If HIV is advanced, the TB tends to present more quickly, as in the case of Mr. B. Doctors should not be surprised by a short history of deterioration in HIV/TB coinfection. Moreover, TB accelerates the progression of HIV infection to AIDS.
- Nearly 40 million people are living with HIV worldwide, and 30 % of those have TB [6]. In the past 15 years, new TB cases have tripled in countries with high HIV prevalence. People with HIV are 50 times more likely than HIV negative people to develop active TB in a given year. Without proper treatment, 90 % of people living with HIV die within months of contracting TB.
- The diagnosis of TB in HIV-positive individuals is hard because sensitive diagnostic tests to detect TB bacteria are lacking. Another problem that exists is that the number with TB who knew their HIV status in low- and middle-income countries is low at 16 %.

Prompt 13: Assess the Interactions That Occur When Treating HIV/TB Coinfection

- TB may be hard to diagnose in people coinfected with HIV. For example, the tuberculin skin test may be negative due to immune response dysfunction leading in the loss of delayed hypersensitivity. Moreover, many people with pulmonary TB are smear negative for AFB. Studies have shown that the problem worsens as severity of HIV increases. People with HIV have a weakened immune system where their bodies produce less sputum. So when they cough, they only produce a few AFB, which is not enough to be detected under a microscope.
- The presentation of pulmonary TB may be atypical, being more severe or unusual in its distribution. Normally, patients with TB demonstrate infiltrates in the upper lungs with or without mediastinal or hilar lymphadenopathy; coinfection HIV/TB patients may have lesions anywhere in the lungs such as lobar and bibasal consolidation. Furthermore, extrapulmonary TB, such as pleural, pericardial, peritoneal, meningeal, renal or spinal TB, or even disseminated TB, is much more common.
- TB treatment in poor countries entails following the WHO DOTS regimen which involved the use of four different TB drugs (the first-line drugs) for 2 months followed by a 4-month continuation phase using the two most potent drugs given in the first 2 months (usually rifampicin and isoniazid). If they have HIV and their CD4 count is low, they are likely to need at least three different types of ARVs. There is increased toxicity from combining anti-TB and anti-HIV drugs.
- Immune reconstitution inflammatory syndrome (IRIS) sometimes occurs when ARV rapidly improves the immune system so much that it raises an inflammatory response to a previous acquired opportunistic infection which causes a paradoxical worsening of their clinical condition. Despite this, the benefit of early ART in coinfected patients, who are prone to other opportunistic infections, outweighs the generally non-life-threatening features of TB-IRIS, and early initiation of ART (with 2–4 weeks of starting TB treatment) is recommended.

Prompt 14: Outline the Emerging Problem of Multidrug-Resistant TB

- If a TB drug regimen is not completed or is taken sporadically, TB bacteria can develop resistance to the drugs. People with HIV/AIDS are at slightly greater risk. Multidrug-resistant (MDR) TB can develop when bacilli become resistant to the two most powerful first-line drugs, i.e., isoniazid and rifampicin. Resistant bacilli can then spread to others. Extensively drug-resistant (XDR) TB occurs when second-line therapies are not used properly and bacteria develop resistance to them as well.

- One of the main challenges in ensuring good TB therapy is compliance. Directly observed treatment, short-course (DOTS) is a major strategy to combat MDR-TB by having an independent observer watching patients swallow their prescribed anti-TB drugs throughout the course of treatment. However, it is not easy to enforce.
- Few new TB drugs have been developed, and the medications used now are the same as those that were used in the 1950s. Massive scale-up in research and development of new TB medication is required to stop TB.

Further Information 3

Mr. B takes all the medications that were prescribed to him under DOTS, and his symptoms get better. After 1 month, however, he stops coming to his follow-up clinics, and he stops taking ART. He says that he lives too far away from the hospital and the drugs are making him feel worse than when he was without them. Within 4 months, Mr. B dies. As a doctor, you do some research to find out how bad the problem of HIV is and what is being done on a global scale to fight it.

Prompt 15: Describe the Epidemiology of the HIV/AIDS Epidemic

- Since the beginning of the epidemic in 1982, more than 60 million people have been infected with HIV and nearly 30 million people have died of HIV-related causes. The greatest burden is in sub-Saharan Africa, South Asia, and Southeast Asia (Fig. 19.1). In 2009, sub-Saharan Africa accounted for approximately 70 % of people living with HIV worldwide and for 72 % of the world's AIDS-related deaths. Most transmission in this region occurs in heterosexual relationships, both in the context of transactional and commercial sex and in long-term relationships, including marriage.
- Globally, AIDS-related illnesses remain one of the leading causes of death, mostly because of inadequate access to HIV prevention care and treatment services. HIV/AIDS is the 6th largest cause of death responsible for 2 million deaths per year. Tuberculosis is the 7th, responsible for 1.5 million deaths per year. HIV also affects people earlier in life imposing a massive burden on the economies and health services of most of the poorest countries in the world to become the 5th largest burden of disease globally [7].
- In 2008, an estimated 33.4 million people were living with HIV (Table 19.3). It is also estimated by WHO and UNAIDS that out of the 15 million people who

Table 19.3 Global summary of the AIDS epidemic

Prevalence – number of people living with HIV	33.4 million (31.1–35.8 million)
Incidence – people newly infected with HIV	2.7 million (2.4–3.0 million)
AIDS deaths	2.0 million (1.7–2.4 million)

Source: UNAIDS, Report on the global AIDS epidemic, 2008 [8]
Notes: The numbers in parentheses are ranges around the estimates that define the boundaries within which the actual numbers lie, based on the best available information

were in need of ART, only 6.6 million people had access to treatment in low- and middle-income countries.

Prompt 16: Discuss International Initiatives for Tackling HIV/AIDS

Treatment 2.0 – A new UNAIDS approach started in 2010 to simplify the way HIV treatment is provided and increasing access to life-saving medicines. It aims to reduce new HIV infections by 33 % and avert an additional 10 million deaths by 2025 [9]. Treatment 2.0 requires progress across 5 areas:

- *Creating a better pill and diagnostics* – Pharmaceutical companies need to develop a "smarter, better pill" that will be less toxic, longer acting, and easier to use. The goal is to develop a simple diagnostic tool to provide viral load and CD4 cell counts at the point of care in order to reduce the burden on health systems.
- *Treatment as prevention* – Effective implementation of ART will result in viral suppression which will reduce the risk of HIV transmission. A study found that HIV transmission rate was 92 % lower than the HIV-positive partner in a heterosexual relationship was on ART [9].
- *Stop cost being an obstacle* – While drugs must continue to be made more affordable, the largest share of costs per person in low- and middle-income countries is from the laboratory, service delivery, procurement, and testing. These costs are currently twice the cost of the drugs themselves.
- *Improve uptake of HIV testing and linkage to care* – An estimated 40 % living with HIV know about their HIV status, as many are afraid of the stigma and discrimination attached to the infection. Community-based approaches are a good solution in improving treatment adherence and prevention practices and reducing stigma.
- *Strengthen community mobilization* – Treatment access and adherence can be improved by involving the community in managing treatment programs. Greater involvement of community-based organizations in treatment maintenance, adherence support, and monitoring will reduce the burden on health systems.

Case Study: HIV/TB Coinfection in Lesotho

Lesotho has the third highest HIV prevalence in the world with just under one in four people living with HIV. The AIDS epidemic paired with widespread poverty has caused the average life expectancy in the country to drop.

TB/HIV coinfection is getting worse, partly due to the impracticalities of adhering to treatment. People diagnosed with HIV/TB have to take a whole battery of medications, which have several side effects, including nausea, vomiting, neuropathy, and hepatitis. Often, these side effects stop them from taking their anti-TB and ART medication, which predisposes them to MDR-TB. One of the main problems cited is that people living in remote rural settings locations find it hard to travel all the way in to hospital to get checkups.

Lesotho has managed to get around this problem by having decentralized care, so care comes to patients rather than the other way around. Patients go to their local clinic to have their blood taken, which is then transported to the hospital laboratory for analysis. A few days later, these results are transported via an outreach vehicle back to the rural village, which saves all the patients coming to the hospital.

References

1. UNAIDS. Report on the global AIDS epidemic. Geneva: Joint United Nations Programme on HIV/AIDS; 2010. Available from: http://www.unaids.org/en/media/unaids/contentassets/documents/unaidspublication/2010/20101123_globalreport_en.pdf. Accessed 22 Aug 2012.
2. Gill GV, Beeching N. HIV infection and disease in the tropics. Lecture notes on tropical medicine. 6th ed. London: Wiley-Blackwell; 2009, Chapter 13.
3. Pantaleo G, et al. New concepts in the immunopathogenesis of human immunodeficiency virus infection. N Engl J Med. 1993;328(5):327–35.
4. WHO. WHO case definitions of HIV for surveillance and revised clinical staging and immunological classification of HIV-related disease in adults and children. 2006. Available at: http://www.who.int/hiv/pub/guidelines/HIVstaging150307.pdf. Accessed 22 Aug 2012.
5. WHO. Antiretroviral therapy for HIV infection in adults and adolescents. Recommendations for a public health approach. 2010 revision. Available at: http://whqlibdoc.who.int/publications/2010/9789241599764_eng.pdf. Accessed 22 Aug 2012.
6. HIV/TB Coinfection: Basic Facts, October 2007. Available at: http://www.eurekalert.org/HIV-TBreport/images/HIV_TB_Coinfection.pdf. Accessed 22 Aug 2012.
7. WHO. The global burden of disease. 2004 update. Available from: http://www.who.int/healthinfo/global_burden_disease/GBD_report_2004update_full.pdf. Accessed 22 Aug 2012.
8. UNAIDS and WHO. AIDS epidemic update. Geneva: WHO; 2009. Available from: http://data.unaids.org/pub/report/2009/jc1700_epi_update_2009_en.pdf. Accessed 22 Aug 2012.
9. UNAIDS. The Treatment 2.0 framework for action: catalysing the next phase of treatment, care and support. Available from: http://www.unaids.org/en/media/unaids/contentassets/documents/unaidspublication/2011/20110824_JC2208_outlook_treatment2.0_en.pdf. Accessed 22 Aug 2012.

Chapter 20
Blinding Eye Diseases

Ed Mew and Clare Gilbert

Learning Objectives

- Understand the basic clinical anatomy of the eye
- Consider differential diagnoses for red eye and visual loss in resource-poor settings
- List relevant features to elicit from history and examination when assessing patients with red eye or visual loss in resource-poor settings
- Outline the etiology, epidemiology, and clinical features of trachoma
- Identify groups at high risk of developing trachoma
- Describe treatment for trachoma
- Understand basic epidemiological terms (incidence, prevalence) and the background of epidemiological assessments of populations
- Outline approaches toward implementing community-based trachoma eradication programs, including budgeting and prioritization
- Explore issues surrounding neglected tropical diseases
- Describe what Vision 2020 is and how to enact its schemes (Fig. 20.1)

Initial Scenario

You are working as a general physician in a small village in rural Nepal. Your remit is ostensibly linked to improving pediatric health, but you hold weekly community clinics for minor presentations. You are struck by the large number of women and

E. Mew, MBBS (✉)
FY2 Doctor, Trauma, Emergency and Acute Medicine (TEAM),
King's College Hospital, Denmark Hill, London, UK
e-mail: eau.mew@gmail.com

C. Gilbert, FRCO phth MD MSc
London school of hygiene and tropical medicine, London, UK

D. MacGarty, D. Nott (eds.), *Disaster Medicine*,
DOI 10.1007/978-1-4471-4423-6_20, © Springer-Verlag London 2013

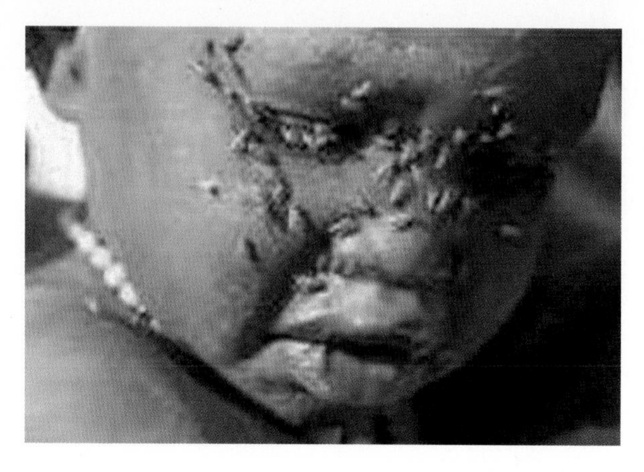

Fig. 20.1 Child with flies in her eyes (Permission courtesy of Sudan Medical Relief) [14]

children who present with eye complaints. Six-year-old Amreet has come to see you today complaining of sore red eyes.

Prompt 1: What Is the Clinical Anatomy of the Eye? (Fig. 20.2)

The cornea and lens are transparent tissues. Their role is to focus light entering the eye onto the retina. The pupil controls the amount of light entering the eye and modifies depth of field.

The retina converts light energy into electrical impulses which are transmitted to the brain via the optic nerve.

In a normal eye:

- The sclera is white.
- The cornea (dome-shaped transparent tissue in front of the iris and pupil) is clear with a bright light reflex.

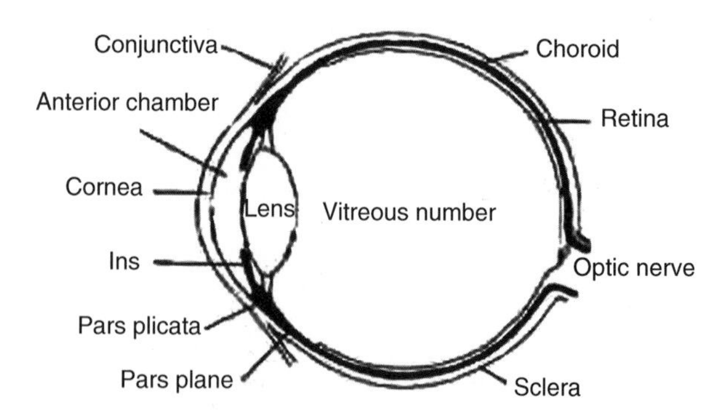

Fig. 20.2 Anatomy of the eye [17]

- No eyelashes touch the eyeball.
- The conjunctiva overlying the inner eyelid (bulbar conjunctiva) is healthy and transparent, with a few faint blood vessels.

Prompt 2: What Are the Commonest Causes of Red Eye and of Visual Loss in Resource-Poor Settings?

- Red eye and visual loss are common ophthalmic presentations. In resource-poor settings, differentials are different to those encountered in developing areas. See Tables 20.1 and 20.2 for details.

Table 20.1 Causes of "red eye"

Etiology	Vision	Common age	Ocular discharge	Special features
Viral conjunctivitis – commonest cause	Normal	Any	Watery	Corneal lesions
Bacterial conjunctivitis	Normal	Any	Purulent	Red/swollen
Ophthalmia neonatorum	Normal	Under 4 weeks	Purulent, particularly in gonococcal infection	Red/swollen, particularly in gonococcal infection URGENT referral is needed
Chlamydia (trachoma)	Normal	Young	Mucopurulent	Follicles on under surface of upper lid. Eyes not very red
Allergic	Normal	Young	Stringy	Itchy with infiltrate round cornea [1]. Eyes not very red
Acute glaucoma	Reduced	Elderly	Nil	Pain + vomiting. Often unilateral
Uveitis	Reduced	Middle age	Nil	Light sensitive. Often unilateral

- Causes of gradual vision loss, especially in a resource-poor setting, should trigger the possibilities listed in Table 20.2.

Prompt 3: What Information Should You Elicit from History and Exam in Cases of Red Eye or Vision Loss in Developing Countries?

History

- Eliciting relevant symptoms and risk factors for your differential diagnoses (see Tables 20.1 and 20.2).
- Any precipitating factor, for example, trauma?

Table 20.2 Gradual visual loss differential diagnosis [1, 2]

Etiology	Age group affected	Clinical features
Cataract	Middle aged or elderly, but can also affect babies and children	Painless, white/gray pupil opacity. So gradual that normally do not present at clinic until significant visual loss
Glaucoma (chronic)	Middle aged or elderly	Chronically raised intraocular pressure causes progressive painless visual loss starting leading to "tunnel vision." The external eye looks completely normal
Refractive errors: reduced distance vision	Any age	Refractive error, especially myopia (nearsightedness), is an increasing problem in children in Asia. The external eye looks completely normal
Age-related macular degeneration (AMD)	Elderly	AMD is a common cause of painless visual loss in the elderly. The external eye looks completely normal
Vitamin A deficiency	Children aged 6–72 months Lactating women	Night blindness, or foamy white conjunctival spots (Bitot spots), or to corneal scarring Exacerbated by measles infection, diarrhea, and malnutrition
Onchocerciasis	Middle aged or elderly	A filarial worm associated with biting blackflies leads to subcutaneous nodules, skin inflammation, and eye disease. Ocular manifestations include night blindness, corneal scars, and uveitis. Only occurs in Africa
Trachoma	Middle aged or elderly	Painful, red eye(s) with mucopurulent discharge and no history of trauma
Posttraumatic	Any age	Poor healing or infection to ocular injuries is likely with poor sanitation and health care

- Enquire about the exact nature of visual change/loss.
- Is this unilateral or bilateral?
- Is there associated discharge or pain?
- Are there any other systemic features that might suggest vitamin A deficiency (night blindness, recurrent infections)?
- Eye hygiene: Are the eyes washed regularly? Is there regular contact with flies or use of dirty towels/rags to wash? Are any others affected in the family? What is the state of local water supply and sanitation? [3]

Examination

- Examine both eyes in turn.
- If examining a child, ensure they are securely held by a parent or wrapped up to prevent wriggling.
- Ideally, you should examine at eye level, in daylight. Detailed advice on the examination process is beyond the scope of this book.
- A "quick and dirty" way to assess vision is to ask the patient to cover each eye in turn, and assess whether they can count the number of fingers you hold up in

front of them, 3 m from their face. Test each eye by showing three different numbers of fingers.
- If any pathology is found, WHO recommends that visual acuity be measured using a standardized Snellen or illiterate "E" chart [3].

Further Information 1

On questioning Amreet's mother, it is clear that he has had problems with both of his eyes which are now sore and gritty. His mother is not sure whether he washes his eyes regularly, but after eating, he wipes his face on a communal rag shared by both of his siblings. His siblings and mother also suffer from similar symptoms. His mother's vision is worsening. His father appears to be unaffected.

On examination, Amreet is an otherwise well, lively child and wriggles when you try to examine him. He frequently wipes at his right eye which is noticeably reddened.

Right eye: The cornea is clear and smooth. On everting the eyelid, multiple follicles are seen in the central tarsal conjunctiva.

Left eye: The cornea is clear and smooth. On everting the eyelid, multiple follicles are seen in the central tarsal conjunctiva.

Conclusion: You conclude that Amreet has trachomatous eye disease.

Prompt 4: What Is Trachoma?

Definition

Trachoma is an eye disease caused by infection of the eyes with a bacterium, *Chlamydia trachomatis*.

Epidemiology

Trachoma is among the commonest preventable cause of blindness worldwide. Globally, over 40 million children suffer from active infection, and over 8 million adults need eyelid surgery to prevent visual impairment. Trachoma affects developing countries with poor standards of sanitation, poor hygiene, and overcrowding. See Fig. 20.3 for the global distribution. The acute stages of the disease are commonest under 9 year olds, in deprived areas with poor water and inadequate sanitation, and also among those with prolonged contact with children – normally women.

The importance of diagnosing trachoma in a child in a clinical setting is that there are highly likely to be other infected children and adults with trichiasis in the community the child comes from.

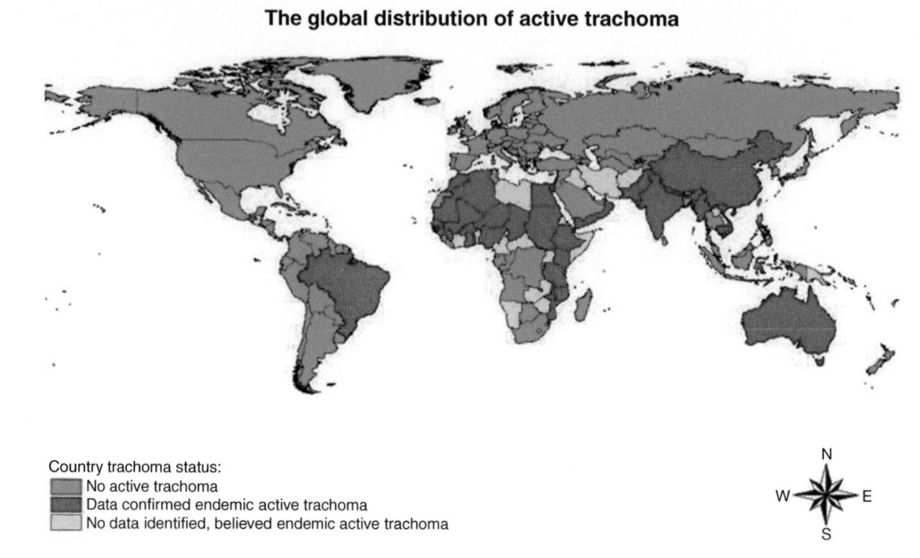

Fig. 20.3 Geographical distribution of active trachoma (Courtesy of WHO) [15]

Etiology

Transmission of the infection is by direct physical transmission of the bacteria through the use of shared bedding, through infected towels and cloths mothers use to wipe their child's face, and through flies.

Clinical Features

Broadly speaking, there are several stages of trachoma.

In children with active infection:

Follicular inflammation (at least 5 pale swellings in the central tarsal conjunctiva. Peripheral follicles may be normal). The eyelid needs to be everted to see signs of trachoma. Later on, this inflammation progresses to upper eyelid thickening. Early symptoms include itchy, sore eyes, and discharge. See Fig. 20.4.

In adults:

- ***Trichiasis***. Scarring from repeated infection leads to inverted eyelashes – at least one eyelash rubs on the eyeball. Symptoms include pain and watering.
- ***Corneal opacification***. This occurs through repeated infection and damage from inverted eyelashes; the cornea becomes opaque, often resulting in visual loss and culminating in blindness.

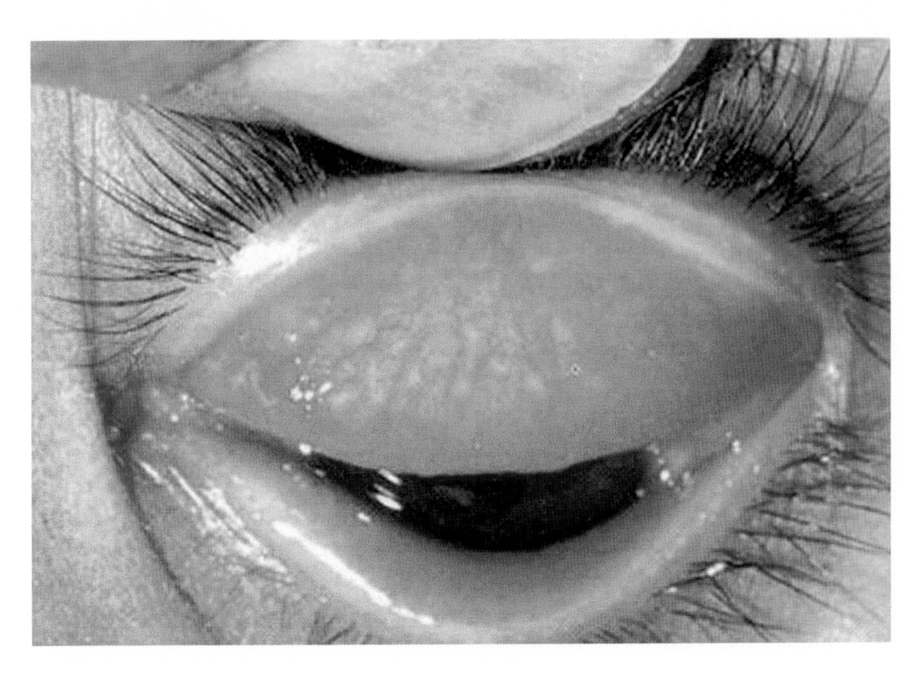

Fig. 20.4 Follicular inflammation (Courtesy of WHO) [16]

Prompt 5: What Is the Treatment for Trachoma?

WHO-endorsed treatment of trachoma comprises the **SAFE** strategy [3], which needs to be delivered to communities affected by trachoma.

Surgery for trichiasis. Surgery is needed to correct trichiasis as the cornea is in danger of opacifying, causing permanent visual impairment.

Antibiotics for active chlamydial infection. Topical 1 % tetracycline is applied twice a day for 6 weeks. Unfortunately, it is unpleasant and is often poorly tolerated. Alternatively, oral azithromycin 20 mg/kg as a single dose is effective and well tolerated but costly.

According to WHO guidelines, communities with prevalence of active trachoma among children of 10 % or more need mass treatment with antibiotics (systemic azithromycin).

Face washing to reduce transmission. As transmission must be literally from face to face, education in good facial hygiene is essential in limiting spread. This usually focuses on encouraging face washing and identifying sharing of towels and poor hygiene with spread of the disease.

Environmental improvement. Improving access to clean water and sanitation is also crucial to reduce transmission by flies. Families can be shown how to do this with only a cup full of water if water is scarce.

Prompt 6: How Do You Estimate the Prevalence of a Disease in a Community?

The prevalence of a disease is an epidemiological term – epidemiology is the study of patterns of diseases in populations. Important epidemiological terms include:

Population = the total number of people in the area in question
Sample = a smaller number of people carefully selected from a population
Prevalence = proportion of the sample who has the condition of interest at a particular point in time
Incidence = the rate at which new cases of a disease occur in a population over a defined time period

The best way to assess the population would be to assess every individual and household in an area, but this is impractical. Therefore, surveys of a population sample (a proportion of the population) can be performed. However, designing a survey requires care if it is to be representative of the population as a whole and to ensure that bias does not occur. For example, a sample of a few households in a badly affected locality may have a disproportionately high prevalence of trachoma compared to the population prevalence. Time of sampling may also have an effect. For example, sampling at a time of day when active (sighted) members of households are out working may alter the recorded proportion of cases in the affected population.

For assessing our population, ideally a detailed survey would necessitate calling in an ophthalmologist and an epidemiologist; however, in reality this may be hard to arrange. You will definitely need a translator if you do not speak the local dialect. It is prudent to survey a population before treating so that we know the burden of disease and, most importantly, how best to target our treatment.

Calculating Numbers of Individuals with Trichiasis and Trachoma

To calculate the number of cases of trichiasis and trachoma in the population, it is expedient to take a sample of the population and extrapolate.

For example: Village A has a total population of 10,000, 30 % of whom are adults aged 30 years and above (i.e., 3,000), and 25 % are children aged less than 10 years (i.e., 2,500). You take a sample of 500 adults and find that 5 have trichiasis (1 %). Therefore (provided your sample is truly representative), 1 % of the 3,000 adults will have trichiasis (30 individuals). If you examine 200 children and find that 10 % of them have signs of active infection, then 250 children in the population will have active infection.

Further Information 2

You speak to an epidemiologist in the capital who details how to estimate the burden of disease in the area. Unfortunately, he will not be able to make it to your village for months due to prior commitments and poor transportation access. You decide to liaise with local health-care professionals and NGO workers who give you access to epidemiological data they have collected in the past. Using these previous epidemiological surveys, you estimate:

Population: 5,000
Trichiasis prevalence in adults: 7 %
Trachoma prevalence: 9 %
Latrines needed: 50
Water sources needed: 5

You sit down and plan how you will organize your trachoma eradication SAFE scheme.

Prompt 7: How Do You Organize a Trachoma Eradication Scheme?

Set Priorities

You may not have the resources, finances, manpower, or time to exhaustively cover the whole SAFE scheme for your village. Therefore, you should be prepared to alter the emphasis of different arms of your SAFE strategy, depending on resources and problems encountered.

High population prevalence of active infection in children – prioritize **A, F, and E**

High population prevalence of trichiasis in adults – prioritize **S**

In reality, active infection and trichiasis usually occur together, so the whole SAFE strategy is needed.

Requirements

- Manpower (surgical staff, educators to spread hygiene messages, labor)
- Materials (surgical, educational, for latrine/water source construction)
- Mobility (vehicles, motorbikes, and bicycles)
- Money
- Management (depending on existing relationships)

Useful questions to ask are the following: Is there a trachoma control program in the country? If so, these are likely to be well organized and coordinated. What existing resources are there? How can I build on these?

Funding and Budgeting

- Funding may come from any agencies. The more support available, the more successful the program will be and the more agencies will want to be involved. To get funding, however, you must ask for it via a funding request.
- Good budgeting will aid funding requests. A detailed budget is useful to ensure that interventions have been fully planned, for personal accountability, and as proof of use of funds for potential funders. It will also show how much money is required for the scheme, giving you a good idea of where to pitch your funding requests.
- Funding from multiple sources may bring conflicts of interest from donors and unwanted bureaucracy.

Prompt 8: How Do You Put a Planned Community-Based Trachoma Eradication Scheme into Effect?

It is useful to consider both key items of your plan and also qualities that you wish to promote.

Items
  Surgical interventions
  Infrastructural development
  Health education and training
Qualities
  Cost-effective and acceptable
  Integrated into existing systems
  Sustainable
  High-quality services to all [3]

So, in real terms, this may translate into the following action points:

Surgical Interventions

- Explore locally whether there are trained surgeons/personnel running eye surgery clinics that you can refer to. If not, explore the possibility of setting up surgical clinics, training, and equipping surgeons.
- You should ensure that surgery is free to maximize uptake.
- You should also ensure that eye surgery is culturally acceptable and wanted by the community.
- Is there appropriate follow-up available if you run surgical camps?

Infrastructural Development

- Assess local access to clean water and safe methods of waste disposal. If inadequate, lobby to improve local access to these amenities.
- Search for other organizations that are working in the area. They may have valuable experience or resources at their disposal.

Health Education

- A prime opportunity for bringing about locally derived improvements in conditions and arguably the most cost-effective intervention.
- You should aim to:
  - Educate locally about trachoma; encourage acceptance of surgery and antibiotics
  - Encourage facial hygiene
  - Increase the demand for sanitation
- To be effective, health education should be planned with the local community and delivered repeatedly to the target audience [3]. It can take the form of plays, informal small group exercises, lectures, leaflets, etc.
- Ideal target areas are community centers like schools, places of worship, community meeting places, and women's groups.
- Lessons should be supported by posters and other media. They should depict the ethnic groups targeted and must be in a language understood by those targeted. Other media include radio messages and jingles, leaflets, pocket-sized cards, and if appropriate television shorts.
- Educators can be anyone with the relevant local knowledge (that does not have to be too detailed or specialized). It is important that health educators are properly trained and assessed to ensure that their knowledge and delivery of information are appropriate and acceptable. Well-placed individuals are dedicated trachoma specialists, health-care professionals like doctors and nurses, teachers, and village elders.

Example Syllabus

- ***Trachoma***: what is it, how it is spread, and how it causes blindness
- ***Surgery***: why it is necessary, what it involves, and availability
- ***Antibiotics***: why they are necessary, what they involve, and availability
- ***Facial cleaning***: how cleanliness helps and how to wash face with small amounts of water
- ***Environmental change***: how improving cleanliness helps reduce disease transmission, latrines [3]

Further Information 3

Amreet's mother has been examined and found to have trichiasis. She is referred to a local hospital for an operation to correct the trichiasis. The district hospital, after a month of phone calls and meetings, has still not agreed to provide any community outreach surgical service in your village as they barely have enough staff to manage the wards, let alone stretch to any outreach work. You have applied to your organi-

zation and the government for extra funding but have been told that your case is not strong enough compared to more pressing public health issues. Meeting with local officials, you are told that sanitation is rudimentary in these remote villages. Waste disposal systems are nonexistent and open sewers run on some streets. Creating new networks of sanitation and providing clean water would take much more money than your organization has.

Prompt 9: How Do You Implement Community-Based Projects with Limited Resources?

- For anything other than very small populations, infrastructural change will require more money, effort, time, and specialist expertise than is usually available.
- An effective way round this is to find out which organizations are already working to improve sanitation and encourage them to give priority to communities endemic for trachoma.
- You could also help communities with high trachoma levels to articulate an increased demand for water and sanitation.

Activities to engage wider support:

- Contact governmental agencies and locally operating NGOs. Ensure you have prepared a fact sheet to raise awareness.
- What methods of feces and waste disposal are there? Contact the Department of Water Supply and Sewerage (if there is one) and local communities to find out. Are any latrines being built in the area? If so, are they being used consistently? Latrines will improve hygiene only if used consistently by a large proportion of the community. Latrine building should ideally be sustainable and so should use local materials. It is important that the type and location of latrines are decided in consultation with communities so that they are acceptable and used.
- What kinds of water sources exist? Water should be available in schools as a priority as children are prone to trachoma. Roof water storage tanks could be built out of local materials.
- How long would it take for each latrine or water source to be constructed? How much would each cost? Ideally, someone should know how to undertake routine maintenance of the water supply if compromised.
- How strong is demand for these interventions? Is there a role for advocacy here?
- Education about the benefit of clean water and sanitation should parallel these endeavors.

Further Information 4

You contact government representatives and hand out preprepared fact sheets on trachoma and how it is affecting rural Nepal. You have included Amreet's story as a case study to generate human interest and papers identifying trachoma as an important neglected tropical disease. You also make enquiries about existing projects to improve sanitation and clean water provision, and the local officials put you in contact with some NGOs that are active in the area. You pay them a visit and find that they maintain a high presence in these rural areas and will consider your case. They suggest you contact the International Trachoma Initiative, which supports trachoma control programs across the developing world, with donation of azithromycin by Pfizer which helps with running schemes related to preventing visual loss.

Prompt 10: What Are Neglected Tropical Diseases?

- Neglected tropical diseases are a group of infectious tropical diseases that are currently de-prioritized in the face of global efforts to control the "Big Three" of tropical medicine: HIV/AIDS, tuberculosis, and malaria. Some people would prefer to call them the "diseases of neglected communities." See Table 20.3.
- As Yamy and Hotez notes, common features of these diseases include:
  - High endemicity in rural or impoverished urban areas of low-income countries
  - An ability to impair childhood growth, intellectual development, and education, as well as worker productivity
  - The propensity for neglected tropical diseases to be poverty-promoting conditions
- Taken together, Hotez et al. calculate that these diseases rank second only to HIV/AIDS as a cause of disease burden – resulting annually in 57 million DALYs (disability-adjusted life year) [5].
- Although previously neglected, Yamy describes a recent revolution in the attitude toward treating these diseases [6]. Realization of the considerable geographical overlap in distribution and pharmacological overlap in treatment has made a "neglected disease package" a possibility. For example, a package of four

Table 20.3 Neglected tropical diseases

Disease	Grouping
Leishmaniasis	Vector-borne protozoan
African trypanosomiasis	
Chagas disease	
Trachoma	Bacterial infection
Leprosy	
Buruli ulcer	
Hookworm	Helminth infections [4]
Ascariasis	
Trichuriasis	
Lymphatic filariasis	
Onchocerciasis	
Drancunculiasis (Guinea worm)	
Schistosomiasis	

drugs (albendazole, ivermectin, azithromycin, and praziquantel) would integrate control of seven major neglected tropical diseases for 500 million people in Africa and could be delivered for about $50 (£25) per person each year [4]. Ivermectin is already being given to more than 90 million people in sub-Saharan Africa, thanks to a donation program by Merk, and volunteers distribute the tablets at community level.

- Furthermore, successful treatment of neglected tropical diseases would eliminate a significant global comorbidity, therefore increasing success of achieving millennium development goals and reducing morbidity and mortality from the "Big Three" [4].

Prompt 11: What Is Vision 2020?

In 2002, there were an estimated 38 million people living with blindness. The net incidence of blindness was estimated to be 1-2 million per year- at least 60% of which is treatable.

At that time, five conditions were responsible for 75 % of all blindness:

Cataract, refractive errors, trachoma, onchocerciasis, and vitamin A deficiency [7].

- The International Agency for the Prevention of Blindness (IAPB) is an umbrella organization of 115 members which represent professional organizations, non-government organizations who support prevention of blindness initiatives, foundations and trusts, and the corporate sector. In 1999 IAPB launched VISION2020: the Right to Sight, in partnership with the World Health Organization (WHO) to tackle the avoidable causes of blindness, of which trachoma is one cause.
- The aim of VISION2020 is to eliminate avoidable blindness by the year 2020. The initiative has brought consensus on priorities and strategies for control, has led to the establishment of national prevention of blindness committees with national prevention of blindness plans in most countries. Advocacy by member organizations at the World Health Assembly has resulted in the control of blindness and visual impairment being an integral part of WHO support to Ministries of Health, and a new Action Plan for the years 2014-2019 is currently being drafted. VISION2020 has led to more resources being allocated for eye health by governments, the non-government and corporate sectors, with increasing outputs, including higher cataract surgical rates. Despite an increasing and ageing world population, the number of individuals in the world who are blind has declined slightly from the last estimate in 2002. Despite these successes, much remains to be done, but global initiatives for the control of trachoma and onchocerciasis are also invigorating programmes and services for control of the other blinding eye diseases such as cataract. World Sight Day, which has taken place every second Thursday in October since 2000, aims to raise awareness about the avoidable causes of blindness and what can be done about them.

Prompt 12: What Other Initiatives to Combat Causes of Visual Impairment Are Being Enacted?

Refractive Errors

- 2005 and 2006 data show that, in some developing countries, up to 94 % of refractive errors go uncorrected – leading to massive morbidity [9, 10].
- The Durban Declaration of March 2007 [11] has called for increased efforts in treating refractive errors, focusing on:

  - Prioritizing refractive services
  - Supporting deployment of human resources, infrastructure, and technology for enhanced refractive services
  - Rationalize tariffs, duties, and taxes imposed on spectacles and optical laboratory equipment [11]

Case Study: Vision 2020 Projects in the Western Pacific Region
The Western Pacific Region is, with a population of approximately 1.7 billion, an enormously geographically disparate, socioeconomically differentiated, and culturally diverse area. Main diseases pertaining to eye health in the region include cataract, uncorrected refractive error, diabetic retinopathy, and vitamin A deficiency. Additionally, trachoma is prevalent in the Pacific Islands, while glaucoma and myopia are relatively common in China, East Asia, and Southeast Asia [13]. There is therefore plenty of need for sight-saving interventions and projects in this complex area.

IAPB, through Vision 2020 programs, has been active in the Western Pacific Region. Special areas of focus include the delivery of capacity-building workshops in the region, the development of a regional website, strengthening regional communication, implementing SAFE to eliminate trachoma in the Pacific Islands, increasing advocacy efforts toward governments and key players in the eye health sector, emphasizing the importance of proper data collection and reporting, and stressing the importance of developing and implementing National Eye Health Plans [13]. In areas of poor resources and stretched transport links, local collaboration and use of existing services are especially important. Trachoma, as a neglected tropical disease, may be treated in the future as part of a package with other diseases.

Cataract

- Cataracts make up as much as 50 % of global burden of visual impairment [2]. Cataract surgery has been identified as a particularly cost-effective solution to improve global visual health.
- Developments to improve treatment of cataract in India include:

- Advance in the manufacture of low-cost but high-technology intraocular lenses at extremely low cost ($4–5)
- Increase in domestic production of equipment such as microscopes
- Increase in training for ophthalmologists, including short (4–8 week) programs in techniques like small incision cataract surgery, a quick, high-quality method that does not require sutures, and phacoemulsification [12]

References

1. Eddleston M, Davidson R, Brent A, Wilkinson R, editors. Oxford handbook tropical medicine. 3rd ed. Oxford: Oxford University Press; 2006.
2. Resnikoff S, et al. Global data on visual impairment in 2002. Bulletin of the World Health Organization. 2004;82(11):844–51. Available at: http://whqlibdoc.who.int/bulletin/2004/Vol82-No11/bulletin_2004_82(11)_844-851.pdf.
3. Trachoma: A guide for program managers. WHO, London School of Hygiene & Tropical medicine & the International Trachoma Initiative. 2006.
4. Hotez P, Molyneux D, Fenwick A, Ottesen E, Sachs S, Sachs J. Incorporating a rapid-impact package for neglected tropical diseases with programs for HIV/AIDS, tuberculosis, and malaria. Public Library of Science Med. 2006;3(5):e102. doi:10.1371/journal.pmed.0030102.
5. Hotez P, Stoever K, Fenwick A, Molyneux D, Savioli L. The neglected epidemic of chronic diseases (letter). Lancet. 2006;366(9496):1514.
6. Yamey G, Hotez D. Neglected tropical diseases. BMJ. 2007;335(7614):269–70. doi:10.1136/bmj.39281.645035.80.
7. WHO action plan. Available online at: http://www.who.int/ncd/vision2020_actionplan/contents/frame.htm. Accessed on 5 Jan, 2012.
8. IAPB Vision 2020 website. Available at: http://vision2020.org/main.cfm?type=IAPBORGHOME. Accessed on 5 Jan, 2012.
9. Patel I, et al. Impact of presbyopia on quality of life in a rural African setting. Ophthalmology. 2006;113(5):728–34.
10. Bourne RR, et al. The Pakistan national blindness and visual impairment survey: research design, eye examination methodology and results of the pilot study. Ophthalmic Epidemiol. 2005;12(5):321–33.
11. The Durban Declaration. www.icee.org/pdf/Final_FINAL_Declaration.pdf. Accessed on 5 Jan, 2012.
12. Aravind S, et al. Cataract surgery and intraocular lens manufacturing in India. Current Opinion in Ophthalmology. 2008;19:60–5.
13. Adapted from 'Who is IAPB' on the IAPB western pacific website, available at: http://www.iapbwesternpacific.org/about-us/who-is-iapb. Accessed on 5 Jan, 2012.
14. Picture of child with flies in her eyes, Courtesy of Sudan Medical Relief, 2009. Accessible via: www.sudanmedicalrelief.org/news/2009_sept/photos/trachoma.jpg. Accessed 3rd September 2012.
15. WHO, distribution of active trachoma. 2006. Accessible via: http://gamapserver.who.int/mapLibrary/Files/Thumbnails/global%20active%20may%202006.jpg. Accessed on 5 Jan, 2012.
16. Photo of follicular inflammation. WHO. Accessible via: http://www.who.int/entity/blindness/causes/TRA%20grading%20TF_small.jpg. Accessed on 5 Jan, 2012.
17. Cross sectional anatomy of the eye, reprinted from original content in Rheumatology and Immunology therapy, 2004, courtesy of Springer-Verlag, accessible via: http://www.springerimages.com/ImageDetail.aspx?id=1-10.1007_3-540-29662-X_1526-0. Accessed on 9 Mar, 2012.

Part V
Public Health

Non-communicable diseases and matters of public health are significant and increasingly appreciated contributors to the global burden of morbidity and mortality. These are often complex, multilayered problems that demand some knowledge of associated medical, economic, socio-political, and gender issues. A broad and multifaceted approach is essential to effective management of non-communicable disease, and this section will adopt an unashamedly interdisciplinary approach to highlight this. Readers therefore will be encouraged to reflect not just on the public health "problem" itself but also on the importance of the particular context in which it finds itself.

The attempt with the choice of chapters in this section is to bring to the reader an appreciation of the key issues in public health. Almost as cogent is the objective to make the reader more at ease with handling topics that require a synthesis of different disciplines. The chapter choices have been made to introduce the reader to certain important or well-publicized examples in public health: Ready-to-Use Therapeutic Foods, Pakistani strategies in sexual health, child soldiers and public health phenomena associated with the demographic transition in the "BRIC" (Brazil, Russia, India, China) emerging economies.

Ed Mew

Chapter 21
Malnutrition

Ed Mew and Kate Godden

Learning Objectives

- Outline the epidemiology and conceptual framework of malnutrition
- Describe the concepts of nutritional requirements for macro- and micronutrients
- Assess individuals suffering from malnutrition
- Understand the model for management and complications of malnutrition and be able to access detailed guidance
- Describe relevant micronutrient deficiencies
- Describe public health strategies for preventing nutritional deficiencies and understand different feeding products currently available
- List other innovative strategies in providing food support to communities

Initial Scenario

You are the new physician working in a small village-based health clinic in rural Malawi. The residents are suffering from recurrent diarrheal diseases – thought to be linked to poor sanitation. You decide to take a quick tour to survey the village. A mother brings her emaciated child to see you.

E. Mew, MBBS (✉)
FY2 Doctor, Trauma, Emergency and Acute Medicine (TEAM),
King's College Hospital, Denmark Hill, London, UK
e-mail: eau.mew@gmail.com

K. Godden, MSc
University of Westminster, London, UK

D. MacGarty, D. Nott (eds.), *Disaster Medicine*,
DOI 10.1007/978-1-4471-4423-6_21,

Prompt 1: How Do You Assess a Patient for Suspected Malnutrition?

Key aims of history and examination should be:

- Confirm malnutrition as a clinical diagnosis
- Establish whether acute or chronic malnutrition
- Assess for complications of malnutrition
- Assess child and family to identify a cause of the malnutrition

History

- The usual diet, last meal, and fluid intake are key features in the history. Birth weight, length of period of exclusive breast-feeding, the timing, and nature of the introduction of any complementary foods (supplements) are important.
- Diarrhea and vomiting may suggest an infective course (e.g., bloody diarrhea) or immunodeficiency (chronic diarrhea, rapid weight loss, multiple infections).
- When was urine last passed? Are they tolerating oral fluids (dehydration may accompany malnutrition)?
- Enquire about vaccinations, past medical history, and sick contacts – especially tuberculosis, measles, pneumonia, and HIV/AIDS.

Examination

- Weight and height/length should be taken. The length of children under 2 years of age (or height < 87 cm if age unknown) is taken lying down, while the height of children over 2 years (height 87 cm or above) is measured standing. The weight for height index is used to diagnose acute malnutrition, and height for age is used to diagnose chronic malnutrition.
- Mid-upper arm circumference (MUAC) is also used to diagnose acute malnutrition (for example of use, see Fig. 21.1). It is the simplest and most reliable indicator but is limited to children of 1–5 years of age [2]. A MUAC of <110 mm is strongly associated with mortality.
- Inspect for edema (swelling) in feet and legs.
- Look for signs of circulatory collapse: cold hands/feet, weak radial pulse, and reduced consciousness. In severe acute malnutrition, nutritional collapse may be accompanied by circulatory collapse.
- The liver should also be palpated as it may become enlarged. Jaundice may be present.
- A general examination may reveal:
    - Pallor: suggests anemia
    - Temperature: hypothermia or fever

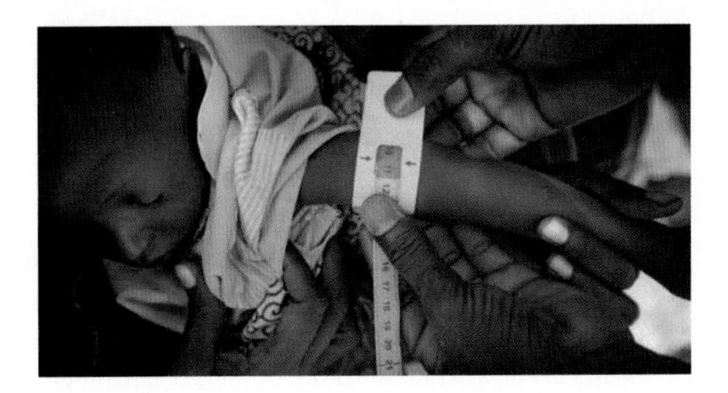

Fig. 21.1 MUAC bands in use, courtesy of Kate Holt and UNICEF [1]

- Eyes: corneal lesions are indicative of vitamin A deficiency
- Ears/mouth/throat: evidence of infection
- Skin: evidence of infection or purpura
- Respiratory: rate, signs of pneumonia, or heart failure

Investigations may not be available but are included for completeness:

- Blood films for malaria.
- Mantoux (for TB) or HIV testing may also be useful. However, WHO notes that these tests are never a substitute for a thorough history and examination [3].
- Blood glucose measurement is useful if the patient is acutely unwell [3].
- Stool analysis for blood or parasitic cysts may diagnose parasitic infestation in patients with diarrheal symptoms.

Prompt 2: Outline Basic Nutritional Requirements

The human body needs macronutrients and micronutrients to survive:

- Macronutrients – carbohydrates, fats, and proteins – provide energy and fuel for muscle and bodily processes, most importantly brain activity. Achieving an adequate energy intake typically ensures an adequate protein intake. Protein is important for adequate growth and development, but its role is often overstated. Severe acute malnutrition (SAM), including kwashiorkor, is treated with a low to moderate protein intake.
- Micronutrients can be categorized as either Type 1 or Type 2 nutrients:
- Type 1 nutrient deficiencies result in specific deficiency diseases, do not always affect growth, but will affect metabolism and immune competence before deficiency signs are apparent. They include vitamins A, B1, B2, nicotinic acid, C, D, as well as iron. Vitamin A deficiency is a major cause of under-5 mortality.

- Type 2 nutrient deficiencies do not show specific clinical signs. They affect metabolic processes and result in growth failure, wasting, increased risk of edema, and lowered immune response. This category of nutrients includes zinc and water [4].

Prompt 3: What Is the Epidemiology of Malnutrition?

- Malnutrition is the largest contributor to global disease and is an underlying factor in over 35 % of the 10–11 million deaths in children under 5 who die each year from preventable causes and 11 % of the global burden of disease [5].
- Malnutrition disproportionately affects the young and restricts their cognitive and physical development. At a population level, this significantly reduces economic development as malnourished people have a diminished capacity for work [6].
- Intrauterine growth restriction and low birth weight are risk factors for developing obesity, hypertension, cardiac disease, and diabetes (the Barker hypothesis) in later life [7].
- Ninety percent of the world's malnourished live in just 36 countries. Despite the focus on sub-Saharan Africa, the most significant problems in undernutrition are found in Asia. In 2011, South Asia had low birth weight (LBW) prevalence of 27 % and stunting at 42 %, whereas sub-Saharan Africa was 14 % and 22 %, respectively [8].

Risk Factors

- The direct causes of malnutrition are inadequate dietary intake and/or excessive disease burden. Various causes of malnutrition are interrelated.
- Disease can lead to increased nutrient requirements, malabsorption, or reduced appetite which may all further affect nutritional status.
- Many underlying factors are involved in malnutrition, including income poverty, access to health services, food insecurity, and deeper sociopolitical issues [5].

Further Information 1

Through an interpreter, you manage to ascertain the following: The child is 4 years old and is called Chisulo. Chisulo eats one small bowl of mashed boiled cassava per day with a small cup of water to drink. He has had this diet for months. He was born at term and was breast-fed for the first 3 months until his mother was told, against WHO guidance, to stop as she is HIV positive. Chisulo has had recurrent bouts of diarrhea over the last two months. He has not been vaccinated. His father left home nine months ago. His two younger brothers have both died from diarrheal disease.

On examination, Chisulo is lethargic and smells strongly of feces. His mucous membranes are moist, CRT = 2 seconds, PR = 100, RR = 20, and skin turgor is normal. His mid-upper arm circumference (MUAC) is 108 mm. There is no edema. His liver is palpable 1 cm below the costal margin.

You conclude that Chisulo is suffering from severe acute malnutrition (SAM) due to insufficient nutritional intake and prolonged diarrheal disease. He is not clinically dehydrated. Chisulo will need refeeding to avoid complications of malnutrition.

Prompt 4: What Are the Clinical Features of Malnutrition?

Marasmus and kwashiorkor are syndromes associated with SAM, as shown in Table 21.1.

Diagnosis

Anthropometry is used to categorize and diagnose different types of undernutrition using *z*-scores (how many standard deviations from the population mean) or % of the median growth standards. Z-scores are preferred and used for surveys and population assessments, while the % of the median is still widely used in clinical practice in many countries.

- Acute malnutrition ("wasting") < −2 *z*-scores weight for height or MUAC 115–125 mm [10].
- Severe acute malnutrition ("severe wasting") < −3 *z*-scores weight for height or <115 mm MUAC. Bilateral edema may be present.
- Chronic malnutrition ("stunting") < −2 *z*-scores height for age.

Acute malnutrition leads to loss of *weight*, while prolonged chronic malnutrition will lead to loss of *height* or "stunting." In general, the pattern, observed by Gill

Table 21.1 Clinical syndromes associated with SAM [9]

	Marasmus	Kwashiorkor
Commonest age	<18 months	>18 months
Theoretic pathology	Simple wasting or starvation	Wasting plus salt/water imbalance Cause is unknown but proven not to be protein deficiency
Features	Wasting (especially thigh, buttock) Irritability, hunger "Old man" appearance	Wasting and edema Hepatomegaly Skin flaking/dermatitis Hypopigmentation
Complications	Dehydration Infection Hepatic and circulatory failure Death 20–30 %	Dehydration Infection Hepatic and circulatory failure Anorexia (refusing food) Death 50–60 %

et al., is for an acute-on-chronic scenario. This often comprises a background of nutritional insufficiency and chronic infections with severe infection precipitating decompensation [11].

Prompt 5: How Do You Treat Acute Malnutrition?

Breast-feeding is the first option and can be enabled by providing food, fluids, and support to the mother. If this is not possible, the child is registered to a feeding program either as an "inpatient" or in the community. Historically, treatment was typically in a hospital setting with associated problems of overcrowding and cross contamination. Nowadays, community-based management of acute malnutrition (CMAM) is accepted as the gold standard treatment [12]. Advances in nutritional science and food packaging have allowed home-based treatment with ready-to-use therapeutic foods (RUTF) of low microbial activity.

Complicated cases of SAM still require stabilization in a clinical setting. Detailed guidance on CMAM is available [13, 14].

Moderate malnutrition: (<–2 *z*-scores or <80 % of median weight/height)

- Patient "well" → outpatient (community) treatment consisting of advice, standard food rations to take home and immunization
- Patient ill or anorexic → inpatient (hospital) treatment

Severe malnutrition: (< –3 *z*-scores weight for height)

- Patient well → outpatient ready-to-use therapeutic food (RUTF) program. As per standard community treatment, using RUTF (explained in detail later) and antibiotics for infection
- Patient ill or anorexic → inpatient (hospital) treatment [9]

Prompt 6: What Features of Decompensated SAM Must Be Considered When Addressing Inpatient Care?

- Inpatient treatment is highly specialized and is largely out of the scope of this book. It starts with initial stabilization of decompensated patients that may be prone to sequelae of malnutrition (hypoglycemia, hypothermia, dehydration, infection).
- Patients are fed with specialized milk products (such as F75) every 3 h round-the-clock to prevent hypoglycemia giving 100 kcal/kg/day. In the absence of F75 or F100, high energy milk can be made up. See Table 21.2 for composition of these.
- On signs of stabilization and recovery (typically at day 1–3), the patient moves to gradual reinstatement of food (F100 or RUTF) to avoid refeeding syndrome (the result of rapid refeeding, characterized by electrolyte derangement, seizures,

Table 21.2 High energy milk formulae [9]

High energy milk formulae	Approximating to F-75	Approximating to F-100
Dried skimmed milk (g)	25	80
Sugar (g)	100	50
Vegetable oil (g)	27	60
Electrolytes (EMS solution)	20	20
Water (ml)	1,000	1,000

Courtesy of Oxford University Press

and cardiac failure) [3]. Recovery can be assessed using the appetite test – the child's ability to eat 75 % of RUTF ration.

- Hypothermia is prevented by ensuring adequate clothing, blankets, skin-to-skin nursing, or using a lamp.
- Dehydration is treated with use of rehydration solution. ReSoMal – a modified oral rehydration solution – is given 10 ml/kg hourly for up to 10 h. IV fluids are only used if the child is in shock due to the risk of precipitating cardiac failure.
- Bacterial infections are eradicated with antibiotics. Other concurrent infections like *Ascaris lumbricoides* (a parasitic roundworm, spread feco-orally) may be treated with anti-helminth drugs like mebendazole. Vitamin A supplementation is given in the acute phase as this lowers mortality especially in cases of measles.
- Once the patient is stabilized, aim for 200 kcal/kg/day. Providing stimulation through play speeds recovery. Also treat other vitamin and mineral deficiencies [3].

Further Information 2

Chisulo is given ready-to-use therapeutic foodstuffs (RUTF) to increase his calorie and nutrient intake. He is also given vitamin A supplements and antibiotics to prevent infection due to his weakened immune system. His mother is encouraged to wrap him in blankets to aid heating and feed him regularly. Having treated Chisulo, you sit down with your colleagues to determine whether you need to start a feeding program. One colleague says that she will try to contact a representative of the World Food Programme to enquire about the availability of appropriate food aid commodities.

Prompt 7: What Is a Feeding Program?

Food aid programs are structured programs designed to provide food relief to areas of famine or reduced food security. Focused on the provision of food, they include:

- Food, health, and hygiene education
- General food distribution

- Supplementary feeding and medical follow-up for vulnerable groups (e.g., children and pregnant women)
- Therapeutic feeding – intensive feeding under close medical supervision

Feeding interventions become more resource and manpower intensive as one goes down the above list. It is cheaper and easier to disseminate education on sanitation than to admit a child to hospital. Issues to consider when planning a feeding program include:

- What is the prevalence of malnutrition or the numbers malnourished? Is there an increase in the numbers presenting with malnutrition at health centers, an increasing mortality rate, or credible reports of malnutrition?
- Who has reduced access to food?
- Are food prices high or have they been rising?
- MUAC (mid-upper arm circumference) measurement is quick and straightforward for rapid assessment.
- Monitor the following as they either cause malnutrition or significantly contribute to mortality in malnourished patients:
  - Diarrheal disease
  - Measles
  - HIV/AIDS

What do you need to sustain food distribution?

- Basic security in the village may ensure equitable allocation of resources
- Adequate staffing and community mobilization
- Food procurement for distribution
- Secure storage space for food supplies
- Setting up a stabilization center for complicated SAM requires the following:
  - An adequate water supply
  - 1 latrine/20 people in therapeutic feeding area (absolute minimum)
  - Buildings or tents to act as the feeding center
  - Food for baby, parents, and staff plus fuel to cook it
  - Staff, ideally including doctors and nurses, or alternatively trained dedicated staff [3]

Prompt 8: What Is the United Nations' Role in Providing Food Relief?

A number of UN agencies are involved in the fight against malnutrition and include:

- WFP (World Food Programme)
- UNICEF (United Nations Children's Fund)

- FAO (Food and Agriculture Organization)
- UNHCR (United Nations High Commissioner for Refugees)

The World Food Programme (WFP) is the food aid arm of the United Nations system. WFP is the largest provider of food aid and is a key player in food logistics and food security analysis. Officially, WFP has the mandate to tackle moderate malnutrition and UNICEF to handle severe malnutrition. FAO has a lower field presence than the UNICEF and WFP, while UNHCR is concerned specifically with refugees.

UNICEF may be able to provide RUTF and F100/F75 alongside medical supplies. They also often support national governments in vaccination campaigns, multiple indicator surveys, and technical advice. WFP may be able to provide fortified foodstuffs.

Further Information 3

Your colleagues reason that villagers are mostly subsistence farmers with few possessions or savings. Most meals consist of boiled mashed cassava, occasionally with a bean-based sauce accompanying. The most recent harvest underperformed. Unfortunately, you have no data concerning death rates. You are informed that diarrheal diseases and measles are both prevalent although you have no actual figures to hand.

You liaise with a local health officer. She has already started up a therapeutic feeding center for children with severe acute malnutrition. While happy to help you, she shares worries about the feasibility of such a scheme relating to issues of staffing and food procurement. She asks you what foodstuffs are available for food relief.

Prompt 9: How Would You Institute a Feeding Program?

Detailed advice can be found in "Community-based Therapeutic Care (CTC): a field manual" [15].

Food Procurement

- Ensure that you are able to obtain and store extra supplies of food. UN agencies like WFP and UNICEF and the local government are useful first points of contact.

Food Targeting

- The scope of your food distribution may depend on the scale of malnutrition, the resources and food you have at your disposal, and the number of cases that you have identified.
- In a village setting, it is unlikely that you will be able to draw on substantial resources or be able to procure large amounts of food in the short term. Therefore,

feeding should be targeted at those at highest risk (typically from conception, that is, pregnant women and children to 2 years of age [16]).

Food Distribution

- Ensure adequate security to maximize fair distribution of food.
- Provide food appropriate to taste, custom, and, if possible, season.
- Involve women in the decision-making process; they often undertake most agricultural labor and yet are excluded from the decision-making processes and are disproportionately affected by malnutrition.

Stabilization Center for Complicated Severe Acute Malnutrition (SAM)

- If one does not exist and there is widespread, SAM sets one up in or as close to a hospital as possible.
- It should provide 24-h care for SAM plus a day center that outpatients can attend.

Education

- Nutrition education and support should be undertaken on the importance of exclusive breast-feeding, appropriate infant and young child feeding, and promotion of hand washing with soap. Breast-feeding with 99 % coverage could reduce deaths in those under 36 months by as much as 9.1 % [6].
- Sociocultural practices may influence education and practice – for example, HIV/AIDS prevalence and breast-feeding.

Prompt 10: What Types of Food Relief Products Are Available?

- Local food: When possible, local foodstuffs should be used for food aid. These will be most familiar to the recipients, have lower transportation costs, and support the local economy.
- Fortified blended foods – Corn Soya Blend (CSB, CSB+): partially cooked staples (like cereals, soya, and pulses), fortified with micronutrient blends. They are used in supplementary feeding programs to support nutritional status in moderate acute malnutrition. They are normally cooked at home as a porridge.
- Ready-to-use therapeutic foods (RUTF): these are ready-to-use foodstuffs that require no preparation. They are usually a relatively costly peanut-based fortified paste designed to treat SAM. See Box 21.1 for an example of RUTF in use.
- Micronutrient powders: micronutrient powders contain the recommended daily intake of 16 essential vitamins and minerals for one person and are therefore useful supplementation tools when individuals are deficient in a large spread of micronutrients. They are sprinkled onto food before eating [17].
- Milk powders are not distributed due to the high risk of microbial contamination through preparation using unclean water.

Box 21.1: Malawi and Plumpy' Nut

Malawi is a low-income country with a high prevalence of malnutrition and associated infant mortality. Traditional therapeutic feeding was unpopular as it kept a parent away from home and productive work for weeks. Plumpy'nut was used to great effect in Malawi. It is a high-energy peanut-based spread fortified with essential micronutrients like vitamin A nutritionally equivalent to F100. It is easy to store, distribute, and eat straight from the packet and is effective in treating SAM. It is simple to administer at home, therefore removing vulnerable children from hospitals where they are likely to contract diseases.

Further Information 4

The feeding program has been implemented. Extra pledged food supplies have failed to materialize. After discussion with local representatives, malnourished children and pregnant women are targeted for supplementary feeding with Corn Soya Blend (a type of fortified blended food) from WFP. Children with complicated SAM are admitted to the local health center for stabilization. You notice that those that survive have manifestations of other dietary deficiencies.

The local health officer comes to speak to you, looking worried. The situation in the village has not improved. Your requests for additional food aid have been rejected due to "prioritization" issues. You decide to brainstorm innovative ways of aid provision that may appeal to stakeholders.

Prompt 11: What Other Important Micronutrient Deficiencies Might Malnourished Patients Suffer From?

Vitamin A Deficiency (Xerophthalmia)

- Vitamin A is a fat-soluble vitamin of a deep orange color found in liver, eggs, and most brightly colored fruits and vegetables. Vitamin A deficiency (VAD) is a huge public health problem and significantly increases mortality from infectious diseases in women and children. It is also a leading cause of blindness worldwide.
- The first manifestation is xerophthalmia: painful dry eyes, scleral spots, and impaired night vision. Vitamin A deficiency has been associated with increased risk of contracting measles and diarrheal diseases. It is also associated with increased mortality in those infected with measles [18].
- The Lancet Maternal and Child Undernutrition series concluded that vitamin A deficiency leads to 600,000 deaths each year [19]. One dose of vitamin A per year reduces all mortality in 6–59 months by 12 %, two doses by 22 %.

- Treatment is with 100,000 IU for those <10 kg and 200,000 IU for >10 kg, given twice per year.

Zinc Deficiency

- Zinc is found in food such as red meats and is important for development. Deficiency leads to poor growth and increased susceptibility to infections – especially diarrheal disease and pneumonia.
- There is currently no direct indicator of zinc deficiency (a proxy of >20 % stunting is used); however, zinc supplementation has been accredited with reducing under 5 mortality rates by 9 % [19].
- Zinc sulfate is used in treatment of diarrhea. Supplementation or fortification of foods with zinc is not yet commonplace.

Iron (Anemia)

- Iron is found in food like red meat, pulses, and green leafy vegetables. Deficiency leads to low hemoglobin levels and iron deficiency anemia which is a significant cause of maternal mortality.
- This manifests as lethargy, shortness of breath, and pallor that is best observed in the conjunctiva and palmar creases. Treatment is with iron – as an oral supplement or by encouraging dietary intake.
- Anemia may also be due to chronic bleeding, infections like malaria or *Ascaris lumbricoides* (roundworm), or hemoglobinopathies like sickle cell disease.

Niacin Deficiency (Pellagra)

- Maize-based diet causes niacin (nicotinic acid, vitamin B3) deficiency. Pellagra is classically described as a triad of dermatitis (photosensitive), diarrhea, and dementia. Pellagra is responsive to supplementation with nicotinamide – a chemical related to niacin.

Vitamin C Deficiency (Scurvy)

- This results from diets deficient in fruits and vegetables such as those highly dependent on food aid. Gingivitis and excessive bleeding are the main clinical features.
- Treatment is with 150 mg vitamin C over 2 weeks or simply by encouraging oral vitamin C intake.

Thiamine Deficiency (Beriberi)

- Beriberi is classically associated with diets heavy in polished rice or alcohol. Two clinical forms exist: "wet" and "dry." "Wet" beriberi has cardiac failure and edema as features and "dry" beriberi is characterized by a painful polyneuropathy.
- Thiamine deficiency also causes the Wernicke-Korsakoff syndrome that features ataxia, ophthalmoplegia, confusion, and amnesia. Treatment is with 100 mg thiamine IV/24 h or alternatively with Pabrinex vitamin complex which contains thiamine.

Vitamin D Deficiency (Rickets)

- Vitamin D is present in foods like fish and egg. Rickets is a disease of developing children characterized by bony malformations, fractures, and faltering growth. It may result from dietary deficiency, reduced exposure to sunlight (especially in those with dark skin), or may be related to renal disease.
- Treatment is usually by supplementation: 400 IU vitamin D orally/24 h and increased sunlight exposure.

Iodine Deficiency

- Iodine is provided by food and plants grown in iodine-rich soil. Deficiency results in a neck swelling called a goiter, short stature, and – if from birth – mental restriction that used to be referred to as cretinism.
- Prevention is tackled using fortified iodized salt, and treatment, for example, in pregnant women, is with iodized oil.

Prompt 12: What Local Schemes Have Proved Successful in Food Support in Resource-Poor Settings?

Voucher Schemes

- In Kenya, Save the Children is giving people vouchers to buy food in local markets. These vouchers are recent but intuitive developments as they boost local businesses and food production while simultaneously diminishing shipping and distribution costs.

Mobile Phone Schemes

- Cash for food can be transferred direct to mobile phones using the popular M-Pesa mobile money system in East Africa. This cuts down on administration costs of transferring cash.

Goat Schemes

- Some areas will identify at-risk families and give them a goat as a way to supply their children with extra milk. The goats are generally very easy to keep themselves.

Food for Work Schemes

- The World Food Programme enrolls people in Food for Work programs. Unemployed individuals are given food for laboring on irrigation or school-building projects. This is presented as a viable alternative in areas of conflict and helps to foster skills and to reduce over-farming.

Case Study: Famine in the Horn of Africa

In 2011, a combination of warfare, drought, and rising food prices provoked the declaration of famine in southern Somalia. Thousands fled to neighboring Ethiopia and Kenya, exacerbating the human disaster. Displacement of peoples created extra strain on an already-struggling system.

The crisis in the horn of Africa provoked a widespread – if arguably delayed – response from the developed world. Large charitable donations ensured that charities like the World Food Programme were able to provide a critical lifeline to vulnerable persons in all three countries, targeting 9.6 million people across the region.

Preexisting school feeding and nutrition programs were scaled up. In Mogadishu, WFP opened hot meal centers and provided food for hospitals as well as general food distributions for internally displaced Somalis. An airlift of 250 metric tons of ready-to-use foods into Mogadishu helped stave off malnutrition for 85,000 young children for a month [20].

These considerable resources and efforts may need to be called on by the horn of Africa in future times. It is unlikely that drought, escalating food prices, political turmoil, or conflict will cease to be pervasive problems in the region – making it a powder keg for further famines. The famine also drew attention to the suboptimal working of international famine prevention. Improvements in early warning systems were not matched by improvements in responsiveness of the international community. Unfortunately, early action (famine prevention) often falls between long-term development and emergency response with similar problems in international aid architecture.

Significantly, in the view of western donors, preventing humanitarian assistance from falling into the hands of Islamist Al-Shabaab was a greater priority than preventing famine [21].

References

1. MUAC band in use, Courtesy of Kate Holt and UNICEF. Accessible via: www.unicef.org.au/discover/what-we-do/survival/malnutrition.aspx. Accessed 3rd September 2012.
2. Myatt M, et al. Technical background paper WHO 2005. A review of methods to detect cases of severely malnourished children in the community for their admission into community based therapeutic care programme. Food Nutr Bull. 2006;27(3 Suppl):S7–23.
3. WHO. Management of severe malnutrition: a manual for physicians and other senior health workers. 1999. Available at: http://whqlibdoc.who.int/hq/1999/a57361.pdf. Accessed on 5 Jan, 2012.
4. World Health Organisation. Vitamin and mineral requirements in human nutrition. 2004. Accessible via: http://whqlibdoc.who.int/publications/2004/9241546123.pdf. Accessed on 5 Jan, 2012.
5. Black RE, et al. Maternal and child undernutrition: global and regional exposures and consequences. Lancet. 2008;371:243–60.

6. The Lancet executive summary on malnutrition. Available at: http://www-tc.iaea.org/tcweb/abouttc/tcseminar/Sem6-ExeSum.pdf. Accessed on 5 Jan, 2012.
7. The Barker Theory. Available at: http://www.thebarkertheory.org/. Accessed on 5 Jan, 2012.
8. UNICEF. State of the worlds children. 2011. Available at: https://www.unicef.org.uk/Documents/Publication.../sowc2011.pdf. Accessed on 5 Jan, 2012.
9. Eddleston M, Davidson R, Brent A, Wilkinson R. Oxford handbook of tropical medicine. 3rd ed. Oxford: Oxford University Press; 2010.
10. Growth Standards, World Health Organisation. 2006. Available at: www.who.int/childgrowth/. Accessed on 5 Jan, 2012.
11. Gill G, Beeching N. Tropical medicine. 6th ed. London: Blackwell; 2009.
12. Community based management of severe acute malnutrition. Joint statement by World Health Organisation, the World Food Programme, the United Nations System Standing Committee on Nutrition and the United Nations Children's fund. May 2007. Available at: http://www.unicef.org/media/files/Community_Based__Management_of_Severe_Acute_Malnutrition.pdf. Accessed on 5 Jan, 2012.
13. Community based therapeutic care (CTC): A field manual. CTC research and development programme, a collaboration between Valid international and Concern Worldwide. 2006. Accessible via: http://www.concernusa.org/media/pdf/2007/10/CTC_Manual_v1_Oct06.pdf. Accessed on 5 Jan, 2012.
14. UNSCN. 2011. http://www.unscn.org/en/gnc_htp/howto-htp.php#howtousehtp. Accessed on 5 Jan, 2012.
15. Detailed guidance can be found in Community based therapeutic care (CTC). A field manual. 2006. Online at: www.validinternational.org. Accessed on 5 Jan, 2012.
16. Victoria CG, et al. Maternal and child undernutrition: consequences for adult health and human capital. Lancet. 2008;371:340–57.
17. Ezzati M, et al. Selected major risk factors and global and regional burden of disease. Lancet. 2002;360:1347–60.
18. WHO vaccination. Available at: http://www.who.int/immunization_delivery/interventions/vitamin_A/en/index3.html. Accessed on 5 Jan, 2012.
19. Bhutta ZA, et al. What works? Interventions for maternal and child undernutrition and survival. Lancet. 2008;371:417–40.
20. Adapted from: http://documents.wfp.org/stellent/groups/public/documents/communications/wfp215812.pdf.
21. Bailey R. Food crises: barriers to early action, Chatham house website, accessible on: www.chathamhouse.org/media/comment/view/183173.

Chapter 22
Sexual and Reproductive Health

Shao Foong Chong

Learning Objectives

- Explore the issues of unsafe abortions in the developing world
- Outline various methods of unsafe abortions
- Describe the clinical features, complications, and management of miscarriage
- Explore common problems in sexual and reproductive health in the low-income countries
- Describe what family planning involves
- Discuss the advantages and challenges of family planning
- Outline the effectiveness of modern contraceptive methods
- Design an effective family planning scheme

Initial Scenario

You are a GP in a busy rural clinic, and a local 18-year-old woman presents to your clinic with acute pelvic pain, bloody vaginal discharge, and rigors. She tells you that she accidentally became pregnant with a boy that she had been seeing but was not ready to have a child especially since they are not married. After building up a good rapport and emphasizing the seriousness of the situation, she admits to having a "back-alley" abortion a couple of days ago, which is illegal in your country. Since then, she has felt extremely poorly. You confirm with a thorough clinical assessment including a vaginal examination that she has had a missed, incomplete miscarriage complicated with sepsis.

S.F. Chong, MBBS, MA (Oxon)
FY2 Doctor, Department of Emergency Medicine,
St George's Hospital, Tooting, London, UK
e-mail: shaofoong@hotmail.com

D. MacGarty, D. Nott (eds.), *Disaster Medicine*,
DOI 10.1007/978-1-4471-4423-6_22,

Prompt 1: What Is the Problem with Unsafe Abortions in Developing Countries?

- An unsafe abortion is "a procedure for terminating an unwanted pregnancy either by persons lacking the necessary skills or in an environment lacking the minimal medical standards or both" [1]. In countries with restrictive laws on abortion, people may go outside the health system to have abortions.
- Unsafe abortion is still a major cause of maternal mortality particularly among young, poor, and rural women. More than 95 % of unsafe abortions occur in developing countries. Every year, an estimated 20 million of the 42 million abortions that occur worldwide are unsafe. 68,000 women die annually of unsafe abortion – 13 % of all maternal mortality [2].
- A woman who is sick, injured, or bled heavily after an abortion may have scars in her uterus that could cause problems with pelvic inflammatory disease and infertility. These reproductive tract infections occur following about 20–30 % of unsafe abortion [3].

Prompt 2: How Are "Back-Alley" Abortions Carried Out?

- Illegal or unsafe abortions are also known as "back-alley," "backstreet," or "backyard" abortions. Various methods have been used (Fig. 22.1):
  - Untrained providers may insert unsterile instruments [4], such as a wire coat hanger or long knitting needle, to perforate the amniotic sac. Such procedures are high risk and frequently lead to uterine perforation, pelvic infection, and infertility through tubal blockage.
  - Natural abortions, using herbal mixtures, minerals, and spiritual preparations, are believed to induce an abortion. However, there is no data on the efficacy of these methods, and they may carry negative side effects, primarily toxicity leading to multiple organ failure.
  - Acquiring abortifacient drugs, such as misoprostol or methotrexate, not under trained medical supervision is another way of inducing miscarriage.

Prompt 3: What Are the Clinical Features of Miscarriage?

- *Miscarriage* – The loss of pregnancy before 24 weeks gestation. Approximately one-third of pregnancies miscarry, mostly in the first trimester. Bleeding of red

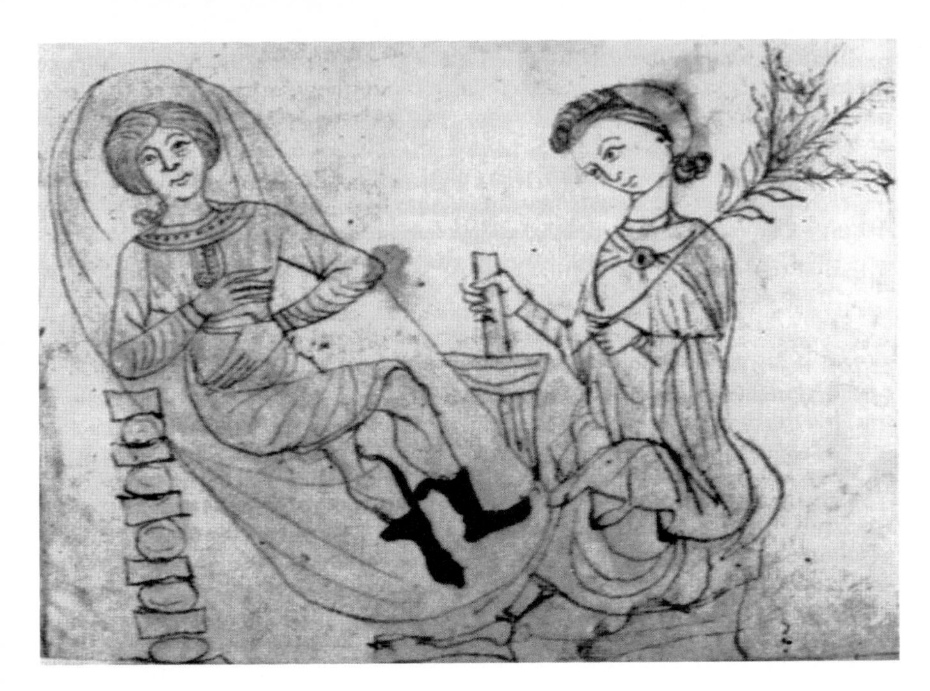

Fig. 22.1 Medieval abortion

blood is usually the first sign followed by a crampy or colicky pain. The uterus is larger and softer, and the cervix patulous or dilated. Pain ceases when the products of conception are expelled.

- *Threatened Miscarriage* – Bleeding, usually painless, occurs, and the cervical os is closed. There is greater risk of preterm rupture of membranes and preterm delivery, especially in the second trimester. Where available, an ultrasound scan should be carried out, and if the fetus is alive, the mother can be reassured. Bed rest is advised, as symptoms will settle 75 % of the time [5].
- *Inevitable Miscarriage* – Symptoms may be severe, and uterine contractions will dilate the cervix. Vaginal examination will show an open os, and ultrasound may demonstrate fetal death.
- *Incomplete Miscarriage* – Substantial bleeding and painful contractions occur while tissue and blood clot may be found in the vagina. An open cervix should be identified, and ultrasound used to exclude the 30 % of women with an open os but with an empty uterus already or those with potentially continuing pregnancy [6].
- *Missed Miscarriage* – The fetus dies but is retained within a "small for dates" uterus. This should be confirmed with ultrasound.

Prompt 4: How Can the Complications of Miscarriage Be Managed?

- *Incomplete Evacuation of the Uterus* – Any delay in evacuation of the retained products of conception may leave it vulnerable to hemorrhagic complications. Originally, first-trimester miscarriage was managed with surgical uterine evacuation with dilatation and curettage. The WHO then primarily recommended manual vacuum aspiration worldwide, as this technique is just as effective but cheaper and fever adverse effects [6]. Unfortunately, in resource poor settings, this technique is not readily available because it requires specialist equipment and training, for example, ultrasonography, sterilization, skilled surgeons, and anesthetists. Therefore, it has now been suggested that a medical evacuation with misoprostol should be used in rural settings for a variety of reasons: high complete evacuation rates of 95–99 % are seen with misoprostol regimen, increased access at secondary or even primary healthcare facilities may occur with nonsurgically trained staff, and it is much cheaper in resource-poor countries [6].
- *Infection* – Sepsis is a severe infection that may occur once the cervix is dilated and unsterile instruments are introduced into the uterine cavity. Unsafe abortions are particularly liable to sepsis due to unsanitary conditions, which are further complicated with background untreated infections such as gonococcus and chlamydia. Retained products of conception are even more likely to become infected, resulting in profuse bleeding pelvic inflammatory disease and subsequent tubal blockage [6]. If sepsis occurs, it is important to take cervical and high vaginal swabs and blood cultures, and then prescribe broad-spectrum antibiotics together with an agent effective against anaerobes [5].
- *Injury Due to Instruments Used During the Procedure* – Trauma may occur by either cervical laceration or uterine perforation. Perforation may lead to injury of the bladder, bowel, or major blood vessels. Surgery is required as soon as possible to avoid fistula formation or hemorrhagic shock [5].

Further Information 1

You start her on broad-spectrum antibiotics (cefuroxime 1.5-g iv TDS and metronidazole 500-mg iv TDS) one hour prior to uterine curettage. The operation is successful – the retained products of conception are removed completely and the bleeding stops. After a few days on intravenous antibiotics and fluids, she recovers. You warn her that using illegal abortion practices is very dangerous. She is lucky that she presented early, as some women come after days of being septic and by that time there is little that can be done to improve their situation. This is not the first case of this you have seen. In fact, this is a recurrent problem in your country. You suggest that greater levels of family planning and greater access to safe abortion services are necessary to meet the Millennium Development Goal (MDG) 5.

Prompt 5: Explore Common Problems in Sexual and Reproductive Health in the Developing World

- Sexual and reproductive health is the state of complete physical, emotional, mental, and social well-being in matters relating to sexuality and the reproductive system; it is not merely the absence of disease, dysfunction, or infirmity [7]. It is a key component of MDG 5 (see Box 22.1).
- Cheap effective interventions are available for early and unwanted childbearing, HIV and other sexually transmitted infections (STIs), and pregnancy-related illness and deaths. Nevertheless, every year, over 120 million couples have an unmet need for contraception; 80 million women have unintended pregnancies; more than half a million die from complications associated with the antenatal, perinatal, and postpartum period; and 340 million people acquire new STIs [4].
- In many developing countries, it is not uncommon for women to have at least 5 children, as very low proportions use a modern method of contraception. Women are poorly informed about their sexual health, resulting in an underutilization of services and inadequate care. This leads to obstetrics and gynecology departments being inundated with treating complications of unsafe abortions. Family planning services are often absent or of poor quality and underused because of cultural sensitivity to issues such as sexual intercourse and sexuality [4].
- The problem is not just for women. There is insufficient engagement of men in promoting good reproductive health for their partners. They need greater levels of information about maternal health and nutrition, STI awareness, and access to contraception.

Box 22.1: MDG 5 – Improve Maternal Health

MDG 5 set a target of reducing maternal mortality by three-fourths by 2015. In 2007, the world's leaders added a second target to achieve universal access to reproductive health [7].

Target 5a: Reduce by Three-Quarters the Maternal Mortality atio

Indicators:

- 5.1 Maternal mortality ratio
- 5.2 Proportion of births attended by skilled health personnel

Target 5b: Achieve Universal Access to Reproductive Health

Indicators:

- 5.3 Contraceptive prevalence rate
- 5.4 Adolescent birth rate
- 5.5 Antenatal care coverage
- 5.6 Unmet need for family planning

Maternal mortality due to complications during pregnancy and childbirth has been reduced by 34 % from 1990 to 2008, from 440 maternal deaths per 100,000 live births to 290 maternal deaths. Progress is notable; however, there are vast disparities especially among developing regions, and this annual rate of decline of 2.3 % is not fast enough to reach the 5.5 % annual rate required for the MDG 2015 target [7]. Adolescent pregnancy rates had decreased globally between 1990 and 2000, but from 2000 to 2008, rates have slowed down or even increased, with 48 births per 1000 adolescent girls aged 15–19 globally. There is a high unmet need for contraceptives especially in sub-Saharan Africa where the prevalence is only at 22 % and inadequate support for family planning remaining at the same moderate to high level in most regions since 2000 [7].

Prompt 6: What Is Family Planning?

- Family planning services provide women and men with the means to prevent unintended pregnancies and time the formation of their families.
- Modern family planning services include:
  - Information and counseling by health personnel about modern contraceptive methods.
  - Provision of contraceptive methods and related surgical procedures, such as IUD insertion or sterilization.
  - Screening and testing for reproductive tract infections, STIs (including HIV), cervical and breast cancer, and other gynecological and urological conditions.

Prompt 7: Why Does Family Planning Matter?

Health Benefits

- Over the past four decades, family planning programs have increased the prevalence of contraceptive practice from less than 10 to 60 % and reduced the number of births per woman in developing countries from 6 to about 3 [8]. However, in many of the low-income countries, contraceptive uptake remains very poor, and greater investment in is required to improve health. Recent estimates indicate that satisfying women's unmet need for family planning could result in a 27 % drop in maternal mortality annually primarily from reducing unintended pregnancies from 75 to 22 million [9].

- Smaller families and wider birth intervals allow families to invest more in each child's nutrition and health, thereby reducing child mortality. Conceptions that occur within 18 months of a previous live birth are at greater risk of fetal death, low birth weight, prematurity, and being of small size for gestational age. One theory on why this may occur attributes the cause to postpartum nutritional depletion, in particular, folate deficiency.
- Greater use of barrier contraception would reduce the transmission of HIV/AIDS, gonorrhea, syphilis, chlamydia, or trichomonas infections.
- Community involvement in family planning would help reduce suffering and stigma due to fistula, infertility, and other reproductive health problems.
- Family planning is considered a "best buy" in global health because of its relative cost-effectiveness, comparatively to other public health interventions, such as antiretroviral therapy, BCG vaccinations, or oral rehydration therapy. It costs a mere $28 in DALYs to avert an unintended pregnancy [4].

Gender Equality, Human Rights, and Education

- In low-income countries in Asia, the burden of domestic chores falls disproportionately on females. By reducing the number of unintended pregnancies particularly among adolescents through family planning, girls would be more likely to complete their education and have greater employment opportunities, which would consequently contribute to the status of women in male-dominated societies [9].
- Countries with rapid population growth have significant problems in providing adequate numbers of teachers, equipment, and classrooms for their increasing number of pupils enrolling in schools. Family planning can have an effect on population growth which has knock on consequences for the quality of education per pupil [8].

Poverty Reduction

- Some people believe that that poor people need many children to help around the house and provide security when they grow older, and thus, family planning promotion may not succeed in very poor countries [8]. However, children from larger families suffer from being poorer, less well nourished, and less well educated than those from smaller families. Smaller families can lead to the provision of more parenting time, greater proportion of income allocated to each child, and hopefully a break from the cycle of poverty.
- In stagnant economies, population growth exacerbates poverty, unemployment, and food shortages. For example, in sub-Saharan Africa where fertility rates are high, the number of individuals living in absolute poverty on less than $1 a day doubled from 164 million in 1981 to 316 million in 2001 [8].

Environmental Sustainability

- The world population has reached 7 billion, and as this rapid rate of population growth, especially in developing world continues, the demand for food, water, and energy increases, which in turn creates major threats to biodiversity and natural habitats.
- Preventing unwanted births through family planning could be one of the most cost-effective ways to reduce the pressure on scarce natural resources and help with the global issue climate change [8].

Further Information 2

In your country, the overwhelming majority of adolescent girls are married and pressured to have a child early, especially in rural areas. Half of all girls in this region are married before their 15th birthday. Of this total, most had not met their husbands until the time of marriage, never used modern contraception, and many are pregnant with their first child between the ages of 15 and 19. Most of these women have little education and few other options in life.

Prompt 8: What Challenges Face Family Planning?

- *Inadequate Funding* – Most low-income countries have appropriate family planning policies, but governments are receiving insufficient financial resources from international and bilateral donors, as their attention is focused on other MDGs. Aid to family planning as a percentage of total aid to health declined dramatically from 8.2 % in 2000 to 2.6 % in 2009 [7].
- *Low Accessibility* – The lack of funding toward reproductive health services means that medical facilities and outreach services are not accessible to many women, especially the poor and those in rural areas. Furthermore, in many developing countries, women lack basic information and social support needed to make informed decisions regarding the sexual health. A lack of public awareness about the effectiveness and safety of modern contraceptive methods may therefore create a barrier to women approaching family planning services.
- *Legitimization* – Unsafe abortions occur in greater numbers in countries where abortion is illegal, and, thus, advocacy is needed to change abortion laws. However, unsafe abortions sometimes occur even in countries where abortions are legal as women are unable to afford medically competent abortion care. Another problem in low-income countries is that child marriage and early childbearing may be socially acceptable; therefore, greater levels of advocacy for smaller families and the use of modern contraception are required.

Prompt 9: Consider the Social and Cultural Barriers That Prevent Men and Women Using Family Planning Products and Services

- *Social and Cultural Norms* – Married women may feel familial pressure to bear children from an early age (see Box 22.2). Great social stigma is often attached to married women who are childless and also to nonmarital sexual relationships. Traditional values may encourage large family sizes and may deem the use of modern contraceptives unacceptable [10]. Thus, encouraging birth spacing as opposed to limiting the final family size may find more support among traditional couples.
- *Gender Roles* – In some cultures, the unequal status of a man prevents a woman from having her opinions heard. The husband's fertility preferences and his attitudes toward family planning may prohibit women in making decisions about the timing of births or use of contraceptives [10]. Furthermore, women may choose not to use health services that are staffed by male health workers. ·
- *Religion* – Some religions discourage and/or forbid the use of contraception. Abortion of a viable fetus is considered a serious crime equivalent to that of murder. This way of thinking may be taught in schools and can also reinforce a country's health policy.

Box 22.2: Adolescents' Vulnerability to Unintended Pregnancy and Abortion [9]

There are some striking statistics regarding adolescents' sexual and reproductive health in the developing world:

-Fifteen percent of females are married before the age of 20, and an estimated 44 % of them want to avoid pregnancy, primarily because they would like to delay their next birth; however, over two-thirds of them do not use any modern contraceptive methods.

-Of unmarried adolescent girls, nearly 17 % in sub-Saharan Africa and 12 % in South America and the Caribbean are sexually active and do not want to get pregnant, but over half of them are not protected by modern contraceptive methods.

-In 2008, adolescents aged 15–19 in the world had an estimated 14.3 million births and accounted for 14 % of all unsafe abortions.

Further Information 3

Access to family planning and reproductive health services is extremely low, resulting in large unmet needs for reproductive health information and services. There is a lack of family planning clinics and family physicians providing contraceptive advice. The international community has finally put sexual and reproductive health back on their agenda. A Family Planning Summit has been arranged in London in July 2012 hosted

Table 22.4 Contraceptive effectiveness, including typical use, 12-month failure rate shown in brackets [8]

Most effective	Effective	Least effective
Sterilization [–]	Oral contraceptive pill (6.9 %)	Withdrawal (15.2 %)
Intrauterine device (1.8 %)	Condoms (9.8 %)	Periodic abstinence (21.6 %)
Implant (1.5 %)		
Injectable (2.9 %)		

by the UK government and the Bill & Melinda Gates Foundation to launch a global movement to provide access to family planning information, services, and supplies to an additional 120 million women in the world's poorest countries (i.e., gross national income ≤£2,500 per year) by 2020. You have been granted the political commitment and resources to design a successful family planning scheme in your country.

Prompt 10: Outline the Effectiveness of Modern Contraceptive Methods in Developing Countries

- Eighty-five percent of couples will become pregnant within one year without contraception.
- Traditional methods that include periodic abstinence and withdrawal have very poor efficacy and are often used by women in poverty and those without education.
- Funds should be directed toward encouraging switching from less effective to most effective ones and increasing adherence to methods to reduce failure rates (refer to Table 22.4). In terms of pregnancies prevented, sterilization and intrauterine devices demonstrate the best value for money, and the need for individual adherence to the method is not an issue. However, these approaches have notably led to unethical coercive pressures in India and China.
- The cultural acceptability of modern contraceptive methods varies between different countries. In Bangladesh, 28.5 % of women rely on the pill; whereas in India, the corresponding figure is only 3.1 %, and sterilization accounts for 38.3 % [11]. In sub-Saharan Africa, birth spacing is valued above family size limitation; thus, injectable contraception has greater acceptability, and the pill is commonly used.

Prompt 11: What Are the Key Components of a Successful Family Planning Scheme?

Phasing

- The early phase of family planning programs should focus on legitimizing modern contraceptive use and the idea of small family sizes. Awareness, accessibility, and affordability of a range of family planning services must also be addressed.

- Later on as programs develop, improvements to service quality should be sought, which includes reaching out to underserved groups like those in rural areas.

Mobilizing Support and Raising Awareness

- Public health interventions should address people from all different backgrounds to sustain health behavior change. Obviously, those at risk of poor health outcomes should be targeted, but also family and influential community members must be engaged to provide support in seeking reproductive and sexual health services. Boosting political support and cooperation among key sectors of society, including religious, secular, traditional leaders, and professional groups, is essential to success.
- The use of media is a powerful and cost-effective way of spreading public health messages about family planning. Street theater shows, radio community talk programs, and television soaps sensitize communities and prompt discussion between spouses about sexual and reproductive health issues like the dangers of child marriage or planning family sizes and birth spacing through the use of contraceptives [8].
- Economic incentives may even be used to reward families financially to not arrange marriages for daughters when they are adolescents, to provide them with the opportunity to complete school and start working which will have a knock on effect in empowering women.

Making Family Planning Methods Accessible and Acceptable

- Usually, sterilizations, intrauterine devices, and injectable contraceptives are available in hospitals, while confidential services that address reproductive tract and sexually transmitted infections or HIV counseling and testing can be provided by family planning clinics. But family planning services need to be available from different types of healthcare facilities to improve accessibility.
- Now, pharmacies, shops, and marketplaces can distribute contraceptive products. The distribution of condoms from these commercial outlets has greatly reduced the risk of HIV and STIs in low-income countries. Outreach and community-based workers who share the language and customs of local women living in rural communities can really help to improve accessibility and acceptability of modern contraceptive methods [12].

Financing and Cost Challenges

- Most government family planning programs worldwide provide family planning services that are free or at very low cost to users.
- But as donor support for family planning has decreased, this strategy is being increasingly questioned as financing needs to be sustainable. There may be movement toward greater cost recovery in health services, which might have knock-on effects on the uptake of modern contraceptive practices particularly for those living in poverty.

Case Study: Increasing Contraceptive Use in Pakistan

Despite years of promoting family planning, Pakistan had one of the highest levels of unmet need in the world through the early 1990s. The government launched a scheme – Pakistan's Lady Health Worker Programme (LHWP) – to increase access to modern contraceptive use among rural women who are cut off from hospitals and health centers by social barriers and distance.

Lady health workers receive several months training in basic health services, such as family planning, immunization, hygiene, and maternal and child health. They then return to the community working in their home villages and provide information on health-related topics, distribute contraceptive supplies like pills and condoms, and refer for other methods like IUD and sterilization.

By 2001, a national program evaluation found that 20 % of rural women in areas served by the lady health workers were using modern contraceptives, compared with 14 % of rural women in areas where the program did not serve [12]. The evaluation of LHWP concluded that doorstep delivery through community-based lady health workers is key to achieving universal access to modern contraceptive methods. In remote areas where there are no doctors and women are often forbidden to work, lady health workers perform an essential role in breaking down social and cultural barriers and improving sexual and reproductive healthcare in rural villages.

References

1. Grimes D, Benson J, Singh S, et al. Unsafe: abortion: the preventable pandemic. Lancet. 2006;368:1908–19.
2. Guttmacher Institute. Facts on induced abortion worldwide [homepage on the internet]. c2007. [updated 2012 January: cited 2012 March 9]. Available from: www.guttmacher.org/pubs/fb_IAW.html.
3. World Health Organization (WHO). Unsafe abortion: Global and regional estimates of the incidence of unsafe abortion and associated mortality in 2008. 6th ed. Geneva: WHO; 2011.
4. Glasier A, Gulmezoglu A, Schmid G, Moreno C, Van Look P. Sexual and reproductive health: a matter of life and death. Lancet. 2006;368:1595–607.
5. Hanretty K. Obstetrics illustrated. 7th ed. Edinburgh: Churchill Livingstone; 2010.
6. Gemzell-Danielsson K, Fiala C, Weeks A. Misoprostol: firstline therapy for incomplete miscarriage in the developing world. BJOG. 2007;114:1337–9.
7. United Nations. The millennium development goals report 2011. New York; 2011.
8. Cleland J, Bernstein S, Ezeh A, Faundes A, Glasier A, Innis J. Family planning: the unfinished agenda. Lancet. 2006;368:1810–27.
9. Singh S, et al. Adding it up: the costs and benefits of investing in family planning and maternal and newborn health. New York: Guttmacher Institute; 2009.
10. Casterline J, Sathar Z, Haque M. Obstacles to contraceptive use in Pakistan: a study in Punjab. Stud Fam Plann. 2001;32:95–110.
11. Population Reference Bureau. Family planning worldwide: 2008 data sheet [homepage on the internet]. c2008 [cited 2012 March 9]. Available from: www.prb.org/pdf08/fpds08.pdf.
12. Douthwaite M, Ward P. Increasing contraceptive use in rural Pakistan: an evaluation of the Lady Health Worker Programme. Health Policy Plan. 2005;20(2):117–23.

Chapter 23
Maternal and Neonatal Health

James Houston

Learning Objectives

- List important conditions to be screened for at antenatal clinics in resource-poor settings
- Detail the epidemiology of maternal deaths around the world
- List common complications of labor in the developing world
- Explore the role of traditional birthing attendants in the provision of pregnancy care
- Detail ways that the WHO is trying to reduce maternal mortality
- Explore key factors that prevent women receiving adequate maternal healthcare in resource-poor settings
- Detail the causes of neonatal deaths in the developing world
- Describe the benefits and controversies surrounding breast-feeding

Initial Scenario

You are a doctor working in a rural health center in a Southeast Asian country. It is Monday morning, and you are running the antenatal clinic. A pregnant young woman comes into the clinic room. Linh is 18 years old. Her last period was 34 weeks ago. This is her first pregnancy, and she came to the clinic because she is anxious about the birth. A family friend died after bleeding during pregnancy. Linh knows another woman who lost her baby when she started fitting during the last

J. Houston, MBBS, MEng
FY2 Doctor, Department of Surgery,
Chelsea and Westminster Hospital,
London, UK
e-mail: jameshouston@doctors.org.uk

D. MacGarty, D. Nott (eds.), *Disaster Medicine*,
DOI 10.1007/978-1-4471-4423-6_23, © Springer-Verlag London 2013

stages of pregnancy. You take a thorough history, perform an examination, and perform some simple investigations.

Prompt 1: What Important Conditions Could Be Screened for at an Antenatal Clinic and How Might This Be Done in Resource-Poor Settings?

Conditions that can affect the mother's or baby's health include the following:

Gestational Diabetes

- The onset of diabetes during pregnancy. Most commonly seen in the third trimester, risk factors include obesity or a family history of diabetes.
- Most women are asymptomatic. Some may have increased thirst, frequent urination, fatigue, or more frequent urine infections.
- Risks in pregnancy are many. High-sugar environment causes large babies (macrosomia), which may cause complications during labor. Babies may also be prone to neonatal hypoglycemia, jaundice, and electrolyte abnormalities.

Preeclampsia

- Defined by a pregnancy-induced hypertension that is associated with protein in the urine with or without edema and end-organ damage. The condition most frequently occurs after 20 weeks. The concern with preeclampsia is that it may progress to eclampsia, which is potentially life-threatening.
- Eclampsia is characterized by tonic-clonic seizures. Magnesium sulfate is the most effective drug for fitting women. Sadly, this medication is in short supply in the developing world, leading to many potentially unnecessary maternal deaths. Worldwide campaigns have been set up to educate healthcare professionals on eclampsia management and to ensure adequate drug supplies [1].

Infections

- Infections such as HIV, syphilis, and malaria are common in the developing world and may have disastrous effects for mother or fetus.
- Malaria in pregnancy increases the risk of profound anemia, stillbirth/spontaneous abortion, and low birth weight [2].
- Women are particularly susceptible to HIV infection for biological and sociocultural reasons [3]. HIV infection will predispose pregnant women to catching further infections. It increases risks to the fetus (low birth weight, preterm labor, premature rupture of membranes). Ultimately, HIV may be transmitted to the fetus (vertical transmission) in 15–40 % of cases of HIV seropositivity without use of antiretrovirals [3].
- Sexually transmitted infections like syphilis are common in some parts of the developing world. Syphilis increases risks of spontaneous abortion or

stillbirth [4]. For live-born infants, it may cause serious neurodevelopmental sequelae [4]. Chlamydia, gonorrhea, and hepatitis B are other important infections that may affect the newborn and cause significant morbidity [5].
- Group B streptococcus (GBS) is common and may cause neonatal infection, especially in premature rupture of membranes.

Anemia

- Anemia is common in developing countries. Reasons for high prevalence are complex, but well-known factors include insufficient diet, hookworm infestations, and malaria. It affects nearly half of all pregnancies worldwide, more so in developing countries [6]. Anemia reduces energy levels in pregnant women and makes any bleeding in pregnancy dangerous due to diminished physiological reserve.

Malposition

- Malposition of the fetus may cause significant difficulties in labor. A common example is breech presentation [5]. Malposition increases the chances of dystocia (difficult labor), which can present as fetal obstruction. Such events drastically increase the chances of death or injury to mother or fetus.

Cheap and helpful tests which can be performed at the antenatal clinic include:

- Examining the mother for fundal height and fetal growth assessment relative to gestational age; also check for the presence of twins or malposition
- Blood pressure
- Urine dipstick for protein, glucose, leukocytes, and nitrates

Resource permitting, you might also consider other tests relevant to this setting such as:

- Hemoglobin
- Blood group and rhesus status
- Rapid diagnostic test or blood films for malaria
- Ultrasound
- Infection serology screens (HIV, syphilis, hepatitis)

The above list is not exhaustive but gives an idea of common investigations that may be appropriate.

Prompt 2: What Is the Epidemiology of Maternal Deaths Around the World?

- Every day 1,500 women and over 10,000 newborn babies die as a result of complications of pregnancy and childbirth [7], roughly 6.3 million a year. 98 % of these deaths occur in the developing world and are largely preventable [8].

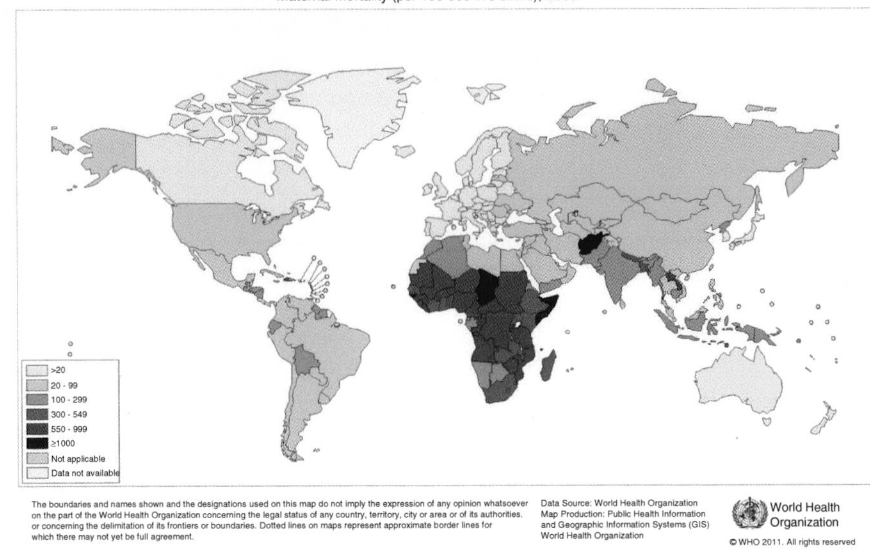

Fig. 23.1 Maternal mortality ratio worldwide (*Source*: WHO, UNICEF)

- More than half of all maternal deaths occur in sub-Saharan Africa, and one-third occur in South Asia [9]. See Fig. 23.1 for a visual representation of the global spread of maternal mortality.
- Maternal mortality is higher in rural areas and among poorer, less educated communities [9].
- According to WHO data, younger mothers face higher risks of death and complications than older women [9]. Indeed, complications in pregnancy and labor are the leading cause of death among adolescent girls in most developing countries [9].

Causes of Maternal Mortality

Causes of maternal mortality are either direct (directly relating to the pregnancy/delivery) or indirect (a condition unrelated to the pregnancy/delivery). The leading causes of maternal mortality are severe bleeding, infections, eclampsia, unsafe abortion, and obstructive labor. These make up 80 % of maternal deaths [9]. The other 20 % of deaths occur due to indirect causes. Preexisting HIV, malaria, and anemia or coexisting malnutrition can prove deadly when pregnancy puts a further strain on an already weakened body.

Causes of maternal mortality also vary considerably between different regions in the developing world, as shown in Table 23.1. To factor in the bias of population

Table 23.1 Causes of maternal deaths by region Source: WHO [10]

Order of prevalence	Africa	Asia	Latin America and Caribbean	Developed
1	Hemorrhage (33.9 %)	Hemorrhage (30.8 %)	Hypertensive (25.7 %)	Other indirect (21.3 %)
2	Other indirect (16.7 %)	Anemia (12.8 %)	Hemorrhage (20.8 %)	Hypertensive (16.1 %)
3	Sepsis (9.7 %)	Other indirect (12.5 %)	Obstructed labor (13.4 %)	Embolism (14.9 %)
4	Hypertensive (9.1 %)	Sepsis (11.6 %)	Abortion (12 %)	Other indirect (14.4 %)
5	HIV/AIDS (6.2 %)	Obstructed labor (9.4 %)	Unclassified (11.7 %)	Hemorrhage (13.4 %)

size and number of pregnant women, maternal mortality ratios (MMRs) are often used when considering maternal health. The MMR is the number of maternal deaths per 100,000 live births. Betran et al. [11] note that the MMR shows a strong association with three factors:

- The proportion of deliveries assisted by a skilled attendant
- The infant mortality rate
- National per capita expenditure on health

Prompt 3: What Are the Important Complications of Labor in the Developing World?

More than 136 million women give birth a year [12]. Labor is a natural process, and the majority of births take place without any complications. However, the WHO estimates that about 20 million women experience pregnancy-related illness after childbirth [12]. Complications include:

- Hemorrhage. This is frequently life-threatening for the mother in the developing world, especially when taking account of the time it takes to access definitive care. In developed countries, almost all women have their third stage of labor (the period between delivery of the child and delivery of the placenta) "actively managed." This refers to the use of drugs such as syntometrine, which causes the uterus to contract strongly and so helps prevent postpartum hemorrhage. This is slowly becoming more available in resource-poor countries.
- Infection: Commonly, untreated genital infections progresses to pelvic inflammatory disease. It may cause chronic pelvic pain or infertility. Swift diagnosis and treatment with antibiotics are key to preventing chronic disease progression.

- Depression is a common complication of pregnancy and labor. Serious depression is encountered by about 10–15 % of women in developed countries and an even greater fraction of women in developing countries [13]. Postpartum depression may cause significant psychological or physical harm to mother and newborn [13].
- Vaginal or perineal trauma may result from a variety of factors including mismanaged fetal malposition, prolonged labor, and cephalopelvic disproportion (especially in young mothers). An example of this is obstetric fistula, where prolonged pressure of the fetus during a protracted labor leads to tissue necrosis and fistula formation. Obstetric trauma can lead to incontinence (urinary or fecal), chronic pain, social stigma, and disability. Poverty and lack of access to obstetric facilities are significant risk factors. The progress of a woman's dilatation can be monitored using a partogram, which indicates when decisions should be made in prolonged labor. Partograms are cheap to use and easy to follow and thus are ideal to use in resource-poor countries. The graph tracks the progress of labor relative to the dilation of the cervix and can indicate to healthcare providers that labour is taking too long and they should act accordingly.

Further Information 1

Routine antenatal history and examination of Linh are unremarkable. Her blood pressure is normal, and she has no glucose or signs of infection on urine dipstick. Linh mentions that her sister had her baby at home with the help of a traditional birth attendant (TBA). You are aware that TBAs are often the only source of assistance that many women get during labor. Linh describes the difficulties her sister had during labor due to the baby being so large, and it was seeing her struggle through the pregnancy that spurred her to visit your clinic. Aware of their potential, you consider setting up a meeting with some local TBAs to discuss labor, management of the neonate, and how and when to refer to medical teams.

Prompt 4: What Are Skilled Attendants and How Do They Differ from Traditional Birth Attendants?

A skilled attendant is someone who has been trained to manage normal (uncomplicated) pregnancies and deliveries. They should:

- Be able to recognize complications of pregnancy
- Know how to refer these cases on to further help
- Have the necessary equipment and medicines to act in an emergency

Traditional birth attendants (TBAs) provide healthcare based upon knowledge that is passed down informally through practice and traditions of their communities. They may:

- Provide a service where other health resources are scarce
- Not receive formal tuition and not be certified by any professional body
- Use traditional herbal medicines and beliefs that do not have an evidence base; although these may be in line with the culture and practices of the region, they can in some cases be harmful

Without training, TBAs may not recognize key complications of pregnancy and may not refer women who are in need of obstetric help. While the vast majority of TBAs have the women's interests at heart, their lack of knowledge may give false reassurance to pregnant women.

Prompt 5: How Important Are TBAs in the Provision of Obstetric Care and What Are the Arguments Surrounding Their Use?

Forty-three percent of births in resource-poor settings are attended by TBAs [14]. It is clear that they are a valuable resource to women who may not otherwise have any help.

The WHO promoted the training of TBAs from the 1970s to 1990s. Unfortunately, this created little improvement in maternal mortality arising as a result of the training. Some, like Kamal et al., argue that this was perhaps due to a lack of support and supervision after the training the TBAs, and their propensity to go back to their traditional roots [15].

A more recent Cochrane review [16] has shown more positive outcomes when TBAs have been better linked to other healthcare resources, resulting in reductions in mortality and morbidity alongside increased rates of referral and breast-feeding [15]. Education has been shown to encourage the feeding of colostrum and also in basic hygiene such as improving rates of washing hands before birth and using clean delivery kits. In some cases, correct referrals to medical staff have increased with associated reduction in maternal mortality.

Controversy surrounds whether it would be better to retrain the TBAs or train new midwives. TBAs may have low levels of formal obstetric education. However, they are rurally based and are easily accessed by pregnant women. Trained midwives may be expensive to keep and may not want to work in the isolated rural places that they are needed most.

In the perfect setting, every birth would be attended by a skilled attendant who could also take care of traditional rituals. In reality, many developing areas are remote and under-resourced with TBAs the only people who have some experience of managing childbirth.

Prompt 6: What Are the Main Areas Where the WHO Has Set Out Strategies to Reduce Maternal Mortality?

Maternal health is the focus of one of the Millennium Development Goals (MDGs), details of which are discussed in another chapter.

MDG 5 involves [17]:

1. Commitments to reduce maternal mortality by three-quarters between 1990 and 2015
2. Commitments to achieve universal access to reproductive health by 2015

Since 1990, maternal deaths worldwide have dropped by 34 % [9]. However, this decline is still far off the original ambitious targets set. Focus on the issue of maternal health has led to the following areas being highlighted as key in controlling the problem [18]:

- Family planning
  - Contraception to avoid unwanted pregnancies
  - Access to safe abortion
- Antenatal Care
  - Folic acid, iron, and calcium supplementation
  - Identification of hypertension (preeclampsia)
  - Identification of macrosomia (GDM)
  - Infection screening
- Delivery
  - Access to skilled care during childbirth
  - Clean facilities to prevent sepsis
  - Use of partograms to predict obstructed labor
  - Preventing and managing postpartum hemorrhage
  - Active third-stage management
  - Resources to perform cesarean sections
  - Thermal care for newborns
- Postnatal care
  - Support of mother and child after birth
  - Extra support for feeding small and preterm babies
  - Antibiotics for treating pneumonia in infants
  - Psychosocial screening

Further Information 2

You host the education session and realize that you would need frequent follow-ups to ensure adequate transmission of information, attitudes, and skills. A better relationship has been formed, and the TBAs enthusiastically take on information regarding clean care and avoiding infection. They also now know where to send patients when they encounter problems.

Two months later, a pickup truck rushes to the hospital, and a man carries Linh into the health center. Linh had her baby at home as the health center was too far away for her to visit while heavily pregnant. No one was available to take her to hospital when things began to prove difficult. The labor took many hours, and Linh has bled postdelivery. She looks pale and is breathing quickly. Her legs are covered in blood.

Prompt 7: Why Is Postpartum Hemorrhage a Major Problem in the Developing World?

Postpartum hemorrhage (PPH) relates to bleeding up to 6 weeks following pregnancy. Causes include:

- **Tone (uterine atony)**. More likely in prolonged labor and multiparity – both of which are prevalent in developing countries. Lack of skilled help in manual compression and administration of drugs to facilitate uterine contraction are also problematic in resource-poor environments.
- **Tissue (retained placenta)**. More likely in absence of attendants with skills to identify retained placenta (analysis of placenta postpartum).
- **Trauma (perineal/genital/uterine)**. More likely with prolonged labor. Also, the lack of skilled attendants to facilitate controlled birthing makes this more likely in areas with poor obstetric cover.
- **Thrombin (coagulopathy)**.

Medicinal Issues with Prevention and Treatment of PPH in Developing Countries

Essential medicines are often restricted due to cost and problems with supply and assured quality [19]. Another issue, that of storage, has made the practice of active third-stage management difficult in some resource-poor environments since oxytocin and ergometrine require refrigeration and must be injected.

An alternative, misoprostol, can be taken as a tablet. While studies show that misoprostol is not as efficacious as oxytocin and has more side effects, in resource-poor settings, it remains a useful drug that reduces PPH when drugs are not available [20].

A study in Nepal [21] based where the majority of women give birth without any skilled healthcare attendants, has shown some success by giving women a misoprostol tablet to take home and administer after they have given birth.

Prompt 8: What Are the Main Factors That Prevent Women Receiving Adequate Maternal Healthcare in the Developing World?

Adequate maternal healthcare requires access to skilled professionals to diagnose and treat the common conditions and complications of pregnancy and childbirth. The WHO estimates that only 46 % of women in developing countries get help from a skilled health worker during childbirth [9]. About a third of women do not have any antenatal health checks. These figures vary widely between developing countries with eastern Africa having some of the worst rates of access [22].

Causes of poor access to healthcare workers include:

- Not enough skilled workers exist in areas of need: This is often attributed to a lack of training [9].
- Distances and terrain: Poor road infrastructure in developing countries makes physical access difficult, especially when a 4*4 vehicle may not be available or affordable.
- Poverty: Patients may not be able to afford treatment and the provision of lifesaving medicines.
- Health beliefs: Maternal health will be influenced by health beliefs; concepts of women's equality and rights to health, attitudes toward obstetric care, and other idiosyncrasies (e.g., examinations by male health professionals).

Further Information 3

One of the nurses inserts an IV line and administers fluids. Bimanual palpation is provided to Linh's uterus. There is no syntometrine in stock. Fortunately, the bleeding stops after prolonged bimanual palpation. Linh recovers, and within three days, she is ready to go home.

During the morning ward round, you take time to sit with Linh and talk about her postnatal care. Linh's baby is lucky to have survived such a long labor. As you discuss her care, she is unsure about whether she should breast-feed after hearing that some substitutes might be better for her baby.

Prompt 9: What Are the Causes of Neonatal Death and How Might These Be Reduced?

A Lancet series investigating neonatal death [23] identified that:

- Roughly 4 million babies die within the first four weeks of life each year
- 99 % of these deaths occur in middle to low-income countries

- Three-quarters of neonatal deaths happen in the first week
- Babies have the greatest risk of dying on the first day of life

The article found the causes of death include [19]:

- Preterm birth (28 %)
- Severe infections (26 %)
- Asphyxia (23 %)
- Neonatal tetanus (7 %)

All of these causes can be effectively reduced with adequate healthcare. While the management of preterm birth maybe resource intensive, infection can be reduced through education, recognition, and access to medicines. Improved perinatal monitoring for the women and child would reduce many cases of asphyxia. Neonatal tetanus is perhaps the most easily prevented of all. See Box 23.1 for further details on neonatal tetanus.

Box 23.1: Neonatal Tetanus

Neonatal Tetanus is a frequently fatal condition where the bacterium *Clostridium tetani* gains access to the infant.

It causes an estimated 60,000 deaths per annum. This figure has been reduced by 92 % since the late 1980s [24]. Infection is largely linked to exposure to contaminants and is thus determined by levels of hygiene and cultural practices. Common means of infection include:

- Through the umbilical stump following nonsterile delivery
- Unsterile circumcision (male and female)
- Rubbing of ghee (clarified butter) or animal dung into the umbilical stump postdelivery-cultural practices

Prevention is by:

- Sterile delivery
- Education of risks of certain traditional practices
- Maternal immunization with tetanus toxoid vaccine

Prompt 10: What Is the Role of Postpartum Care of the Infant and Mother in Resource-Poor Settings?

Postpartum care refers to care provided to mother and infant after the delivery of the child. In the developing world, many mothers do not routinely see any skilled healthcare professionals after delivery, with an estimated 70% not receiving any postpartum care[25].

The majority of deaths (both maternal and neonatal) happen in the first week postpartum [8]. Thus, focus should be made on improving postpartum services to pick up complications. Mridha and Koblinsky [26] refer to integrated community-based postpartum care, which offers a group of services that should not only pick up complications but also offer counseling and services for the promotion of healthy behaviors.

While similar issues, such as low numbers of staff and difficulties with physical access can cause barriers, a timely visit, especially if birth has happened with unskilled attendant, has been shown to decrease perinatal mortality [27].

A mother check may look for signs of shock or sepsis as well as perineal tears. A baby check may involve asking how it is feeding, examining for signs of postnatal illness or congenital deformities, and recording its weight.

Mothers can be encouraged to exercise healthy behaviors for the baby including exclusive breast-feeding, clothing and shelter, and immunizations. Likewise, advice on contraception can be explained to help with birth spacing. Continuing care can be provided by giving the mother details on where to go should she experience any longer term complications, such as fistula, or require advice planning a future pregnancy. Insecticide treated bed nets can also be provided to prevent vector borne diseases such as malaria.

Prompt 11: Should Breast-Feeding Be Encouraged?

Exclusive breast-feeding should be encouraged up to six months. After this period it can be continued along with additional supplementation. The WHO recommends commencing breast-feeding within an hour of birth (feeding the colostrum) and states that a lack of exclusive breast-feeding contributes to over a million avoidable child deaths each year [28].

Benefits include [29]:

- A natural and free source of nutrition for the child
- A safe source of food and reduction in diarrheal disease and pneumonia
- Immune protection by providing antibodies in milk
- Providing a bond between mother and child
- When done correctly, it may provide a natural form of contraception

HIV and Breast-Feeding

- While HIV can cross to the baby in breast milk, the WHO still supports the use of breast-feeding in HIV-positive mothers. Studies have shown that the risk of perinatal mortality is still greater in those who have not had breast milk than those who have been fed with breast milk from an HIV-positive mother.
- For infant feeding in maternal HIV seropositivity, discuss options with the parents and provide antiretroviral medications where possible. If chosen, milk formulas must be acceptable, feasible, affordable, sustainable, and safe (AFASS criteria) [30].
- To help improve the coverage of breast-feeding, education must be given to mothers about its benefits. Breast-feeding counselors [31] have been made available to new mothers to help them through common concerns. Communities must be encouraged to help progress those interventions as well.

Case Study: Vietnam

Maternal mortality has decreased by about 70 % in Vietnam between 1990 and 2010 [32]. Training has been improved, and 86 % of births are now attended by trained health workers. In 2002, a Health Care Fund for the Poor was established to provide free care to close to 20 % of the population, and in 2009 close to 55 % of the population were covered by some form of health insurance. The national assembly increased the healthcare section of the budget from 8 to 10 %. Many national strategies have been put in place such as the National Plan on Safe Motherhood and the National Action Plan for Child Survival [33]. Improvements have been made in vaccination for tetanus and contraceptive use. Achievements have been made by the expansion of reproductive healthcare service to a provincial level. Still the maternal mortality rate is nearly double in rural areas; 145/100,000 compared to 79/100,000 in urban areas. This disparity is likely attributable to geographical factors, the educational level of mothers and traditional practices. Likewise, it is difficult to persuade professionals trained in urban areas to go out and work in remote rural communities. Where other countries have not been so successful, Vietnam appears to have reduced its maternal mortality by increasing funding and focusing improvement on a local scale.

References

1. Engender Health. Balancing the scales: expanding treatment for pregnant women with life-threatening hypertensive conditions in developing countries. 2007. http://www.engenderhealth.org/files/pubs/maternal-health/EngenderHealth-Eclampsia-Report.pdf. Accessed 18 May 2012.
2. WHO. Malaria in pregnancy. http://www.who.int/malaria/high_risk_groups/pregnancy/en/index.html. Accessed 18 May 2012.
3. WHO. HIV in pregnancy: a review. 1998. http://www.unaids.org/en/media/unaids/contentassets/dataimport/publications/irc-pub01/jc151-hiv-in-pregnancy_en.pdf. Accessed 18 May 2012.
4. Genç M, Ledger WJ. Syphilis in pregnancy. Sex Transm Infect. 2000;76(2):73–9. Review.
5. Collier J, et al. Oxford handbook of clinical specialities. Oxford: Oxford University Press; 2009.
6. WHO. Iron deficiency anemia: assessment, prevention, and control. Geneva: WHO; 2001.
7. UNICEF. Maternal and newborn health. New York; 2009.
8. WHO. The world health report 2005 – make every mother and child count, Geneva. Available at URL: http://www.who.int/whr/2005/en. Accessed 30 Oct 2011.
9. WHO. Maternal mortality fact sheet. http://www.who.int/mediacentre/factsheets/fs348/en/index.html. Accessed 19 May 2012.
10. Khan KS, et al. WHO analysis of causes of maternal death: a systematic review. Lancet. 2006;367:1066–74.
11. Betrán AP, Wojdyla D, Posner SF, Gülmezoglu AM. National estimates for maternal mortality: an analysis based on the WHO systematic review of maternal mortality and morbidity. Biomed Central Public Health. 2005;5:131.
12. WHO. 10 facts on maternal health. http://www.who.int/features/factfiles/maternal_health/maternal_health_facts/en/index.html. Accessed 19 May 2012.

13. UNFPA. Surviving birth but enduring chronic ill health. http://www.unfpa.org/public/mothers/pid/4388. Accessed 19 May 2012.
14. MacArthur C. Traditional birth attendant training for improving health behaviours and pregnancy outcomes: RHL commentary (last revised: 1 June 2009). The WHO Reproductive Health Library. Geneva: World Health Organization.
15. Kamal IT. The traditional birth attendant: a reality and a challenge. Int J Gynaecol Obstet. 1998;63 Suppl 1:S43–52. Review.
16. Sibley L, et al. Traditional birth attendant training for improving health behaviours and pregnancy outcomes. Cochrane Database Syst Rev. 2007;18.
17. WHO. MDG 5: improve maternal health. http://www.who.int/topics/millennium_development_goals/maternal_health/en/index.html. Accessed 17 May 2012.
18. WHO. Essential interventions, commodities and guidelines for reproductive, maternal, newborn and child health. http://www.who.int/pmnch/topics/part_publications/201112_essential_interventions/en/index.html. Accessed 19 May 2012.
19. WHO. Medicines: essential medicine fact sheet. 2010. http://www.who.int/mediacentre/factsheets/fs325/en/index.html. Accessed 19 May 2012.
20. Derman R, et al. Oral Misoprostol in preventing postpartum haemorrhage in resource-poor communities: a randomised controlled trial. Lancet. 2006;368(9543):1248–53.
21. Rajbhandari S, Pun A, Hodgins S, Rajendra P. Prevention of postpartum haemorrhage at homebirth with use of Misoprostol in Banke District, Nepal. Int J Gynecol Obstet. 2006;94:S143–4. Print.
22. Campbell OM, Graham WJ. Strategies for reducing maternal mortality: getting on with what works. Lancet. 2006;368(9543):1284–99.
23. Lawn JE, et al. 4 million neonatal deaths: When? Where? Why? Lancet. 2005;365(9462): 891–900.
24. WHO. Maternal and neonatal tetanus (MNT) elimination. http://www.who.int/immunization_monitoring/diseases/MNTE_initiative/en/index.html. Accessed on 19 May 2012.
25. USAID (Measure Demographic and Health Surveys). Postpartum care: levels and determinants in developing countries. Baltimore; 2006, http://www.measuredhs.com/publications/publication-CR15-Comparative-Reports.cfm. Accessed 19 May 2012.
26. Mridha MK, Koblinsky M. Integrated community-based postpartum care for mother and newborns: a crucial intervention to achieve MDG 4 and 5. http://www.jhsph.edu/gra/Research/Maternal_Neonatal_Health/Maternal_and_Neonatal_Publications/MotherNewBorNet_Publications/MotherNewBorNet_Policy_brief_Community-Based_Postpartum_Care_Revised.pdf. Accessed 19 May 2012.
27. Baqui AH, et al. Effect of timing of first postnatal care home visit on neonatal mortality in Bangladesh: a observational cohort study. BMJ. 2009;339:b2826. doi:10.1136/bmj.b2826.
28. Betran AP, De Onis M, Lauer JA, Villar J. Ecological study of effect of breast feeding on infant mortality in Latin America. BMJ. 2001;323(7308):303–6.
29. WHO. Infant and young child feeding: model. Chapter for textbooks for medical students and allied health professionals. Geneva: World Health Organization; 2009.
30. UNICEF. HIV and infant feeding. http://www.unicef.org/nutrition/index_24827.html. Accessed 19 May 2012.
31. WHO. Community-based strategies for breastfeeding promotion and support in developing countries. Geneva: World Health Organization; 2003. Print.
32. Bale B. Achieving the millennium development goals: UNFPA's responses to the needs of safe motherhood and newborn care in Viet Nam. Ha Noi, Viet Nam: UNFPA; 2007.
33. MDG-5: improve maternal health report represented by Vietnam. Available at URL: www.aipasecretariat.org/wp-content/uploads/2011/03/8-CR-Vietnam.pdf. Accessed 19 May 2012.

Chapter 24
Mental Health Following Armed Conflict

David MacGarty and Rachel Brand

Reviewed by Jane Gilbert

Learning Objectives

- Investigate the global prevalence of child soldiers in conflict and outline international policy regarding the use of child soldiers
- Determine the impact of conflict on the mental health of individuals and communities
- Outline priorities in psychosocial interventions following armed conflict
- Explore cultural differences in the understanding and treatment of mental health
- Explore the importance of PTSD in the postconflict setting
- Outline the evidence for mental health intervention following conflict
- Consider the wider context of mental health provision in low-income countries
- Consider new approaches to mental health intervention in conflict zones

Initial Scenario

The same old routine, the never-ending red tape, the cold winter; you are becoming weary with your psychiatry training. You peruse a global health magazine and become immediately engrossed in a story from Central Africa describing the rehabilitation of escaped child soldiers abducted by a rebel militia.

D. MacGarty, MBBS, BSc (✉)
FY2 Doctor, Department of Obstetrics and Gynaecology,
St Peter's Hospital, Chertsey, Surrey, UK
e-mail: dmacgarty@hotmail.com

R. Brand,
Doctorate in Psychology (Dclinpsy),
BSc St Georges Mental Health NHS Trust, London, UK

D. MacGarty, D. Nott (eds.), *Disaster Medicine*,
DOI 10.1007/978-1-4471-4423-6_24,

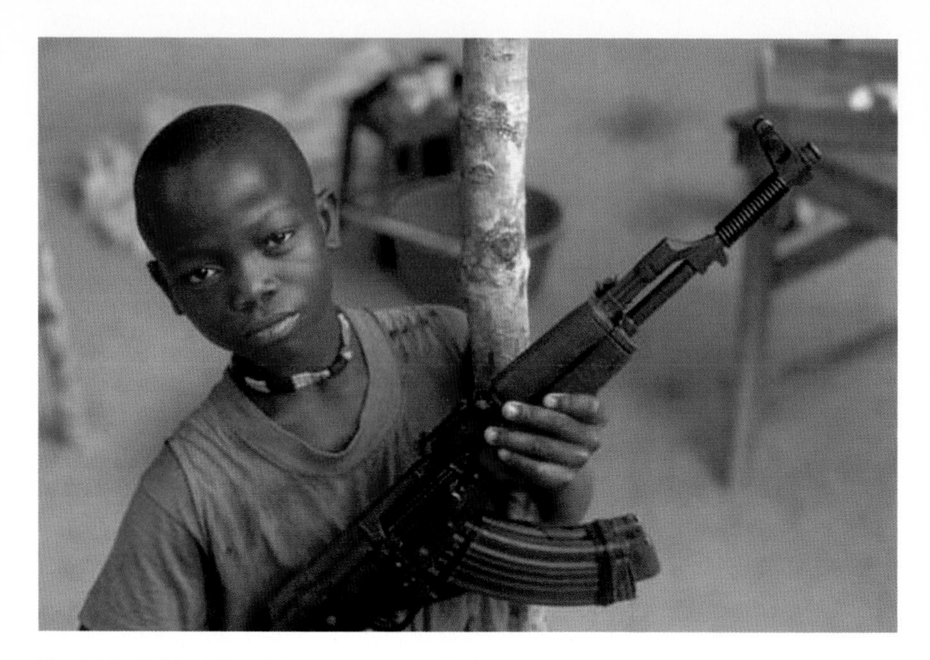

Fig. 24.1 Child soldier with gun (Reproduced with permission from UNICEF)

These abducted children take part in raids on their home villages and aid the militia in battles against government forces. Unsurprisingly, the escaped children return to their communities showing signs of physical and psychological trauma. The article prompts you to consider the impact these experiences will have on the long-term mental health of affected children.

On impulse, you note down the author and contact details for the rehabilitation center and promise yourself to act on it when you get home.

Prompt 1: What Is a "Child Soldier" and Why Are They Recruited?

- UNICEF defines a "child soldier" as "any person below 18 years of age who is recruited or used by an armed force or armed group in any capacity, as fighters, cooks, porters, spies or for sexual purposes" (see Fig. 24.1). It does not only refer to a child who has taken a direct part in hostilities [1]. It is estimated that 1/3 of child soldiers are girls [2].
- In a bid to reduce the recruitment of 16- and 17-year-olds into government armed forces, the definition of a child soldier was raised from 15 to 18 years, therefore implicating many armed forces in the Western world.

- Children are easier to recruit and train than adults and are used to keep numbers high in lengthy conflicts with many casualties [3]. Increased trafficking of small arms and light weapons means that children are more able to serve as effective soldiers since these weapons require little training and are light to carry.
- Girls are often recruited as wives for men in the militia and are required to carry out domestic chores and meet the sexual needs of their "husbands" [4].

Prompt 2: What Is the Extent of Child Recruitment for Conflict Globally?

- UNICEF estimate there are 300,000 child soldiers worldwide. The majority of child soldiers are in nongovernmental military groups, but there are also children under the age of 18 in governmental military groups across the world.
- As of 2007, as many as 26 countries continued to recruit 16- and 17-year-olds into their peacetime armies including Australia, Austria, Canada, the Netherlands, the United Kingdom, and the USA. Children were actively involved in armed conflict in 19 countries between 2004 and 2007 in Africa, Asia, and South America [6].
- A number of international treaties and conventions have attempted to limit the participation of children in armed conflicts. Most recently, the Paris Commitments and Principles (2007) guided international policy. The principles are concerned with the protection of children from recruitment or use in armed hostilities and their release and successful reintegration into civilian life. The principles outline the need for long-term prevention strategies in order to end child involvement in armed conflict. As of September 2010, 95 countries have endorsed the Paris Commitments and Principles [1].

Prompt 3: What Are the Effects of Disaster and Conflict on Mental Health?

- Palmer (2007) suggests that emotional resilience in the face of great adversity is underestimated by mental health professionals, and the pathologizing of normal cognitive, emotional, and behavioral reactions should be avoided. Everyone experiencing psychological trauma is changed by it, but recovery is the norm [7].
- WHO research on the conflict in Darfur (and following the tsunami in Indonesia) produced estimates on the effect of psychological trauma on populations [8]:
  - 20–40 % of people will have mild psychological distress which resolves within a few days or weeks and will not need any specific intervention.

- 30–50 % of people will have either moderate or severe psychological distress that resolves with time or mild distress that may remain chronic. This group would benefit from social and basic psychological interventions.
- 15–20 % of people will have mild and moderate mental disorders (e.g., depression and anxiety disorders, including PTSD). General population prevalence rates of mild and moderate common mental disorders are about 10 % [9].
- 3–4 % of people will have a severe mental disorder (psychosis, severe depression, severely disabling anxiety, severe substance abuse, etc.) which will severely disable daily functioning. In general, population prevalence rates for severe mental disorders are 2–3 % [9].
- Trauma and loss may exacerbate previous mental illness (e.g., it may turn moderate depression into severe depression) and may cause a severe form of trauma-induced common mental disorder in some people.

Further Information 1

Two months later, you arrive to a warm welcome at the rehabilitation center. You are impressed with what you see. The children are engaging in a group drama activity relating to their experience in captivity. The rehabilitation staff are affectionate with the children, and the message is clear that whatever happened during abduction, it is not the child's fault.

You ask about the prevalence of PTSD and depression among returning children. The manager tells you the center focuses on reintegrating children into their communities rather than providing specific mental health intervention. While group therapy sessions are given, there are no tailored individual therapies. Education programs and cultural reconciliation ceremonies have proved to be the most important community interventions.

A new boy named "Okello John" has been brought to the center following escape from the militia. You ask if you can meet him. Okello John has been given new clothes and is eating a feast but is too quiet and despondent to engage with.

Prompt 4: What Are the Initial Priorities in Psychosocial Interventions Post Conflict?

Palmer (2007) suggests that the most important initial management is social and practical [7]:

- Providing a safe place with food, water, shelter, and basic comfort is the first step.
- Separation from loved ones is a major stressor; therefore, providing information to help people find family and loved ones is high priority. Family tracing is one of the first activities undertaken in child rehabilitation centers [10].

- Returning the victim to normality and normal daily routine, for example, schooling for children and work for adults.
- When the social and practical considerations are dealt with, help may then be given for specific mental health disorders. In child rehabilitation centers, counseling is generally given in groups [11].

Williams et al. (2010) emphasize the importance of the community in initial management [12]:

- Intervention from aid agencies or other nonlocal organizations will only be appropriate if they integrate with existing community support mechanisms. All work must be in collaboration with local colleagues to ensure the response is sensible and sensitive which may oblige adaptation of normal Western treatment approaches or engagement with traditional local practices.
- Information and activities that normalize reactions, protect social and community resources, and signpost access to additional services are fundamental to effective psychosocial responses. Access to mental health services (in general very limited) will be required by a substantial minority of survivors. The aim is to reduce individual symptoms and improve ability to function in the community.
- The specifics of the situation must guide intervention. Different stressors (conflict or disaster) create different challenges to societal, community, and individual coping.

Prompt 5: What Cultural Differences Are There in the Understanding of Mental Health Difficulties?

- Cultural differences in the understanding of mental health problems are rooted in the assumptions different cultures have for making sense of experience. Cultural understanding of experience shapes the way in which individuals make sense of their own distress.
- Western conceptualizations of mental health difficulties tend to be based on diagnostic classifications which focus primarily on the individual and follow a "medical model," that is, identification of symptoms and a diagnosis.
- Non-Western models of mental health difficulties tend to be rooted in a more interdependent view of self which places the community at the heart of life. Thus, the attribution of mental health problems tends to be located outside the individual, for example, mental distress might be considered a sign of bad spirits or to be a result of an individual having lost the context of their traditional social hierarchy.
- Many people in non-Western countries consult traditional healers rather than "medical" health-care providers for treatment. Traditional healers are therefore a central part of mental health care in many parts of the world [13].
- Manifestations of emotional distress which exist in other cultures but do not exist within Western classification systems have been labeled "culture-bound syndromes." For example, "Zar" is a term applied in North African cultures to the experience of spirit possession. From a Western perspective, the symptoms of

"Zar" include episodes of shouting, laughing, hitting the head against a wall, singing, or weeping. Individuals may show apathy and withdrawal, refusing to eat or to carry out daily tasks, or may develop a long-term relationship with the possessing spirit [14].
- Caution is needed in directly transposing Western mental health classification systems to other cultures. Western classifications are based on the Western ideology of health care which often has little relevance to communities with traditional conceptualizations of mental health experience. Any successful attempt at Western mental health intervention requires understanding of traditional belief systems.
- In considering problems with mental health intervention in low-income countries, it is important to be mindful of concerns with our own Western conceptualizations of mental health. Some academics believe that there are inherent weaknesses in Western DSM-based diagnoses on which most Western interventions are based [15].

Further Information 2

Your sleep is broken by piercing screams from the children's dorm. You rush through the entrance to find the children cowering and complaining of nightmares. Okello John is covered in sweat and shivers as you approach. During your stay, you have noticed some of the children find it hard to sleep at night, particularly when they first arrive. Many of these same children are also seen avoiding social activities and group exercises. You suspect that Okello John and some of the other children are suffering from PTSD. The literature suggests that levels of PTSD are particularly high in former child soldiers, and you decide to discuss possible interventions with the manager.

The manager is agitated when you mention PTSD, and he complains that many Western doctors say the same thing. He explains that his people believe nightmares and strange behavior are caused by unsettled spirits, the only cure for which is time, reconciliation, and spiritual healing ceremonies in the community. All the communities in the area share the same belief.

Prompt 6: What Is PTSD, and How Is It Treated in Western Cultures?

- Western classification systems conceptualize posttraumatic stress disorder (PTSD) as a type of anxiety disorder, which can occur after an individual witnesses or experiences a traumatic event involving threat of injury or death.
- The key symptoms are "reliving" (flashbacks, nightmares, and upsetting memories), "avoidance" (emotional numbing, avoiding people and places, memory

loss), and "arousal" (problems concentrating, hypervigilance, and sleep disturbance) [16].

- In the West, PTSD is treated with trauma-focused cognitive behavioral therapy (CBT) which is an individual therapy offered at weekly intervals. Through CBT, the victim is helped to reduce avoidance and to process traumatic memories. Unhelpful thoughts and appraisals about the event are also reevaluated in order to reduce distress. Antidepressant medications are often used to manage symptoms if psychological treatment is refused or is unsuccessful.

Prompt 7: Are Western Conceptualizations of PTSD Applicable in Non-Western Postconflict Situations?

- Individuals in conflict situations are experiencing extreme events in which emotional distress is a normal and expected reaction. It has been argued that using a diagnosis to explain these emotional consequences of traumatic situations may be medicalizing and pathologizing a "normal" response to abnormal situations. Indeed, applying models of diagnosis developed in Western populations not experiencing war can lead to pathologizing whole communities who live with the consequences of war every day [17].
- War and conflict are generally experienced on a community level rather than an individual level, and suffering is experienced and resolved in a social context. Using psychiatric labels in this context can overly focus on individual reactions, rather than social meanings [17].
- Focusing on symptoms which Western models deem to be problematic, for example, nightmares, may divert the focus from experiences that individuals from different cultures see as more distressing, for example, family breakdown [17].

Prompt 8: What Mental Health Interventions Are Recommended Following Conflict?

- In non-Western countries, community-based healing and cleansing rituals are generally valued highly with the majority of the population believing in the power of such rituals. Traditional healers are often able to provide very appropriate and effective treatments for mental distress. It is important that any Western intervention offered incorporates these culturally valued practices [13].
- In conflict zones, entire communities respond and adjust to multiple, enduring traumas. In this situation, focusing on individual therapies can be inappropriate as it separates the individual from their community. Intervention focused on

rebuilding and strengthening community support structures can be more meaningful and effective in reducing suffering.

- A review by Patel and colleagues (2007) demonstrates that there is evidence in favor of treatment for Western classification mental health problems in non-Western communities. Evidence supports the use of antidepressants, counseling, and psychological interventions in the treatment of depression and the use of antipsychotic medications and psychoeducation in the treatment of schizophrenia [18].
- When appropriately adapted, individual (one-on-one) Western developed therapies (e.g., KIDNET – see Box 24.1) can also be useful for many former child soldiers experiencing symptoms of PTSD [19].

Box 24.1: KIDNET

Narrative exposure therapy for traumatized children and adolescents (KIDNET) is an individually delivered therapy which aims to reduce PTSD symptoms in refugee children who have experienced trauma.

KIDNET is an eight-session therapeutic approach based on cognitive behavioral principles. It is based on an understanding of PTSD primarily as a difficulty in the processing of traumatic memories [20], which leads to reexperiencing symptoms.

Therapy Process

A therapist works with the young person to construct a detailed biographical narrative. This narrative focuses on traumatic events experienced throughout the child's life, specifically when they were involved with the militia. To facilitate this process, the therapist gives the child a piece of string to symbolize his or her life. The therapist encourages the child to place stones along the rope to represent sad or difficult events and flowers to represent joyful or happy events. The therapist then explores these events with the child to investigate current and past emotional, physiological, cognitive, and behavioral reactions to the events. At the end of therapy, children are encouraged to unwind some of the unused section of the string to explore imagined future hopes and fears.

The child receives a written biography at the end of treatment.

Evidence Base

KIDNET has been shown to significantly reduce PTSD symptoms and improve functioning in refugee children [19, 21] and former child soldiers [22].

Further Information 3

Okello John gradually begins to sleep better and becomes more open to interaction. After 2 months of rehabilitation, it is time for him to be returned to his community. You are given permission by Okello John's family to attend the reconciliation ceremony in the village.

During a powerful community ceremony involving both the offender and the victim's families imbibing a bitter drink together, you meet with a local health official.

He tells you that mental health provision in the region is appalling and people with severe mental health problems are either locked up in an asylum in town or are cared for by their families (see Fig. 24.2*). There are no mental health professionals working in the region and no medicines to treat the mentally ill. He says that many of the children returning from the rehabilitation centers do not fare well in the community.*

Prompt 9: What Does Long-Term Follow-Up of Rehabilitated Child Soldiers Show?

- Positive social outcomes have been reported, with most former child soldiers successfully achieving normal social "milestones," such as getting married and having children [14]. However, in some areas (such as Uganda) under 60 % of

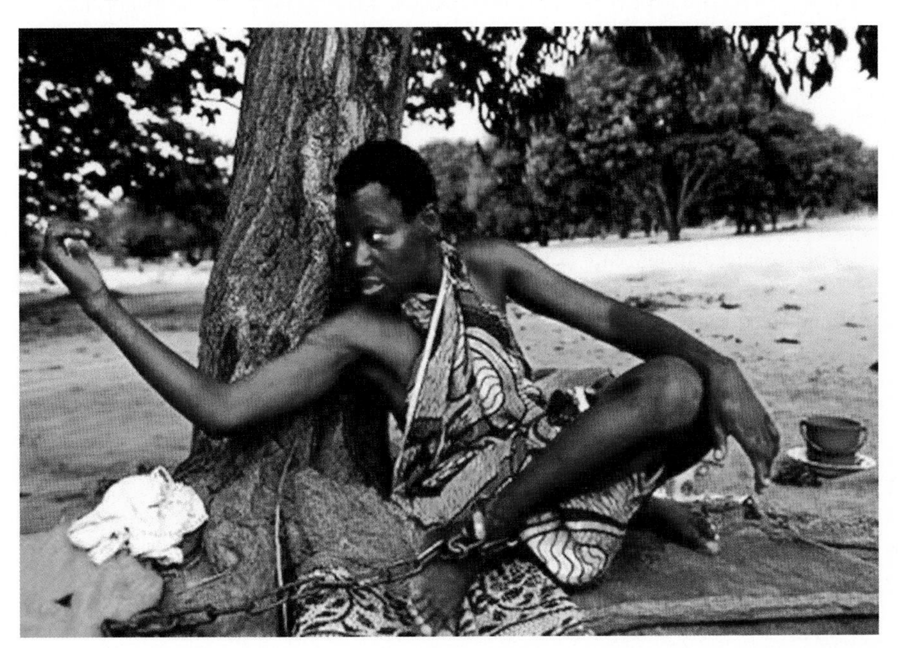

Fig. 24.2 Mentally ill patient chained to tree (Reproduced with kind permission from Grégoire Ahongbonon)

former child soldiers have been reported to have been fully reintegrated into their community and family [23].

- A significant minority of former child soldiers show emotional and behavioral difficulties in adult life [14] with many former child soldiers experiencing strong feelings of revenge following their return [24]. This needs attention as it may be a contributing factor to the cycles of violence seen in many war-torn countries.
- When children are returned to their local communities, it is common for them to be re-recruited into a militia group or into government armed forces. Due to their military training and inside knowledge of the militia group, they are attractive recruits [25].
- Economic difficulties often mean that children return to impoverished living situations. This has an ongoing impact on their physical health and also means that they are not able to use the occupational skills learned in rehabilitation centers [14]. Children frequently attempt to reenter rehabilitation centers from the community.

Prompt 10: What Is the Wider Context of Mental Health Care in Low-Income Countries?

- Mental health remains a low priority in most low-income and middle-income countries [18]. In many countries, the prevailing public health priority agenda supports funding for communicable diseases such as HIV and malaria [26].
- Increased acceptance of the importance of mental health, especially in countries with low and middle incomes, has not been met with increased allocation of financial resources [27]. There are approximately 1800 psychiatrists for 702 million people in Africa compared to 89 000 psychiatrists for 879 million people in Europe [28].
- Much of the tertiary mental health care set up in non-Western countries is a throwback to colonial times. There is growing evidence favoring a paradigm shift toward primary care community-based approaches to mental health [29].
- Opinion differs on the outcome of severe mental health difficulties in developing countries. Large-scale studies conducted by the World Health Organization found that outcomes for schizophrenia were better in developing countries [30, 31]. Possible reasons put forward for this were more social cohesion, more opportunities for integrating people back into work roles, and less segregation and stigmatization. This finding has been criticized by Burns (2009), who suggests poorer outcomes for schizophrenia in developing countries due to common experiences of stigma, lack of service provision, and human rights abuses, as well as increased poverty and higher mortality rates among sufferers [32].

Prompt 11: How May the Investigation of Mental Health Intervention in Conflict Be Improved?

Jordans et al. (2009) conducted a systematic review of the evidence and treatment approaches for children affected by war. The main findings were as follows [29]:

- There is a lack of rigorous studies evaluating psychosocial care for children affected by war. Review of the literature exposed a lack in both evidence-supported interventions and the presentation of applications of treatment approaches.
- The field at large seems to have moved away from a narrow "diagnosis"-based approach toward a broad "well-being, mild distress, and psychopathology"-based approach.
- Community-based rehabilitation models are increasingly favored as a low-cost and integrative framework for care, but there is a lack of evidence about effectiveness of such interventions [18].
- The literature presents consensus on a number of treatment-related issues, yet the application of these treatments remains limited across interventions.

Jordans et al. (2009) suggest clearer objectives should be set for dealing with the psychosocial and mental health care of children. Setting these objectives will be challenging given the lack of developed theory in broad "well-being"-based approaches to mental health intervention.

In order to develop the evidence base from which these interventions can be scaled up, innovative methods for measuring the success of community-led intervention must be developed. Measuring community interventions in a systematic way is problematic in practice. For instance, reconciliation ceremonies are personal affairs where outside interference from academics would not be tolerated. Investigation into the shared characteristics of successful communities emerging from conflict is required.

Case Study: The Rehabilitation of Child Soldiers in Uganda

Between 1986–2008, civil war raged in northern Uganda between the Joseph Kony led Lord's Resistance Army (LRA), and the governmental forces of Yoweri Museveni. Joseph Kony mobilized his army through the violent abduction of children from villages, with upward of 90 % of LRA ranks populated with abducted children. World Vision estimates that between 30,000 and 66,000 children were abducted during the war. The children and adolescents were forced to kill, mutilate, torture, raid, and burn villages in addition to committing atrocities against each other and against their communities [33].

Studies suggest that up to 97 % of children returning from the LRA showed posttraumatic stress reactions of clinical significance [23, 34]. Children also exhibited a variety of other emotional and behavioral difficulties.
Since 1994, Gulu Support the Children Organisation (GUSCO) has been operating in the northern Ugandan district of Gulu. This organization provides center-based rehabilitation for formerly abducted children. This center works with local communities to raise awareness of the needs of former child soldiers and facilitates the reintegration of the children through traditional rituals. The center also offers counseling and medical support to the children as well as education and vocational training. By 2010, an estimated 8,900 children and young people had passed through the various services offered by GUSCO [25].

Recent assessments of the outcomes of GUSCO's rehabilitation efforts have been mixed, with under 60 % of children being found to be reintegrated with their family and community and even less fully participating in community activities. Particular difficulties have been found in the rehabilitation and reintegration of former child soldiers who spent more than 5 years in the LRA or held positions of seniority in the LRA. Similarly, less than 60 % of former child soldiers report having good health. If full rehabilitation and reintegration is considered to involve good outcomes in community integration, good health, livelihood, and education, just over a quarter of children achieve this [25].

References

1. UNICEF. Paris principles and guidelines on children associated with armed forces or armed groups. Paris: UNICEF; 2007.
2. McKay S, Mazurana D. Where are the girls? Girls in fighting forces in Northern Uganda, Sierra Leone, and Mozambique: their lives during and after war. Montreal: International Centre for Human Rights and Democratic Development; 2004.
3. Human Rights Watch. Facts about child soldiers; 2008 (http://www.hrw.org/news/2008/12/03/facts-about-child-soldiers).
4. Machel G. Promotion and protection of the rights of children: impact of armed conflict on children. United Nations; 1996.
5. Coalition to Stop the Use of Child Soldiers. Child soldiers global report. 2008 (http://www.childsoldiersglobalreport.org/files/country_pdfs/FINAL_2008_Global_Report.pdf).
6. Palmer I. Psychological aspects of providing medical humanitarian aid. In: Redmond AD, Mahoney PF, Ryan JM, Macnab C, editors. ABC of conflict and disaster. Oxford: Blackwell Publishing Limited; 2006.
7. WHO Report. Mental health assistance to the populations affected by the Tsunami in Asia. 2011. (Accessed 2012 @ http://www.who.int/mental_health/resources/tsunami/en/index.html).
8. Boothby N, Crawford J, Halperin J. Mozambique child soldier life outcome study: Lessons learned in rehabilitation and reintegration efforts. Glob Public Health. 2006;1(1):87–107.
9. Jareg E. Crossing bridges and negotiating rivers – rehabilitation and reintegration of children associated with armed forces. Norway: Save the Children; 2005.

10. Williams R, Bisson J, Ajdukovic D, Kemp V, Olff M, Alexander D, Hacker Hughes J, Bevan P. NATO guidance: psychosocial care for people affected by disasters and major incidents. 2010.
11. Gilbert J. Responding to mental distress: cultural Imperialism or the struggle for synthesis? Development in Practice. 1999;9(3):287–95 (see also www.janegilbert.co.uk).
12. Trujillo M. Multi-cultural aspects of mental health. Primary Psychiatry. 2008;15(4):65–71.
13. Lopez SJ, Edwards L, Teramoto-Pedrotti J, Prosser EC, LaRue S, Spalitto SV, Ulven JC. Beyond the DSM-IV: assumptions, alternatives, and alterations. J Counsel Dev. 2006;84:259–67. e-Publications@Marquette.
14. Linda JV, David BM, David Z. Post-traumatic stress disorder. In: A.D.A.M. medical encyclopedia. A.D.A.M.: Atlanta; 2011.
15. Summerfield D. War and mental health: a brief overview. Br Med J. 2000;321:232.
16. Patel V, Araya R, Chatterjee S, Hosman C, McGuire H, Rojas G, Van Ommeren M. Treatment and prevention of mental disorders in low-income and middle income countries. Lancet. 2007;370:991–1005.
17. Onyut PL, Neuner F, Schauer E, Ertl V, Odenwald M, Schauer M, Elbert T. Narrative Exposure Therapy as a treatment for child war survivors with posttraumatic stress disorder: Two case reports and a pilot study in an African refugee settlement. BMC Psychiatry. 2005; 5:7.
18. Ehlers A, Clark DM. A cognitive model of posttraumatic stress disorder. Behav Res Ther. 2000;38:319–45.
19. Ruf M, Schauer M, Neuner F, Catani C, Schauer E, Elbert T. Narrative exposure therapy for 7- to 16-year-olds: a randomized controlled trial with traumatized refugee children. J Trauma Stress. 2010;23(4):437–45.
20. Ertl V, Pfeiffer A, Schauer E, Neuner F, and Elbert T. Follow up of a randomized controlled trial Narrative Exposure Therapy: a disseminable, community-based treatment approach for former child soldiers. In: 24th ISTSS annual meeting, terror and its aftermath, Chicago, 2008.
21. GUSCO. Reintegration of returnees, ex-combatants and other war-affected persons in the communities of Gulu and Amuru districts, Northern Uganda: a research report. Gulu: GUSCO; 2010.
22. Derluyn I, Broekaert E, Schuyten G, De Temmerman E. Post-traumatic stress in former Ugandan child soldiers. Lancet. 2004;363(9412):861–3.
23. Okeny R. Reintegration of formerly abducted persons in Northern Uganda, Gulu: a case study of Gulu Support the Children Organization (GUSCO). The Hague: International Institute of Social Studies; 2009.
24. Saraceno B, Van Ommeren M, Batniji R, Cohen A, Gureje O, Mahoney J, Sridhar D, Underhill C. Barriers to improvement of mental health services in low-income and middle-income countries. Lancet. 2007;370:1164–74.
25. Saxena S, Thornicroft G, Knapp M, Whiteford H. Resources for mental health: scarcity, inequity, and inefficiency. Lancet. 2007;370:878–89.
26. World Health Organisation. Mental health atlas. Geneva: World Health Organisation; 2005.
27. Jordans MJ, Tol WA, Komproe IH, De Jong JVTM. Systematic review of evidence and treatment approaches: psychosocial and mental health care for children in war. Child and Adolescent Mental Health. 2009;14(1):2–14.
28. Jablensky A, Sartorius N, Ernberg G, et al. Schizophrenia: manifestations, incidence and course in different cultures. A World Health Organization ten-country study. Psychol Med. 1992;20:1–97.
29. World Health Organization. International pilot study of schizophrenia. Geneva: WHO; 1973.
30. Burns J. Dispelling a myth: developing world poverty, inequality, violence and social fragmentation are not good for outcome in schizophrenia. Afr J Psychiatry. 2009;12(3):200–5.
31. Amone-P'Olak K. Mental states of adolescents exposed to war in Uganda: finding appropriate methods of rehabilitation. Torture. 2006;16(2):93–107.
32. Derlyn I, Broekaert E, Schuyten G, de Temmerman E. Post traumatic stress in former Ugandan child soldiers. Lancet. 2004;363:861–3.

Chapter 25
The Global Crisis in Noncommunicable Disease

Will Barker and Jessi Tucker

Learning Objectives

- Define noncommunicable diseases (NCDs)
- Learn what is meant by the noncommunicable disease crisis
- Understand the significance and key findings of the Global Burden of Disease study
- Describe the main risk factors for noncommunicable disease and their interrelationships
- Understand how and why NCDs affect the developing world as well as the developed world
- Outline priority actions in reducing noncommunicable disease, both at the level of government and on a global scale (Fig. 25.1)

Before We Start…

A word on how we measure the effect of disease on a population:

Two ways in which the effect of a disease is measured on a population are (i) the overall (crude) number of deaths it causes and (ii) the burden of disease it places on a population, measured in disability-adjusted life years (DALY – see Box 25.1).

W. Barker, MBBS, MPhys (✉)
FY2 Doctor, St Thomas' Hospital,
Westminster Bridge Road, London, UK
e-mail: willbarker@doctors.org.uk

J. Tucker
Emergency Medicine Department, Royal London Hospital,
Whitechapel, London, UK
e-mail: jessicatucker@doctors.org.uk

D. MacGarty, D. Nott (eds.), *Disaster Medicine*,
DOI 10.1007/978-1-4471-4423-6_25,

Box 25.1: Calculating DALYs to Measure Burden of Disease [1]

- Disability-adjusted life years (DALYs) are thought to give a more accurate calculation of the burden of disease than crude mortality figures alone. They take into account the age at which people die as well the years of "healthy life" lost due to disease or disability. One DALY is equivalent to one lost year of "healthy life" [1].
- DALYS are worked out as follows:
- Disability-adjusted life years (DALYs) = YLL + YLD
- YLL = years life lost (number of years lost due to early mortality compared to living to old age)
- YLD = years lost due to disability (calculated by number of disease episodes * duration of episodes * disability weighting)
- Disability weighting is an arbitrary measure of the disability caused by a disease. All diseases are ranked between 1 = perfect health and 0 = death. Disability weightings are controversial as they may be misconstrued as devaluing the life of a disabled person.
- The burden of disease is therefore a measurement of the gap between the current health status and an ideal situation where everyone lives to old age in good health.

Initial Scenario

You are doing a surgical placement in Indonesia, and you peruse your surgical list for the day. First up is a patient named Wayan, a 45-year-old man with an infected foot. You complete the consent form with him, and you ask him some general questions about his health.

Wayan grew up in a farming village but moved to the city to work as a tuk-tuk driver aged 15 (Fig. 25.1). *He works long hours, smokes heavily, and his diet is composed of fast food and sugary drinks. He has long-term problems with diabetes and high blood pressure but he receives no treatment owing to prohibitive costs. He recently suffered a heart attack and is losing vision in his right eye.*

In theater, you observe the circulation in his foot is very poor. As you debride, you see pus penetrating deep into the fascia and know his second toe is necrotic and amputation is the only option.

Prompt 1: What Are Noncommunicable Diseases and What Is Their Significance Globally?

> About 100 million people died from (diseases caused by) smoking in the 20th century – twice as many deaths as Stalin, Hitler, and Pol Pot together were responsible for [2].

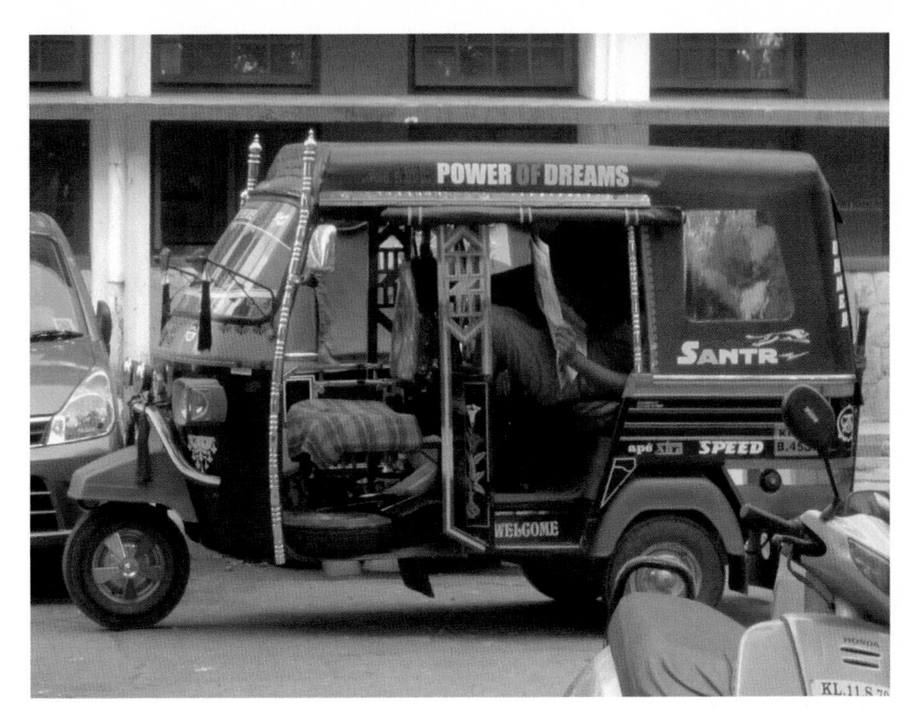

Fig. 25.1 An urban tuk-tuk driver. Photo by Will Barker

- Noncommunicable disease (NCD) includes all forms of noninfective disease. Cardiovascular disease (especially ischemic heart disease and stroke), diabetes, cancer, chronic respiratory disease, and mental illness are the leading players in the NCD global crisis [1].
- Globally, out of every ten deaths, six are due to noncommunicable diseases; three to communicable, reproductive, or nutritional conditions and one to injuries [1].
- Cardiovascular disease is the world's leading cause of death; figures from 2004 for causes of death in all age groups globally show ischemic heart disease (IHD) as the number one cause of death, accounting for 12.2 % of all deaths, followed by cerebrovascular disease accounting for 9.7 % of all deaths [1].
- Chronic obstructive pulmonary disease is the 4th biggest global killer, accounting for 5.1 % of all deaths [1].
- Various cancers, diabetes, hypertensive heart disease, and suicide make up a further 6 of the top 20 global leading causes of death [1].
- Burden of disease figures highlight the significance of NCDs, with unipolar depression the leading noncommunicable burden of disease, coming third out of the top 20 overall, with other NCDs (IHD, stroke, COPD, diabetes, hearing loss, and suicide) also ranking in the top 20 [1] (see Fig. 25.2).
- Mental health problems (such as depression) are a significant yet often overlooked category of NCD. It is estimated that mental health disorders affect 120 million people globally with fewer than 1 in 4 of those affected having access to treatment [1].

Fig. 25.2 Leading causes of burden of disease (DALYs), all ages, 2004 [1]

	Disease or injury	DALYs (millions)	Per cent of total DALYs
1	Lower respiratory infections	94.5	6.2
2	Diarrhoeal diseases	72.8	4.8
3	Unipolar depressive disorders	65.5	4.3
4	Ischaemic heart disease	62.6	4.1
5	HIV/AIDS	58.5	3.8
6	Cerebrovascular disease	46.6	3.1
7	Prematurity and low birth weight	44.3	2.9
8	Birth asphyxia and birth trauma	41.7	2.7
9	Road traffic accidents	41.2	2.7
10	Neonatal infections and other	40.4	2.7
11	Tuberculosis	34.2	2.2
12	Malaria	34.0	2.2
13	COPD	30.2	2.0
14	Refractive errors	27.7	1.8
15	Hearing loss, adult onset	27.4	1.8
16	Congenital anomalies	25.3	1.7
17	Alcohol use disorders	23.7	1.6
18	Violence	21.7	1.4
19	Diabetes mellitus	19.7	1.3
20	Self-inflicted injuries	19.6	1.3

- Hearing loss and blindness also cause great morbidity and have the potential to end careers prematurely. Often they could be easily preventable through the use of hearing and eye protection and or may be easily treatable through simple interventions such as cataract operations [1].

Prompt 2: NCDs Mainly Affect Developed, High-Income Countries, Right?

- Wrong! Traditionally, a huge emphasis has been placed on infectious/parasitic disease and/or nutritional problems as needing the focus of health-care prevention and treatment in the developing world. While this remains pertinent, it does not give the

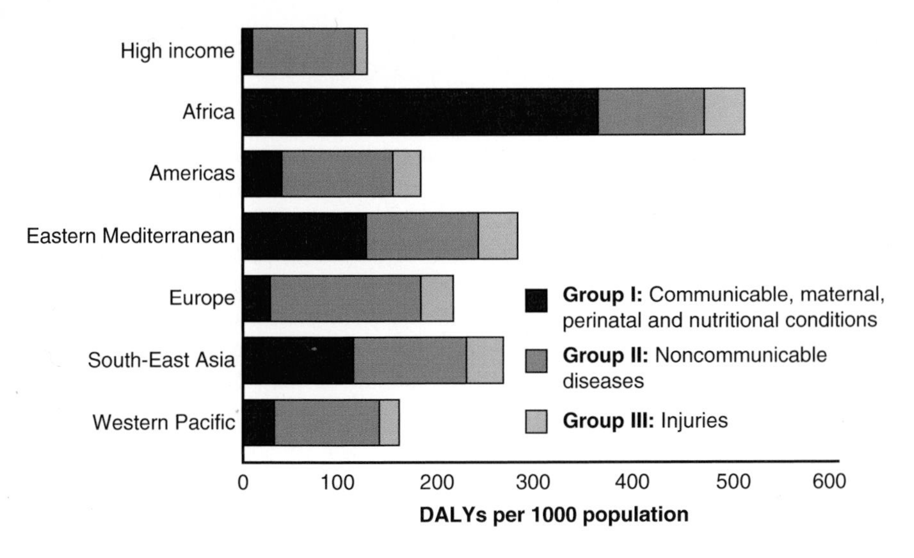

Fig. 25.3 Mortality rates among men and women aged 15–59 years, region and cause of death group, 2004 [1]

full picture. In 2004, ischemic heart disease was actually the second leading cause of death in low-income countries, with stroke and COPD being fifth and sixth out of the top 10, respectively (the rest being either infectious diseases or childbirth complications) [2]. In middle-income countries, NCDs were the top three leading causes of death (stroke, IHD, and COPD, respectively) [1].

- In high-income countries, NCDs accounted for 9 out of the top 10 leading causes of death in 2004 [1].
- To put it bluntly in low-income countries, you are more likely to die young of infectious disease, whereas in high-income countries, you are more likely to die over 70 of an NCD. However, for those that survive past childhood in low and middle income countries, now nearly 45 % of the adult disease burden is due to NCD [1] (Fig. 25.3). WHO states this increasing disease burden is attributable to changes in the distribution of risk factors and population aging.
- With regard to the world's leading cause of death, more than 80 % of the global cardiovascular disease burden now occurs in low and middle income countries [3].

If adjusted for age, NCD risks are actually higher in low and middle-income countries than high-income countries, mainly due to the burden of cardiovascular disease and the higher burden of visual impairment and hearing loss [1]

Note: The classification of countries into low income, middle income, and high income is a World Bank definition. This chapter uses references which are based on 2004 data. For more information as to how the World Bank categorizes countries, please follow this link: http://data.worldbank.org/about/country-classifications/country-and-lending-groups

Prompt 3: What Is the Global Burden of Disease Study and Why Is It Significant?

- The Global Burden of Disease (GBD) study began in 1991 as a collaboration between WHO and the World Bank to compile global statistics for health, producing morbidity and mortality rates for disease and injury, and risk factors contributing to them [1, 4]. It also introduced the concept of the disability-adjusted life year [1] as a unit of measurement of the burden of disease.
- Its goal was to provide a comprehensive assessment of the burden of 107 diseases and injuries and ten selected risk factors for the world and eight major regions in 1990. In effect it was the first attempt to quantify global disease and injury burden, using a common framework, which allows us to directly compare data from all over the world.
- From this initial study, priorities have been determined with regard to further research, development, policy, and funding.
- After the initial 1990 GBD project, further updates have been undertaken by WHO based on extensive databases and information from member states for 2000–2002. The most recent update of the 1990 GBD study, published in 2008 by WHO, undertook "comprehensive, comparable and consistent estimates of mortality and burden of disease by cause for all regions of the world in 2004" [1]. This 160-page comprehensive WHO report has been referenced widely throughout this chapter.
- A new GBD 2010 study, funded by the Bill & Melinda Gates Foundation and the first comprehensive effort since the original in 1990, is currently underway.
- The GBD study highlighted disparities in disease burden between high- and low-income countries. In higher income countries, people not only live longer but also remain healthy for longer; a child born in Africa can expect to live 15 % of its life disabled but in developed countries this is just 8 % [1] (Fig. 25.4).
- There are also large regional differences in health. For example, Africa and India represent 26 % of the world's population but 40 % of those suffering ill health. DALY rates are at least twice as high in Africa than any other region [5].
- Furthermore, the GBD study is able to predict future trends. It predicts that non-communicable disease will represent 75 % of all deaths in 2030. Tobacco-associated deaths will continue to increase by 5.4 million to 8.3 million in 2030, representing 10 % of all deaths [1].
- In the future, Africa is still expected to bear the largest relative burden of disease globally, but this will be comprised increasingly of noninfective diseases. As Chapter 10 has shown, the impact of global warming, population growth, and financial crisis will play a major role in shaping future mortality and morbidity.

Prompt 4: How Does the GBD Study Reflect Wayan's Situation?

- As a 45-year-old man living in a lower middle-income country with IHD, hypertension, and diabetes with complications, Wayan is, unfortunately, fitting fairly

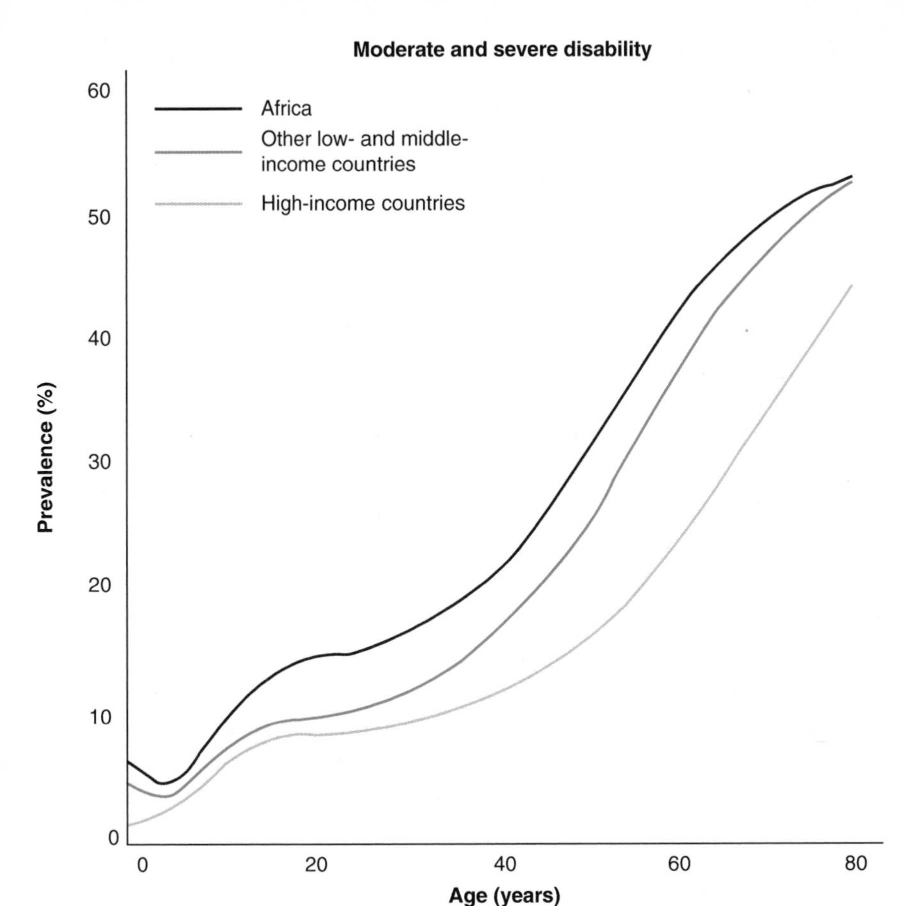

Fig. 25.4 Estimated prevalence of moderate and severe disability by region and age, global burden of disease estimates for 2004 [1]

neatly into statistics. Nearly half of all the disease burden in low- and middle-income countries is carried by those aged 15–59 [1]. Out of that disease burden, we have already seen that IHD is the second biggest cause of burden of disease (with depression being the first).

- Diabetes and hypertensive heart disease are not in the top 10 causes of burden of disease in a country like Indonesia; however, they *are* in the top 10 leading causes of death, with stroke and IHD being first and second, respectively [1].
- In middle-income countries, nearly half of all people live to 70, and NCDs are still the major killer. Looking at Wayan's risk factors (more on which later), his heavy smoking means, if he survives long enough, he is also at increased risk of developing COPD and smoking-related cancers.
- To calculate Wayan's DALY, assuming Wayan is affected by diabetes aged 45 and lives 10 years with moderately severe disability (disability weight 0.5), before dying prematurely aged 55:

– His YLL against a reference age of 75 would be 75–55 = 20.
– His YLD would be 1*10 *0.5 = 5.
– And so, his total burden of disease would equal 20 + 5 = 25 DALYs.

Further Information 1

After the operation, you talk to Wayan about his medical problems, and you discuss the medications he will need in order to stay healthy. Wayan is overwhelmed. He says he wished he had AIDS instead of diabetes because then he would receive free treatment and that already he is disabled more than people with HIV [6].

He tells you diabetes medications are too expensive for him. He would no longer be able to pay school fees for his daughter if he regularly bought the suggested medications.

However, his work is becoming increasingly dangerous due to his failing vision. He tells you his position is impossible. You worry about the increasing numbers of patients like Wayan in your clinic and wonder about the global problem this presents.

Prompt 5: What Are the Risk Factors for NCDs?

- Risk factors can be split into non-modifiable risk factors (e.g., age, family history, and ethnicity) and modifiable risk factors (e.g., tobacco use, diet, alcohol intake, and obesity).
- For the purposes of this chapter, we will be focusing on modifiable risk factors for the NCDs causing the largest global burden of disease and death, namely, IHD, stroke, cancer, chronic respiratory disease, and diabetes.
- Risk factors can be both a risk for developing disease and a disease in itself, e.g., insulin resistance and high blood glucose lead to diabetes and are also risk factors for IHD.
- WHO compiled a report in 2009, based on their 2004 Global Burden of Disease update, entitled Global Health Risks [5]. This identified the "five leading global risks for mortality in the world as being high blood pressure, tobacco use, high blood glucose, physical inactivity and overweight and obesity."
- Risk factors can also have a combined/cumulative effect, with more than one leading to the same disease. For example, according to the same WHO report (2009) [5] "45 % of cardiovascular deaths among those older than 30 can be attributed to raised blood pressure, 16 % to raised cholesterol and 13 % to raised blood glucose, yet the estimated combined effect of these three risks is about 48 % of cardiovascular diseases."

- There are also risk factors for risk factors, e.g., high dietary salt intake can cause high blood pressure.
- Given their dominance in affecting the morbidity and mortality of high-income countries, traditionally, knowledge of risk factors has been based on population data from those same high-income countries.
- The INTERHEART study was an attempt to rectify this. Published in the Lancet in 2004, it established a standardized case–control study of acute MI in 52 countries on every continent in the world [3].
- Their results showed that nine potentially modifiable risk factors account for over 90 % of the risk of an initial acute MI, consistent across different countries, ethnicities, and sex.
- Those nine risk factors are abnormal lipids, smoking, hypertension, diabetes, abdominal obesity, psychosocial factors, poor consumption of fruits and vegetables, increased alcohol consumption, and physical inactivity [3].
- The same risk factors for cardiovascular disease not only have a cumulative effect for IHD if occurring together but can also – individually or together – be a risk for other, different, NCDs, e.g., poor consumption of fruit and vegetables can also cause gastrointestinal cancer [5].
- To muddy the water still further, risk factors beget risk factors, e.g., obesity causes IHD and stroke in itself, but it also causes hypertension and type 2 diabetes which in themselves cause cardiovascular disease.
- The bottom line is high blood pressure, high blood glucose, abnormal lipids, tobacco use, poor diet (be it too much salt or alcohol or too little fruit and vegetables), physical inactivity, and being overweight/obese all, individually and cumulatively, account for the majority of NCD burden of disease and deaths around the globe.
- Ultimately, what people actually do – smoke; drink too much alcohol; eat high-salt, high-sugar, low-fruit and -vegetable diets; and avoid exercise – underpins the major risk factors for the major NCDs in the world today.

Prompt 6: Why Have NCDs Become Such a Global Problem?

- As nations advance, child deaths are prevented by public health measures (e.g., vaccinations), sanitation, and improved medical care. The population as a whole therefore ages. NCDs affect older populations at a greater rate than younger populations, thereby shifting the dominant disease pattern from communicable disease to NCDs. As we have seen, high-income countries are furthest along this shift [5].
- The risk pattern also changes. Communicable disease risks (e.g., undernutrition, poor sanitation) are slowly replaced by NCD risks such as smoking, inactivity, and obesity. In a 2011 Lancet paper [7], Beaglehole et al. refer to this as the "globalisation of risks, particularly tobacco use."

- The poorest populations continue to be exposed to "traditional risks" such as undernutrition, as well as increasing NCD risks such as smoking, thereby having to fight the battle on both fronts.
- It is easy to blame personal choices, yet agricultural subsidies and market liberalization have led to decreased prices and increased availability of unhealthy foods high in saturated fats, salt, and sugar. The consumption of unhealthy foods has subsequently increased which has resulted in a rapid rise in global obesity. It is estimated that 38,000 people die every day as a result of obesity-related causes.

Prompt 7: What Simple Interventions Can Be Made to Reduce Wayan's Health Risks on His Recovery from Surgery?

- The goal of treatment in Wayan's case is to reduce his risk of death from cardiovascular disease and to reduce the morbidity associated with diabetic complications such as blindness, renal failure, and infection. Important initial steps include:
  - Stop smoking
  - Weight loss
  - Diet: eat fewer calories and eat healthier (less salt, sugar, and fat; more fruit and vegetables)
  - Regular exercise (30 min of moderate exercise daily)
- Given Wayan is already experiencing the negative consequences of his increased NCD risk, i.e., has already had an MI and has complications of poorly controlled diabetes, lifestyle advice alone will not reduce his cardiovascular risk sufficiently. Medication is also needed such as aspirin and a B-blocker as secondary prevention for his MI. Other proven cost-effective interventions are a statin to lower cholesterol and an ACE inhibitor to reduce blood pressure. Oral hypoglycemic agents such as metformin will also reduce his risk of further diabetic complications of blindness and renal failure. These medicines typically cost relatively more to people in developing countries due to insufficient supply and inefficient markets. Much lower disposable incomes make them even more unaffordable and therefore underused. Furthermore, access to reliably manufactured drugs in the first place can be a problem [8].
- An affordable combination polypill has been proposed as a solution to combined risk factors and has been trialed with some success in India [9].

Further Information 2

Following up your interest in NCDs, you gain permission to attend a national conference to discuss the issue of preventative approaches to health. Large numbers of delegates from multinational companies, including pharmaceutical, food, and tobacco firms, are present. They argue the best way to improve health is through voluntary agreements.

You have seen this rhetoric before with little change, and so you seek a government advisor. He is sympathetic to your concerns but says the economy is precarious and there are genuine worries that forced intervention will scare off international investment.

Prompt 8: How Can the Noncommunicable Disease Crisis Be Addressed?

Prevention of disease can be broken down into:

- Primary prevention: Healthier lifestyles to reduce risk factors and development of disease.
- Secondary prevention: Once people have disease, treat it, e.g., b-blockers after MI.
- Tertiary prevention: Prevent the complications of disease, e.g., aspirin, statins, and antihypertensives for people with diabetes.
- Since risk factors for NCDs are multifactorial, overlap, and can be culturally ingrained, government should be best placed to tackle them. Policies to reduce demand for unhealthy choices such as education initiatives and high pricing (cigarettes) are generally favored by governments since this infringes liberty less and allows tax revenues.
- Regulation of advertising to children has been shown to be a more effective prevention strategy than education, and targeting children leads to long-term health gains.
- Reducing supply of unhealthy choices is traditionally not used; however, agriculture could be reformed to subsidize healthy food over unhealthy [7]. A notable example of this is Mauritius, which changed its important edible oil policy and reduced LDL cholesterol levels by about 0.8 mmol/L [10].

Further Information 3

You read around the subject area and find that the global management of NCDs is as much a political issue as a medical one. Such is your newfound passion for the topic you consider putting down your surgical knife and commencing a career in public health and politics.

Despite evidence of a noncommunicable disease crisis you find that most Western donors still focus their attention on easily publicized infective or nutritional crises rather than tackle NCDs.

Prompt 9: What Are the Global Intervention Priorities for Managing Noncommunicable Disease?

- In a Lancet article, Beaglehole et al. (2011) identified five priority interventions: tobacco control, salt reduction, improved diets and physical activity, lower alcohol consumption, and better access to essential drugs. The economic benefits of intervention easily outweigh the costs as these interventions would be cheap, with most costing < $100 per DALY averted [7].
- Tobacco control is the most urgent priority. Currently, one billion people smoke or chew tobacco, and 15,000 die every day as a result. Tobacco consumption is actually rapidly increasing in poor countries.
- Policies must also target disadvantaged populations throughout the world to address the social determinants of health, even in developed countries. For example, UNITAID is developing strategies for innovating affordable fixed-dose combination medicines to treat cardiovascular disease [11].

Prompt 10: What Are the Key Challenges in Addressing NCDs?

- Addressing NCDs requires coordination between all sectors within society including agriculture, education, employment, social planning, and taxation [11]. Inertia and vested interests maintain the status quo despite overwhelming evidence for intervention. There is likely to be continued resistance from tobacco, alcohol, and food companies [6].
- The failure to address NCDs globally could be viewed as a political failure rather than a technical failure; the technology and science has been available for decades [12]. For sustained success, the misconception that NCDs primarily affect rich nations, the old, or the overindulgent must be challenged.
- Rather than leading progress, the USA, Canada, and the European Union have been blocking proposals on NCDs [13].
- Current trade agreements are constructed to benefit corporations, which limit government control of alcohol and food markets. Global firms heavily push advertising and sales.
- The current system of intellectual property is blocking access to medicine for most of the world's population. Intellectual property rules obstruct access to essential medicine through prohibitive pricing, such as when a medicine is in patent, pharmaceutical firms charge monopoly prices [8]. In developing countries, public pharmacies often only have one-third of available essential medicines and may cost 2.5 times international prices [14].
- Growth in health systems cannot be relied upon to ensure that greatest health needs are met. In the USA, health care costs 15 % of GDP compared with just 8 % in the UK, and yet in the USA, 17 % are uninsured and many others forced

into poverty by part payments [15]. To insure a family of 4 for a year in the USA costs on average $14,000 a year [16].

- Lack of epidemiological evidence on NCDs in lower income countries masks the scale of the problem.

Case Study: India (Currently Classified as a Lower Middle-Income Economy by the World Bank) [17]

India accounts for one-fifth of the world's population and has experienced a massive societal shift toward industrialization and urbanization, yet profound societal inequalities remain.

Deaths in India from NCDs are expected to double from 4.5 million in 1998 to 8 million in 2020. The number of years lost due to premature heart disease will increase from 7.1 million to 17.9 million in 2030, a greater number than is projected for China, Russia, and the USA combined [17].

Traditional risk factors still play a role in health; more than 80 % of the Indian population uses solid fuel for cooking, which contributes to high levels of respiratory disease. Modern risk factors are becoming more widespread – 36.7 % of men smoke, and there is a trend for increasing use of tobacco in young people. Like elsewhere in the world, smoking contributes to health inequalities in India, with higher smoking rates in low-income and in rural populations.

World class health-care services are available in India, but there is a price to pay. Most health-care costs are paid out of pocket with little social support and are consequently very expensive, crippling the families of those affected. Although there are cost-effective primary and secondary interventions available, coverage is low, especially in poor and rural populations.

In Conclusion

- The NCD crisis has been likened to the HIV crisis 10 years ago: an emerging epidemic that has been neglected for a significant period, with disease that disproportionately affects the poor alongside a stigma of "moral hazard" where perceived poor lifestyle choices have caused the disease [18]. Smoking, lack of exercise, poor diet, and high sugar and alcohol intake contribute to two-third of the new cases of NCDs. Poor social conditions compound the problem, making it harder for the disadvantaged to make healthy choices. There is also a sizeable funding gap as seen with HIV 15 years ago, where the medicines exist and could be made affordable, but currently remain prohibitively expensive for the poor.

- The scale of growth in NCDs is setting back progress toward the millennium development goals. As we have seen, NCDs disproportionately affect the poor, and this challenges broad development goals such as health equity, poverty reduction, and economic stability. The World Economic Forum ranks NCDs as one of the top threats to economic development (Fig. 10.3)
- In response, the UN high-level meeting on noncommunicable diseases met in September 2011 to make NCDs a high priority in the development agenda (The last high-level meeting for health was held in 2001 for HIV/AIDS). Emerging countries are now obliged to split their limited resources between infective disease and NCDs.
- Most recently, at the 65th World Health Assembly in May 2012 in Geneva, world leaders agreed to cut deaths from NCDs by a quarter by 2025 [19].

The BMJ reports [19]:

> "... this voluntary target came eight months after world leaders signed an agreement to tackle the causes of the four main NCDs – cardiovascular disease, lung disease, cancer and diabetes - at the United Nations General Assembly….. The governing body of WHO also agreed to set targets to reduce the four main risk factors – high blood pressure, tobacco smoking, dietary salt and physical inactivity…… WHO's director general, Margaret Chan, told delegates at the end of the assembly that the organisation was giving its responsibilities on non-communicable diseases its 'highest priority.'"

References

1. Mathers C, Boerma T, Ma Fat D. The global burden of disease: 2004 update. Geneva: WHO; 2008.
2. Delamothe T. Deaths from smoking: the avoidable holocaust. BMJ. 2012;344:e2029. doi:10.1136/bmj.e2029.
3. Yusuf S, Hawken S, Ounpuu S, Dans T, Avezum A, Lanas F, McQueen M, Budaj A, Pais P, Varigos J, Lisheng L, INTERHEART Study Investigators. Effect of potentially modifiable risk factors associated with myocardial infarction in 52 countries (the INTERHEART study): case–control study. Lancet. 2004;364(9438):937–52.
4. Institute for Health Metrics and Evaluation. Global burden of disease study. 2012. Available from: http://www.globalburden.org/index.html. Accessed on 1 Apr 2012.
5. Mathers C, Stevens G, Mascarenhas M. Global health risks: mortality and burden of disease attributable to selected major risks. Geneva: WHO; 2009.
6. Cohen D. Will industry influence derail UN summit? BMJ. 2011;343:d5328. doi:10.1136/bmj.d5328.
7. Beaglehole R, Bonita R, Horton R, Adams C, Alleyne G, Asaria P, Baugh V, Bekedam H, Billo N, Casswell S, Cecchini M, Colagiuri R, Colagiuri S, Collins T, Ebrahim S, Engelgau M, Galea G, Gaziano T, Geneau R, Haines A, Hospedales J, Jha P, Keeling A, Leeder S, Lincoln P, McKee M, Mackay J, Magnusson R, Moodie R, Mwatsama M, Nishtar S, Norrving B, Patterson D, Piot P, Ralston J, Rani M, Srinath Reddy K, Sassi F, Sheron N, Stuckler D, Suh I, Torode J, Varghese C, Watt J. Priority actions for the non-communicable disease crisis. Lancet. 2011;377:1438–47.
8. Brook K, Baker JD. Patents, pricing, and access to essential medicines in developing countries. Am Med Assoc J Ethics. 2009;11(7):527–32.

9. Yusuf S, Pais P, Afzal R, et al. Effects of a polypill (Polycap) on risk factors in middle-aged individuals without cardiovascular disease (TIPS): a phase II, double-blind, randomised trial. Lancet. 2009;373(9672):1341–51.
10. Uusitalo U, Feskens E, Tuomilehto J, Dowse G, Haw U, Fareed D, Hemraj F, Gareeboo H, Alberti K, Zimmet P. Fall in total cholesterol concentration over five years in association with changes in fatty acid composition of cooking oil in Mauritius: cross sectional survey. Br Med J. 1996;313:1044–6. doi:10.1136/bmj.313.7064.1044.
11. UNITAID. The medicines patent pool initiative [Internet]. Geneva: UNITAID; 2009. [cited 2012 Apr 1]. Available from: http://www.who.int/hiv/amds/unitaid_patent_pool2_2009.pdf.
12. Geneau R, Stuckler D, Stachenko S, McKee M, Ebrahim S, Basu S, Chockalingham A, Mwatsama M, Jamal R, Alwan A, Beaglehole R. Raising the priority of preventing chronic diseases: a political process. Lancet. 2010;376(9753):1689–98. PubMed PMID: 21074260.
13. NCD Alliance. Media Release – Thursday, 18 Aug 2011 [cited 2012 Apr 1]. Available from: http://ncdalliance.org/takeaction.
14. MDG Gap Task Force. Millennium development goal 8. Delivering on the global partnership for achieving millennium development goals. Geneva: WHO; 2008 [cited 2012 Apr 1]. Available from: http://www.who.int/medicines/mdg/MDG8EnglishWeb.pdf.
15. WHO. World Health Statistics 2009. Geneva: WHO; 2009 [cited 2012 Apr 1]. Available from: http://www.who.int/whosis/whostat/2009/en/index.html.
16. Wolf R. Number of uninsured Americans rises to 50.7 million. McClean; USA today; 2010 Sep 17. [cited 2012 Apr 1]. Available from: http://www.usatoday.com/news/nation/2010-09-17-uninsured17_ST_N.htm.
17. Patel V, Chatterji S, Chisholm D, Ebrahim S, Gopalakrishna G, Mathers C, Mohan V, Prabhakaran D, Ravindran RD, Reddy KS. Chronic diseases and injuries in India. Lancet. 2011;377(9763):413–28. Epub 2011 Jan 10. PubMed PMID: 21227486.
18. Stuckler D, Basu S, McKee M. Commentary: UN high level meeting on non-communicable diseases: an opportunity for whom? BMJ. 2011;343:d5336. doi:10.1136/bmj.d5336.
19. Gulland A. World leaders agree to cut deaths from non-communicable diseases by a quarter by 2025. BMJ. 2012;344:e3768. Available from: www.bmj.com.

Index

D. MacGarty, D. Nott (eds.), *Disaster Medicine*,
DOI 10.1007/978-1-4471-4423-6, © Springer-Verlag London 2013

S

T